PRAISE FOR *JOHNS HOPKINS EVIDENCE-BASED PRACTICE FOR NURSES AND HEALTHCARE PROFESSIONALS, ...*

"The latest edition of Johns Hopkins Evidence-Based Practice for Nurses and Healthcare Professionals *remains an essential resource for advancing evidence-based practice in healthcare. As the foundation of our DNP Project Process, the JHEBP framework and tools provide a structured, accessible approach to implementing high-quality practice change. The model's clarity and practical guidance support students while also facilitating faculty development, offering effective strategies to critically appraise and translate research into needed practice change. Across acute care, primary care, and specialized practice environments, this framework empowers healthcare professionals to implement evidence-based solutions that drive meaningful improvements in patient outcomes across organizations of varying size. A must-have book for educators and clinicians dedicated to excellence in evidence-based practice and transformative change."*

–Sara L. Hubbell, DNP, APRN, PMHNP-BC, FNP-C
Clinical Associate Professor
Program Coordinator, DNP
Co-Lead to the Well-Being & Resilience Collaborative (WRC)
School of Nursing, UNC Wilmington

"The JHEBP model and guidelines are the most comprehensive and user-friendly tools for busy healthcare professionals and students who strive to deliver evidence-based care. Each chapter clearly, logically, and simply describes some typically time consuming or intimidating components of the EBP process. The enhancements in the fifth edition have really 'moved the needle' of evidence-based practice by modifying language through a pragmatic reconceptualization of the EBP process and its purpose: to make evidence-based decisions with efficiency, effectiveness, and confidence."

–Angela M. Cecil, PhD, MBA, OTR/L, FNAP
Program Director, BS in Occupational Science
Department of Occupational Science and Occupational Therapy
Saint Louis University

"The JHEBP model is dynamic and easy to follow, making it an ideal model used in coaching and guiding clinical nurses to develop and implement EBP projects. The updates and evolution outlined in this fifth edition have further simplified the process, which will be welcomed by clinical nurses who are often overwhelmed and intimidated by the complexity of an EBP project. The text provides clear explanation of the contents, and the appendices are user-friendly and great supplemental documents to ensure robust projects that are meaningful, impactful, and sustainable."

–Marga Kasim, DNP, RN, CNS, AGCNS-BC, CNML, EBP-C
Manager, Nursing Research Department
Loma Linda University Health

"I wholeheartedly endorse Johns Hopkins Evidence-Based Practice for Nurses and Healthcare Professionals, *Fifth Edition*. *The shift from PICO to an EBP question enhances clarity, making it accessible for nurses across all settings. The readily available EBP tools and the common-sense approach to grading literature, with a focus on the quality of evidence, make this book invaluable for healthcare professionals. An excellent guide for practical, evidence-based practice designed for every nurse.*"

–Perry M. Gee, PhD, RN, NEA-BC, FAAN
Enterprise Director of Nursing Research and Evidence-Based Practice
Nurse Scientist and Associate Professor of Research
Intermountain Health

"*I sincerely commend* Johns Hopkins Evidence-Based Practice for Nurses and Healthcare Professionals, *Fifth Edition, as an indispensable resource for nursing students and nurses seeking to learn about and integrate EBP into their daily work. This edition streamlines the EBP process while maintaining its integrity, making it more accessible and efficient for frontline practitioners. I appreciate the reimagined approach to question formulation and the simplified ways of making best-evidence recommendations and guidance for real-world implementation.*"

–Julie Peila Gee, PhD, MSN Ed, RN
Associate Professor
College of Nursing, University of Utah

"Johns Hopkins Evidence-Based Practice for Nurses and Healthcare Professionals *is a comprehensive guide for understanding, teaching, and applying evidence-based practice in healthcare. This book equips practitioners with the knowledge to effectively implement EBP initiatives, driving clinical and organizational improvements. The JHEBP model and tools have consistently demonstrated their ability to enhance outcomes.*"

–Viji George, DNP, MA, RN, RNC-NIC, NEA-BC
Clinical Excellence Program Manager
Nursing Professional Practice
Texas Health Resources
Magnet Program Director
Texas Health Presbyterian Hospital Plano

"Johns Hopkins Evidence-Based Practice for Nurses and Healthcare Professionals: Model & Guidelines, *Fifth Edition, provides modernized and practical modifications. As both technology and healthcare continue to evolve, the processes to evaluate information continue to change. The updates to the model will enhance the EBP process, supporting improvements and optimal outcomes.*"

–Gale Shalongo, DNP, RN, NEA-BC, NPD-BC
System Director of Nursing Research/EBP and Policy
Geisinger Health

FIFTH EDITION

JOHNS HOPKINS EVIDENCE-BASED PRACTICE
FOR NURSES AND HEALTHCARE PROFESSIONALS

Model & Guidelines

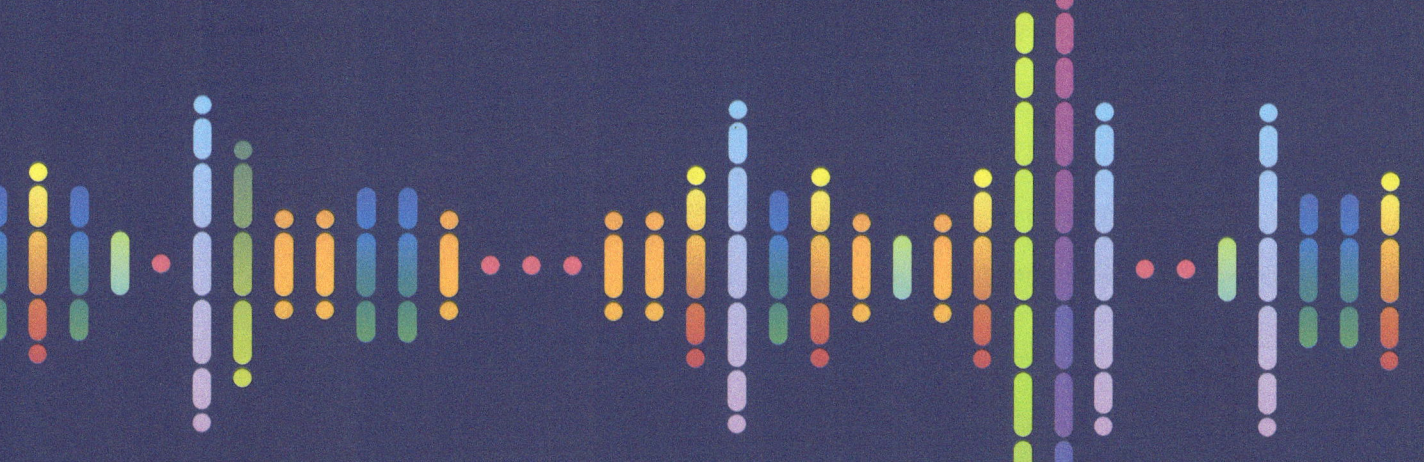

Kim Bissett, PhD, MBA, RN
Judith Ascenzi, DNP, RN
Madeleine Whalen, MSN/MPH, RN, CEN, NPD-BC

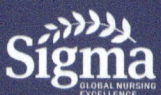
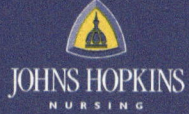

Copyright © 2025 by Sigma Theta Tau International Honor Society of Nursing

All rights reserved. This book is protected by copyright. No part of it may be reproduced, stored in a retrieval system, or transmitted in any form or by any means, electronic, mechanical, photocopying, recording, or otherwise, without written permission from the publisher. Any trademarks, service marks, design rights, or similar rights that are mentioned, used, or cited in this book are the property of their respective owners. Their use here does not imply that you may use them for a similar or any other purpose.

This book is not intended to be a substitute for the medical advice of a licensed medical professional. The author and publisher have made every effort to ensure the accuracy of the information contained within at the time of its publication and shall have no liability or responsibility to any person or entity regarding any loss or damage incurred, or alleged to have incurred, directly or indirectly, by the information contained in this book. The author and publisher make no warranties, express or implied, with respect to its content, and no warranties may be created or extended by sales representatives or written sales materials. The author and publisher have no responsibility for the consistency or accuracy of URLs and content of third-party websites referenced in this book.

Sigma Theta Tau International Honor Society of Nursing (Sigma) is a nonprofit organization whose mission is developing nurse leaders anywhere to improve healthcare everywhere. Founded in 1922, Sigma has more than 80,000 active members in over 100 countries and territories. Members include practicing nurses, instructors, researchers, policymakers, entrepreneurs, and others. Sigma's 600 chapters are located at more than 700 institutions of higher education throughout Armenia, Australia, Botswana, Brazil, Canada, Chile, Colombia, Croatia, England, Eswatini, Finland, Ghana, Hong Kong, Ireland, Israel, Italy, Jamaica, Japan, Jordan, Kenya, Lebanon, Malawi, Mexico, the Netherlands, Nigeria, Pakistan, Philippines, Portugal, Puerto Rico, Saudi Arabia, Scotland, Singapore, South Africa, South Korea, Spain, Sweden, Taiwan, Tanzania, Thailand, the United States, and Wales. Learn more at www.sigmanursing.org.

Sigma Theta Tau International
550 West North Street
Indianapolis, IN, USA 46202

To request a review copy for course adoption, order additional books, buy in bulk, or purchase for corporate use, contact Sigma Marketplace at 888.654.4968 (US/Canada toll-free), +1.317.687.2256 (International), or solutions@sigmamarketplace.org.

To request author information, or for speaker or other media requests, contact Sigma Marketing at 888.634.7575 (US/Canada toll-free) or +1.317.634.8171 (International).

ISBN: 9781646481859
EPUB ISBN: 9781646481873
PDF ISBN: 9781646481880

Library of Congress Control Number: 2024061342

Publisher: Dustin Sullivan
Acquisitions Editor: Emily Hatch
Development Editor: Jillmarie Leeper Sycamore
Cover Designer: Rebecca Batchelor
Interior Design/Page Layout: Rebecca Batchelor
Indexer: Larry D. Sweazy

Managing Editor: Carla Hall
Publications Specialist: Todd Lothery
Project Editor: Todd Lothery
Copy Editor: Todd Lothery
Proofreader: Todd Lothery

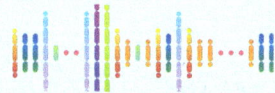

DEDICATION

This book is dedicated to nurses and healthcare professionals everywhere in whatever setting they practice—who are committed to excellence in patient care based on the best available evidence.

ACKNOWLEDGMENTS

We would like to acknowledge the insight and expertise of the authors of the first edition (2007) of *Johns Hopkins Nursing Evidence-Based Practice: Model and Guidelines*:

Robin P. Newhouse, PhD, RN, NE-BC, FAAN

Sandra L. Dearholt, DNP, RN

Stephanie S. Poe, DNP, RN

Linda C. Pugh, PhD, RNC, CNE, FAAN

Kathleen M. White, PhD, RN, NEA-BC, FAAN

Additionally, we would like to thank Deborah Dang, PhD, RN, NEA-BC, whose dedication to investigation and lifelong learning continues to inspire us.

The foundational work of these experts transformed evidence-based practice into a process that promotes autonomy and provides frontline nurses with the competencies and tools to apply the best evidence to improve patient care. The profession as a whole is indebted to them.

ABOUT THE AUTHORS

Kim Bissett, PhD, MBA, RN, is a nurse educator and Director of EBP at the Institute for Johns Hopkins Nursing. She has been involved with the JHEBP model for many years including as an EBP Fellow, a hospital-based EBP Coordinator, and a workshop facilitator. She has extensive experience in EBP education, presenting and consulting on evidence-based nursing practice nationally and internationally. Bissett assisted with developing and publishing previous editions of the *Johns Hopkins Nursing Evidence-Based Practice: Model and Guidelines*. She also teaches part time in the Johns Hopkins University School of Nursing's Doctor of Nursing Practice Program. Her research interests include self-compassion and fostering nurse well-being.

Judith Ascenzi, DNP, RN, is the Director of Pediatric Nursing Programs for Education, Informatics, and Research at the Johns Hopkins Children's Center. She also teaches part time in the Johns Hopkins University School of Nursing's Doctorate of Nursing Practice Program. Ascenzi has presented and consulted nationally on the topic of evidence-based practice. She has served as expert facilitator on many evidence-based practice projects in her pediatric practice setting as well as with her adult colleagues at the Johns Hopkins Hospital. Ascenzi acts as a project advisor and organizational mentor for many doctoral students utilizing the JHEBP model as the foundational model for their projects.

Madeleine Whalen, MSN/MPH, RN, CEN, NPD-BC, is the Evidence-Based Practice Program Coordinator for the Johns Hopkins Health System. In this role she educates and supports frontline nurses in completing robust and actionable EBP projects rooted in bedside experience. She began her nursing career in the emergency department while earning her master's degrees in nursing and public health. She is a Joanna Briggs Institute Scientific Writer and a member of the *Journal of Emergency Nursing* editorial board. She continues to work clinically part time and serves as adjunct faculty at the Johns Hopkins University School of Nursing and the Johns Hopkins Medicine Center for Global Emergency Care. Her professional interests include global health, evidence synthesis, and empowering nurses to advance the profession and science of nursing through inquiry.

CONTRIBUTING AUTHORS

Chapter 1 – Evidence-Based Practice: Past, Present, and Future

Dörte Thorndike, DrPh, MSN, RN, NEA-BC, currently serves as a Nursing Coordinator for the Office of Nursing Professional Practice at the Johns Hopkins Hospital, where she leads and supports various nursing initiatives. A pediatric nurse by training, she has 15 years of clinical nursing experience and has held leadership positions in both Switzerland and the United States for the past 14 years. In addition to her institutional impact, including chairing the CUSP-XT committee and working on projects related to Chronically Critically Ill Children, Thorndike has contributed her expertise to international initiatives through Johns Hopkins Medicine International. She has served as a content expert in nursing operations, leadership development, performance management, and patient experience. Thorndike has also collaborated on several multidisciplinary, evidence-based research projects, co-authoring publications that document their findings.

Lisa Grubb, DNP, MSN, BSN, RN, CWCN, CPHQ, C/DONA, is an Assistant Professor at the Johns Hopkins University School of Nursing, where she coordinates and teaches in the DNP/AP project courses. She uses the Johns Hopkins Evidence-Based Practice model as a foundation for all DNP project courses. Before her current role, she was the Senior Director of Quality and Patient Safety at the Johns Hopkins Howard County Medical Center, where she focused on using evidence-based practices to improve patient outcomes, including reducing length of stay, decreasing readmissions, and enhancing patient satisfaction and value-based care. Additionally, she has collaborated with the Institute for Johns Hopkins Nursing and the Johns Hopkins Nursing Administration to support nurses in evidence-based practice, knowledge translation, and quality improvement research projects. Grubb has a strong interest in promoting EBP in both clinical settings and academic environments.

Kim Bissett, PhD, MBA, RN. See Kim Bissett's bio earlier.

Chapter 2 – The Johns Hopkins Evidence-Based Practice (JHEBP) Model for Nurses and Healthcare Professionals (HCPs) Process Overview

Kim Bissett, PhD, MBA, RN. See Kim Bissett's bio earlier.

Judith Ascenzi, DNP, RN. See Judith Ascenzi's bio earlier.

Special acknowledgment to previous author Sandra L. Dearholt, DNP, RN, NEA-BC. Dearholt is Assistant Director of Nursing for the Departments of Neurosciences and Psychiatry Nursing at the Johns Hopkins Hospital. Dearholt has written numerous articles on EBP and has extensive experience in the development and delivery of EBP educational programs. Her areas of interest focus on strategies for incorporating EBP into practice at the bedside, the development of professional practice standards, promoting healthcare staff well-being, and fostering service excellence. She is a co-author of the first edition of *Johns Hopkins Nursing Evidence-Based Practice: Model and Guidelines* and a contributing author to *Johns Hopkins Nursing Evidence-Based Practice: Implementation and Translation*.

Chapter 3 – Practice Question Phase: The Problem

Kim Bissett, PhD, MBA, RN. See Kim Bissett's bio earlier.

Lisa Klein, MSN, RN, AGCNS-BC, CNRN, is a certified Adult-Gerontology Clinical Nurse Specialist on two acute and intermediate care medical-surgical neuroscience units at Johns Hopkins Hospital. Klein received her bachelor of science in nursing in 2005 and master of science in nursing in 2014 from the Johns Hopkins University School of Nursing. She has championed efforts to increase patient mobility, decrease patient falls, and improve patient outcomes by leading evidence-based practice projects, mentoring staff, enhancing nursing education, and advancing quality improvement initiatives. Klein has published as a primary author and co-author on articles focusing on promoting mobility in the inpatient hospital setting and implementation of stroke centers. She has presented nationally and internationally on nursing stroke care and mobility promotion.

Chapter 4 – Practice Question Phase: The EBP Question

Lisa Klein, MSN, RN, AGCNS-BC, CNRN. See Lisa Klein's bio earlier.

Kim Bissett, PhD, MBA, RN. See Kim Bissett's bio earlier.

Chapter 5 – The Interprofessional Team

Julia Krzyzewski, MAS, RRT, RRT-NPS, is the Respiratory Therapy Clinical Supervisor in the Neonatal Intensive Care Unit and Emergency Center at Johns Hopkins All Children's Hospital in St. Petersburg, Florida. She supports frontline respiratory therapists in providing patient and family centered care and collaborates with the medical team to plan for the respiratory care needs of patients both in the hospital and beyond. She is on faculty for the Johns Hopkins Neonatal-Perinatal Medicine Fellowship Program and has been a long-time member and leader of shared governance councils within the organization. She began her respiratory therapy career in the United States Air Force, eventually earning a master's degree in Patient Safety and Healthcare Quality from the Johns Hopkins Bloomberg School of Public Health. Her professional interests include evidence-based practice, promoting interprofessional collaboration, and improving safety and quality across the healthcare continuum.

Judith Ascenzi, DNP, RN. See Judith Ascenzi's bio earlier.

Jenna Spencer, DNP, APRN, ACCNS-P, CPEN, is a pediatric emergency department clinical nurse specialist with a special focus in suicide prevention, sepsis awareness, and patient safety. Her passions include quality improvement, implementation science, and mentoring, whether it be in patient care or evidence-based practice. Outside of work, Spencer enjoys exploring new countries, trying different foods, and playing games.

Chapter 6 – Evidence Phase: Introduction to Evidence

Martha Abshire Saylor, PhD, RN, is an Assistant Professor at the Johns Hopkins School of Nursing. Her clinical experience in cardiac and critical care has been the foundation of her research and teaching. Her research interests include an emphasis on psychosocial sequelae of advanced illness, advanced heart failure management, shared decision making, and patient-reported outcomes. Saylor has taught data analysis courses for DNP students for many years and has methodological expertise in using mixed quantitative and qualitative methods to understand complex phenomena including multi-component interventions.

Deborah W. Busch, DNP, CPNP-PC, IBCLC, CNE, FAANP, FAAN, is an Associate Professor, Certified Pediatric Nurse Practitioner, and Licensed Lactation Consultant with over three decades of nursing experience. She currently serves as the Director of the DNP/PNP Track at the Johns Hopkins School of Nursing, teaching advanced pediatric and doctoral-level nursing courses full-time. Busch remains clinically active, with her research centered on pediatric care, lactation, and educational methodologies in healthcare and nursing academia. Her work has been featured in numerous peer-reviewed journals, book chapters, and webinars. As a recognized expert, Busch has presented at national and international conferences on pediatric primary care, breastfeeding/lactation, and nursing education topics. Busch's commitment to the field extends beyond her professional roles. She actively volunteers in various local, state, and national professional organizations, including the Peace Corps, where she is dedicated to improving healthcare outcomes for the maternal-child dyad.

Madeleine Whalen, MSN/MPH, RN, CEN, NPD-BC. See Madeleine Whalen's bio earlier.

Kim Bissett, PhD, MBA, RN. See Kim Bissett's bio earlier.

Chapter 7 – Evidence Phase: The Evidence Search and Screening

Madeleine Whalen, MSN/MPH, RN, CEN, NPD-BC. See Madeleine Whalen's bio earlier.

Stella Seal, MLS, is the Lead Informationist for the School of Nursing, Hospital, and Health Systems Services of the Welch Medical Library, Johns Hopkins Medical Institutions. With over 20 years of experience, Seal provides formal and informal instruction in finding and using library resources, conducting systematic and other evidence-synthesis projects, and providing bibliometric and scholarly publishing support. Her professional interests include research ethics, information-seeking behavior, and methods to combat the spread of misinformation.

Marcus R. Spann, MLIS, is an Informationist at the Welch Medical Library of the Johns Hopkins Medical Institutions, with 20 years of public, academic, and medical library experience. He provides formal instruction through library resources while also conducting systematic reviews and evidence-synthesis projects, plus database searching, citation management, and information retrieval for faculty, staff, and students in various clinical departments including nursing and medicine. Through his diverse professional background, Spann has led various academic initiatives for underserved communities while taking part in library assessment and leadership programs.

Elisheva Wecker, MLIS, is an Informationist at the Welch Medical Library of the Johns Hopkins Medical Institutions. She provides formal and informal instruction in finding and using library resources, conducting systematic reviews and evidence-synthesis projects, database searching, and citation management for Johns Hopkins Hospital nurses and faculty, staff, and students in various departments across public health and medicine.

Chapter 8 – Evidence Phase: Appraising the Evidence

Madeleine Whalen, MSN/MPH, RN, CEN, NPD-BC. See Madeleine Whalen's bio earlier.

Martha Abshire Saylor, PhD, RN. See Martha Abshire Saylor's bio earlier.

Deborah W. Busch, DNP, CPNP-PC, IBCLC, CNE, FAANP, FAAN. See Deborah Busch's bio earlier.

Chapter 9 – Evidence Phase: Summary, Synthesis, and Best-Evidence Recommendations

Katherine Thompson, DNP, APRN, ACCNS-P, CCRN, is the Clinical Nurse Specialist for the Blalock-Taussig-Thomas Pediatric and Congenital Heart Center at Johns Hopkins Hospital. As the CNS, she supports evidence-based nursing practice, systems optimization, collaboration across departments, and provides expert specialty patient care. She earned her DNP from Johns Hopkins School of Nursing, where she now serves part-time as an advisor. Her areas of interest include proactive risk assessment for harm prevention, comprehensive neonatal care for patients with congenital heart disease, and empowering nurses through education and experience to function at the top of their scope.

Madeleine Whalen, MSN/MPH, RN, CEN, NPD-BC. See Madeleine Whalen's bio earlier.

Chapter 10 – Translation Phase: Translation

Carla Aquino, DNP, MSN, BA, RN, is the Nursing Program Director of Nursing Quality at Johns Hopkins Hospital. She leads nursing programs, projects, and initiatives to improve nurse-sensitive patient outcomes such as pressure injuries, falls, CAUTI, CLABSI, and others and the automation of data collection and reporting of Nurse Sensitive Indicators for the Johns Hopkins Health System to support data-driven quality improvement work. Aquino has previously worked with entities such as the Joint Commission Center for Transforming Healthcare Collaborative and Applied Physics Laboratory in quality improvement collaborations to prevent pressure injuries. She is a board member of the National Pressure Injury Advisory Panel. She mentors DNP students as an adjunct faculty at the Johns Hopkins University School of Nursing. She has been a nurse for almost 30 years, with experience in pediatric nursing, informatics, and nursing leadership. Aquino received her diploma in registered nursing from DePaul School of Nursing, BS in nursing from the University of Virginia, MS in nursing management, policy, and leadership from Yale University, and DNP from Johns Hopkins University.

Judith Ascenzi, DNP, RN. See Judith Ascenzi's bio earlier.

Holley Farley, DNP, RN, has worked as a registered nurse at the Johns Hopkins Hospital since 2012. Farley graduated with her DNP from the Johns Hopkins University School of Nursing. In her current role in Nursing Clinical Quality, she provides operational leadership in establishing processes and structures that support the improvement of Nurse Sensitive Indicators. She has made contributions to advance nursing knowledge through publications in the *Journal of Nursing Care Quality, Workplace Health & Safety, Journal of the American Geriatrics Society, American Journal of Physical Medicine & Rehabilitation,* and *International Journal of Nursing Studies.* She is well-known as a subject matter expert for fall prevention throughout the Johns Hopkins Health System and was recognized for her outstanding achievements in EBP at the 2022 SHINE Conference.

Chapter 11 – Translation Phase: Implementation

Carla Aquino, DNP, MSN, BA, RN. See Carla Aquino's bio earlier.

Judith Ascenzi, DNP, RN. See Judith Ascenzi's bio earlier.

Holley Farley, DNP, RN. See Holley Farley's bio earlier.

Chapter 12 – Ongoing Considerations: Communication and Dissemination

Madeleine Whalen, MSN/MPH, RN, CEN, NPD-BC. See Madeleine Whalen's bio earlier.

Sowmya Kumble, MPT, PT, NCS, is an Assistant Professor in Physical Medicine and Rehabilitation, Johns Hopkins School of Medicine and Clinical Resource Analyst at Johns Hopkins Hospital, Baltimore, Maryland. She began her career as a physical therapist in acute and critical care. She is passionate about promoting safe patient mobility of all hospitalized patients and early rehabilitation of critically ill patients. She collaborates with the fall prevention, safe patient handling, and other safety/quality taskforces to integrate and promote safe patient mobility. She has published several articles on early mobility and rehabilitation in peer-reviewed journals. She also serves as the Program Director of the Johns Hopkins Hospital and University of Delaware Neurologic Physical Therapy Residency Program that trains PTs in the area of neurological physical therapy.

Erik Hoyer, MD, is an Associate Professor in physical medicine and rehabilitation at the Johns Hopkins University School of Medicine, with a joint appointment in the Department of Medicine. He specializes in hospital-based rehabilitation, musculoskeletal and neurological rehabilitation, and electrodiagnostic medicine. As Vice Chair for Quality, Safety, and Service, Hoyer leads efforts to improve patient safety across Johns Hopkins Health System. He is also the co-founder and Director of Innovation for the Johns Hopkins Activity and Mobility Promotion program, which promotes safe patient mobility in hospitals. In addition to his clinical and administrative roles, Hoyer is actively involved in research focused on quality improvement and health services, with over 50 peer-reviewed publications and extramural funding supporting his work.

Chapter 13 – Exemplars

Nadine Rosenblum, MS, RN, IBCLC, NPD-BC, is the Central Nursing Program Coordinator – Lactation and Baby Friendly Programs at the Johns Hopkins Hospital. She was previously a Nursing Inquiry Coordinator for the JHH Center for Nursing Inquiry, where she provided training and support for nurses pursuing inquiry work throughout the Hopkins healthcare system. In that role, she served as principal investigator for nurse-led research studies, lead multiple unit-based quality improvement projects, and guided several EBP projects. Rosenblum has a strong interest in human lactation and supporting nurse-led activities that bring best practices to the bedside.

FACILITATOR GUIDE & WORKBOOK AVAILABLE

A facilitator guide and workbook for this book are available for sale from most retailers. Ask your book seller or simply search for this book title with added keywords of "facilitator guide" or "workbook" to purchase one or both. You can also email our Marketplace team for bulk orders at solutions@sigmamarketplace.org.

SPECIAL NOTE TO READERS

Here at Sigma, we realize that language is constantly evolving. The meaning of a word often changes over time, some words become obsolete, and some terms that were once acceptable may become controversial or even offensive, depending on the context or circumstances. We have made every effort to make language choices that are inclusive and not offensive. Should you identify words in this book that you believe negatively impact a group or groups of people, please reach out to us at Publications@SigmaNursing.org.

Recently we were made aware of the fact that the word *stakeholder* is objectionable to some individuals. In this book, the term refers to people with a vested interest in practice change—either decision makers or those directly affected by decisions. Although the term is widely used in healthcare research and literature, it strikes some audiences as untenable because of its use in colonial times, when a stakeholder was the person who drove a stake into the ground to demarcate the land that the stakeholder was occupying—essentially stealing—in Indigenous territories. Therefore, in our books we have decided to limit the use of the word and use alternative terms (such as impacted groups) where it makes sense to do so.

TABLE OF CONTENTS

About the Authors vii
Contributing Authors ix
Foreword xix
Introduction xxi

PART I EVIDENCE-BASED PRACTICE OVERVIEW 2

1 Evidence-Based Practice: Past, Present, and Future 4
Introduction 6
Information Explosion 6
EBP Defined 6
The Past 7
The Present 8
The Future: Emerging Trends 9
Summary 12
References 13

2 The Johns Hopkins Evidence-Based Practice (JHEBP) Model for Nurses and Healthcare Professionals (HCPs) Process Overview 16
Introduction 18
Differentiating Between Quality Improvement, Research, and EBP 18
Essential Components of The JHEBP Model for Nurses and HCPs:
  Inquiry, Practice, and Learning 19
Description: The JHEBP Model 24
JHEBP PET Process: Practice Question, Evidence, and Translation ... 27
Ongoing Considerations 34
Summary 37
References 37

PART II PRACTICE QUESTION, EVIDENCE, TRANSLATION (PET) 40

3 Practice Question Phase: The Problem 42
Introduction 44
Explore the Problem 44
Describe the Problem 44
Develop the Problem Statement 51
Summary 52
References 52

4 Practice Question Phase: The EBP Question 54
Introduction 56
Previous Approaches to EBP Questions 56
The Updated EBP Question 57
Additional Considerations 61
Summary 62
References 62

5 The Interprofessional Team 64
Introduction 66
The EBP Team... 66
Effective Teamwork: Competencies of an Interdisciplinary Team 70
Summary 74
References 74

Overview of the Evidence Phase 76

6 Evidence Phase: Introduction to Evidence 78
Introduction 80
Evidence Defined 80
Types of Evidence 81
Summary 89
References 90

7 Evidence Phase: The Evidence Search and Screening 92
Introduction 94
Searching the Literature 94
Systematic Literature Screening 109
Minimizing Bias in Literature Search and Screening 113
Summary 115
References 115

8 Evidence Phase: Appraising the Evidence 118
Introduction 120
Overview of the Appraisal Process 120
Appraisal Process by Type of Evidence 122
Summary 129
References 129

9 Evidence Phase: Summary, Synthesis, and Best-Evidence Recommendations 132
Introduction 134
Evidence Summary 134
Organization/Preparation 137
Synthesis 138
Best-Evidence Recommendations 139
Summary 142
References 144

10 Translation Phase: Translation 146
Introduction 148
Context in the EBP Project 149
Assess the Risk, Fit, Feasibility, and Acceptability of the Best-Evidence Recommendations 149
Additional Tools to Guide Organizational Considerations for the Translation Phase 152
Identify Practice Setting-Specific Recommendations 153
Summary 154
References 154

11 Translation Phase: Implementation 156
Introduction 158
Identifying an Implementation Framework or Model 158
Create an Implementation Action Plan 165
Monitor Sustainability and Identify Next Steps 168
Summary 169
References 169

12 Ongoing Considerations: Communication and Dissemination 170
Introduction 172
How to Create a Dissemination Plan 172
Internal Dissemination 173
External Dissemination 177
Future Considerations 184
Summary 185
References 185

PART III EXEMPLARS ... 188

13 Exemplars ... 190
Introduction ... 192
Strategies in Promoting and Increasing Certification Among Perianesthesia Nurses ... 192
Manila Doctors Hospital Evidence-Based Culture of Nurse Retention ... 194
RN-Driven High Flow Nasal Cannula Guidelines: Using Evidence to Change Practice Management ... 196
Set Sail for Home: A Nurse-Driven Initiative Promoting Early Ambulation in Post-Operative Neurosurgical Patients ... 198
Reducing Nurse Burden Related to Limited Care Partner Visitation ... 200
Transforming the Landscape of Gender-Affirming Care for Transgender Youth Through Acute Rehabilitation Provider Empowerment ... 202

PART IV APPENDICES ... 204

A EBP Project Steps and Overview ... 206

B Question Development Tool ... 210

C Searching and Screening Tool ... 216

D Appraisal Tool Selection Algorithm ... 224

E1 Pre-appraised Evidence Appraisal Tool ... 228

E2 Single Study Evidence Appraisal Tool ... 234

E3 Anecdotal Evidence Appraisal Tool ... 243

F Evidence Terminology and Considerations Guide ... 248

G1 Best-Evidence Summary Tool ... 264

G2 Individual Evidence Summary Tool ... 271

H Summary, Synthesis, & Best-Evidence Recommendations Tool ... 276

I Translation Tool ... 284

J Implementation and Action Planning (A3) Tool ... 288

Index ... 295

FOREWORD

I am thrilled to present the fifth edition of *Johns Hopkins Evidence-Based Practice for Nurses and Healthcare Professional: Model & Guidelines*. This new edition is not just a revision—it is an enhancement that anticipates the needs of frontline teams in healthcare delivery and education.

Healthcare has undergone rapid change since the beginning of the global pandemic. Most of these changes have stemmed from the need to change our care delivery models, focusing on redesign and implementation strategies to deliver high-quality and efficient care. Unlike many transformative approaches in the past, the changes are organic and come from the very front line of where healthcare is delivered—our nurses and other healthcare professionals on the care team. We have transformed how we work to care for complex and vulnerable people, with a continued focus on shared decision-making and quality outcomes with the patient at the center. Striving to keep our teams healthy, we have created flexible work schedules, integrated clinical support staff into primary nursing teams, and leveraged technology to enhance workflow and time with our patients. All these approaches to support our teams and patients have required EBP expertise and creativity but also the invaluable feedback from our frontline teams.

As with past editions, the feedback received from diverse end-user groups from practice and academia impacted the revisions in this edition. The authors have always valued the collaborative spirit that inspires this work. This edition highlights the expansion of the model to include an interprofessional approach to care coordination that builds capacity of all team members to discern best practices from common practice that will inform healthcare policies. The fifth edition hones with precision the strategies and tools to enhance the EBP process. The reader will benefit from the expanded focus on strategies to develop a problem statement and learn a new approach to EBP projects that includes the PET process and new evidence searching strategies. This new edition launches practical and precise approaches to enhancing EBP. Soon, there will be a companion Workbook and Facilitator Guide to enhance teaching and coaching of this fresh approach to providing quality, evidence-based care.

Johns Hopkins Evidenced-Based Practice for Nurses and Healthcare Professionals: Models & Guidelines assists interprofessional teams in creating a supportive infrastructure for building a contemporary and relevant EBP healthcare environment. I am humbled and honored to introduce this edition, which highlights nursing excellence and innovation.

–Deborah Baker, DNP, AG-ACNP, FAAN

INTRODUCTION

"Progress lies not in enhancing what is, but in advancing toward what will be."
–Khalil Gibran

Welcome to the fifth edition *of Johns Hopkins Evidence-Based Practice for Nurses and Healthcare Professionals: Model & Guidelines*. Originally developed to guide clinical nursing inquiry, the Johns Hopkins Evidence-Based Practice (JHEBP) Model for Nurses and Healthcare Professionals (HCPs) has evolved to make it easy for frontline nurses, health professionals, and students to use the best evidence in everyday practice. The book is arranged according to the EBP process using the Practice Question, Evidence, Translation (PET) process.

For more than 20 years, the model has been continuously evaluated and revised based on the honest, frank, and generous feedback we receive from frontline users across the globe. We continue to be grateful to those healthcare professionals who have taken the time to offer input, suggestions, and insights to improve the model's clarity and usability in various clinical and academic settings.

Experience shows us that there are many barriers to EBP in healthcare, including lack of time, resources, knowledge, and support to complete complex EBP projects. Thus, our overarching goal in the 2025 revision was simplicity. Our planning and brainstorming explored eliminating inefficiencies and unnecessary granularity from the process without losing model integrity. We looked for ways to enhance the current model to provide more direction and support. Through investigation into the current EBP landscape, as well as discussions and interactions with users, we identified several important areas for improvement.

First, we recognized, as many others have, the ineffectiveness of PICO as a question structure in EBP. Completing the PICO components is a time-consuming endeavor filled with many questions. In addition to the need to write "not applicable" to at least one of the four components of the PICO for background (best practice) EBP questions, teams may struggle to decide what terms should be listed under "C" or "O" when developing a background question or prematurely select an intervention, "I," to complete the structure. Chapter 4 addresses the problems with PICO and provides an alternative approach to developing both a broad (background) and an intervention (foreground) question. Using the new question structure saves teams valuable time and energy by avoiding the need to assign terms to an arbitrary letter. The Question Development Tool (Appendix B) has been updated to reflect these changes.

Next, we identified a need to improve our approach to evidence, in terms of hierarchy and quality.

In previous versions, the JHEBP model used a five-level hierarchy of evidence based on study design and intent. Research evidence occupied levels one through three and non-research evidence levels four and five. Teams were spending a great deal of time and energy trying to identify very specific details about the evidence that ultimately had no bearing on the support for practice change. Over the years we added decision trees and algorithms to help make this decision process easier. However, there was still a great deal of wasted energy—for example, determining if a piece of non-research evidence constituted a literature review or an expert opinion when both offer the same level of support for practice change. With this revision, we wanted to remove some of the unnecessary granularity and simplify this process while maintaining attention to evidence type and methodology. We also wanted to move away from static hierarchies as the judge of best information. We progressed from a five-level hierarchy to broader categories of evidence grouped according to the degree of decision-making confidence that evidence affords. For example, quality improvement (QI), with the intention of improving practices on the local level, was previously considered the lowest level of evidence, level five, regardless of methods or rigor. With the changes, QI evidence is now categorized based on the methodology. For example, a QI project that employs a formal study design may fall into the same broad category of moderate support for decision-making as a quasi-experimental study. Chapter 6 provides an updated overview of what constitutes evidence and how these broad categories are defined.

In addition to categories of evidence, we recognized the need to simplify the way we viewed the quality of the evidence. Traditionally, evidence quality was determined to be high quality (A), good quality (B), or low quality (C). Using the appropriate appraisal tool, teams checked boxes to indicate whether that article met predetermined criteria. From there, the team decided if the quality was high, good, or poor. There was no established number of "yeses" to garner a high rating or "noes" to earn a low-quality rating. Teams would spend time trying to come to consensus, often struggling between an "A" or "B" and sometimes compromising at an "A–" or "B+." Ultimately, these nuances make little difference in subsequent steps to generate recommendations. What is important is whether the evidence is good enough to use or not. Should it be included in the evidence summary or excluded? The revised evidence appraisal tools (Appendices E1, E2, and E3) guide this decision-making, helping the team consider the piece of evidence as a whole. Chapter 8 has been fully revised to cover this new and improved process.

The third area for elimination of inefficiency and simplification was deciding when a comprehensive literature review is necessary, specifically identifying when EBP questions have already been answered in existing literature. With the fourth edition of the JHEBP model, we introduced the decision tree to determine the need for an EBP project. This was a step in the right direction but did not seem to go far enough. This fifth edition includes an improved "Evidence Phase Decision Tree" to place more emphasis on using suitable pre-appraised evidence (clinical practice guidelines, literature reviews with a systematic approach, evidence summaries) in place of an exhaustive EBP when such evidence answers all aspects of the EBP question. This step saves a great deal of time and energy, allowing teams to more quickly move into translation.

This fifth edition represents some of the biggest changes to date, and we are excited to share them. We believe that our model was not meant to be static but progressive. Just as EBP resists relying on tradition and historical practices, our model must also resist stagnation. We are confident these changes, born from both practical and experiential knowledge, strengthen the model and make the process even more manageable. We hope this edition provides a catalyst for change in your practice or that of your organization.

Other key updates include:

- A brief discussion of the impact of COVID-19 on EBP and emerging issues such as artificial intelligence

- A new chapter highlighting the interprofessional team and the important considerations for impacted groups (formerly known as stakeholders)

- A separate chapter for the problem with an expanded focus on strategies to develop a problem statement

- More direction for searching and screening to streamline the process
- New ways of characterizing best-evidence recommendations
- A chapter specific to implementation and greater direction on real-world implementation models
- New exemplars showcasing the JHEBP model in action

We also enhanced the appendices by including more flowcharts, decision supports, and specific directions. In general, we wrote this edition to better serve as a step-by-step how-to manual for EBP projects. For downloadable versions of the appendices/tools, go to Hopkins.org/tools. For other resources, go to Hopkins.org/resources.

The fifth edition continues to honor the imperative first established by M. Adelaide Nutting, Assistant Superintendent of Nurses at the Johns Hopkins Hospital, Principal of the Johns Hopkins School of Nursing, and pioneer in the development of nursing education:

"We need to realize and affirm a view that 'medicine' is one of the most difficult of arts. Compassion may provide the motive, but knowledge is our only working power . . . surely we will not be satisfied with merely perpetuating methods and traditions; surely we should be more and more involved with creating them."

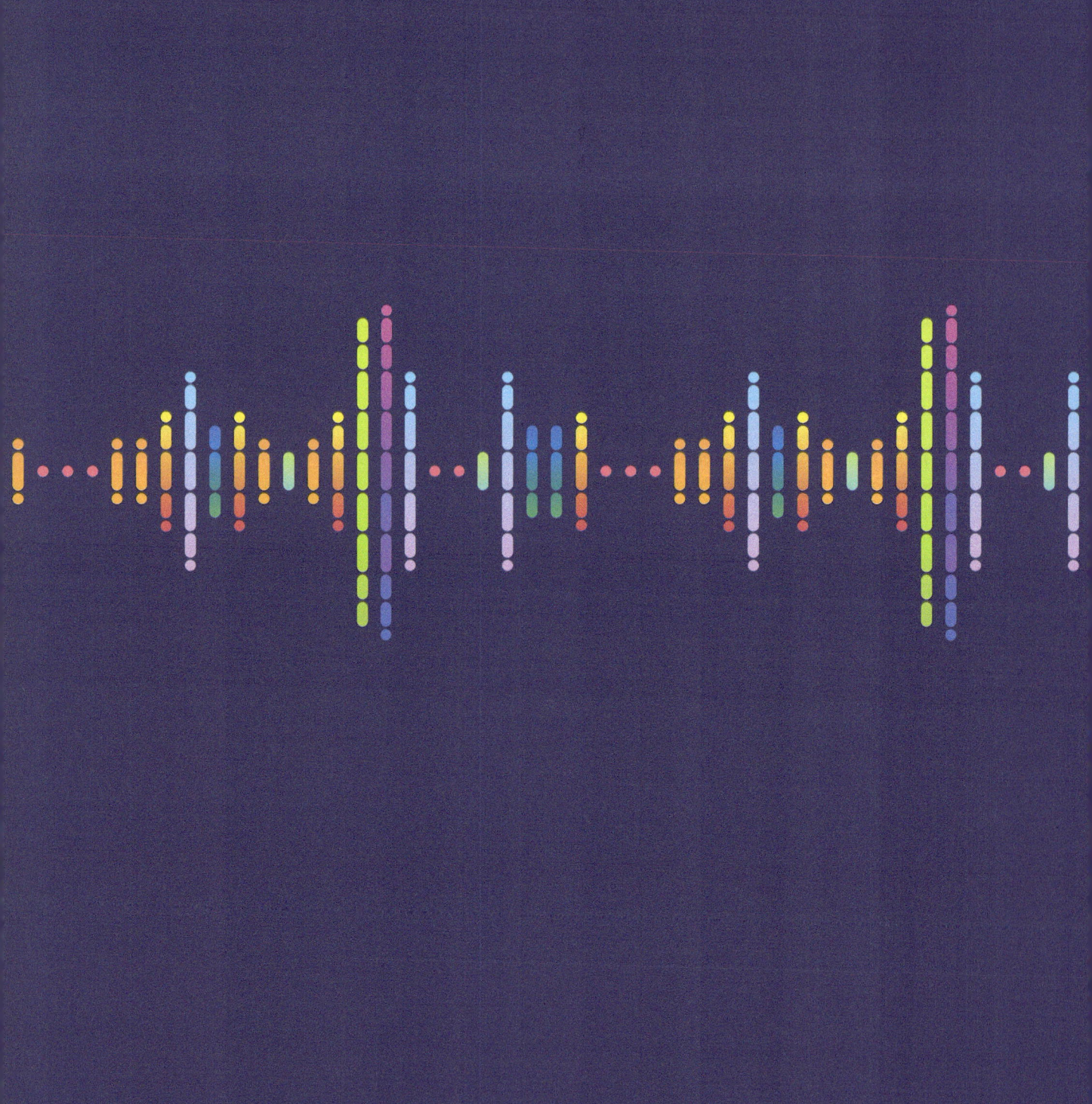

PART I
EVIDENCE-BASED PRACTICE OVERVIEW

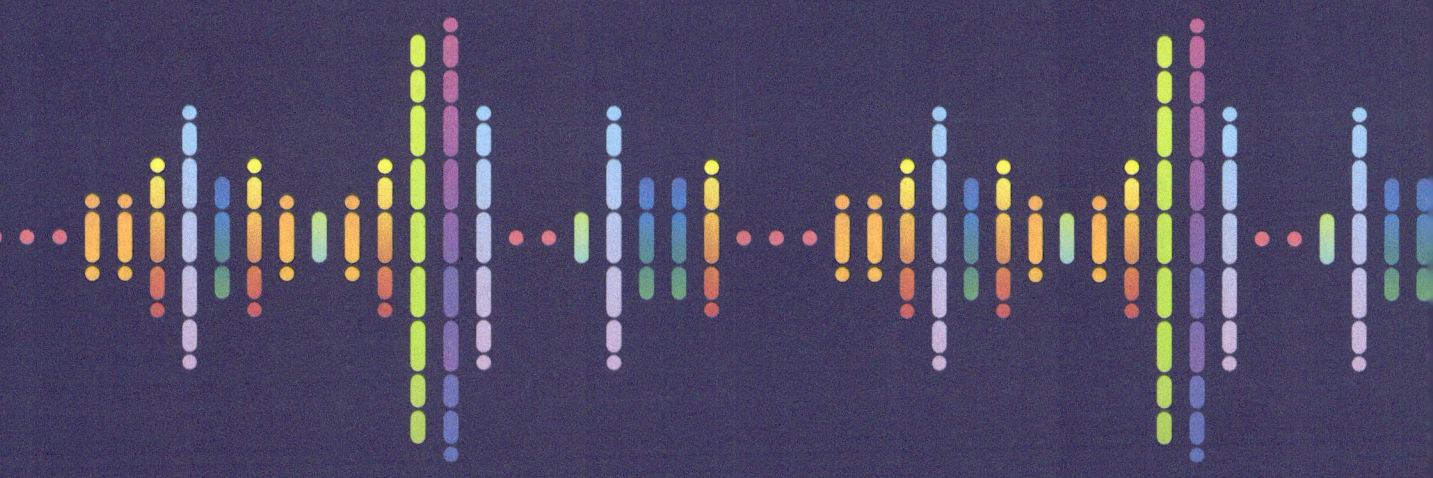

1. Evidence-Based Practice: Past, Present, and Future 4

2. The Johns Hopkins Evidence-Based Practice (JHEBP) Model for Nurses and Healthcare Professionals (HCPs) Process Overview ... 16

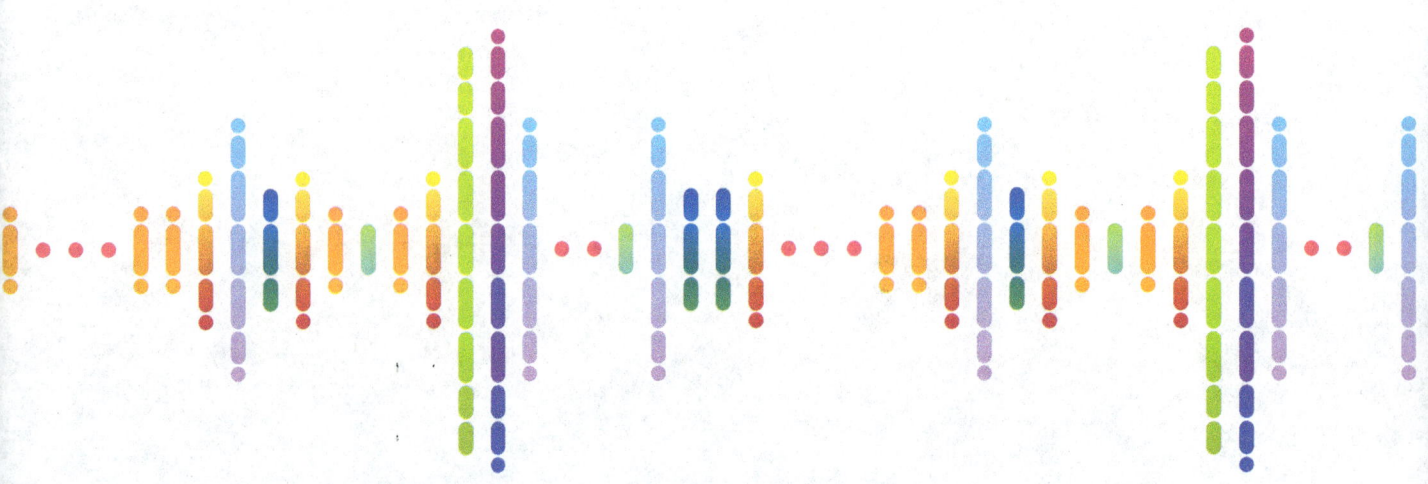

OBJECTIVES

- Define EBP
- Describe the evolution of EBP in healthcare
- Discuss the current state of EBP
- Highlight healthcare clinicians' role in EBP
- Discuss emerging concepts and challenges that impact the EBP process

EVIDENCE-BASED PRACTICE: PAST, PRESENT, AND FUTURE

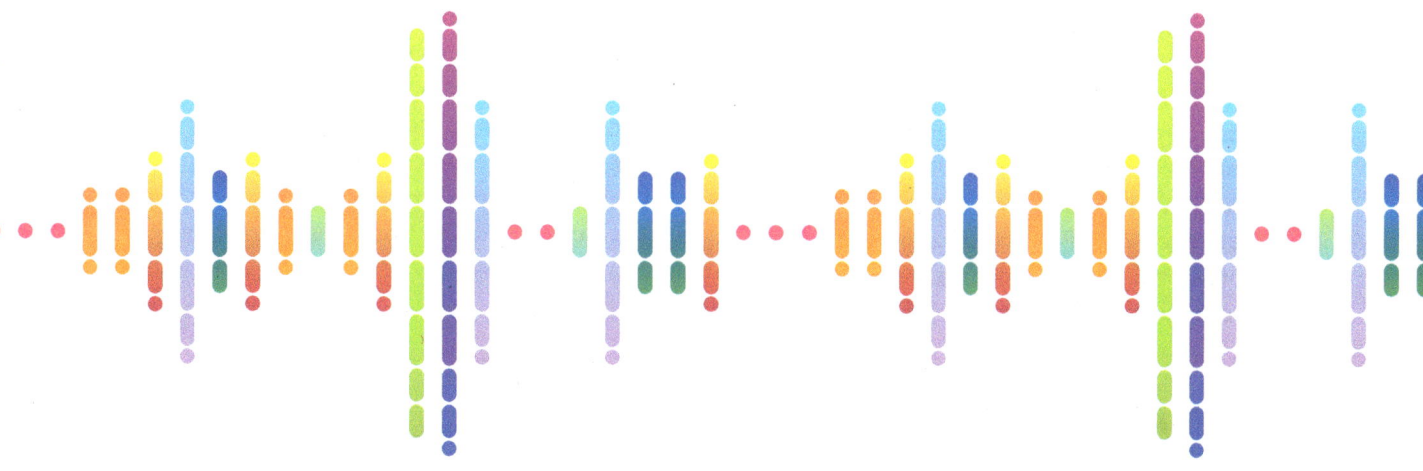

KEY POINTS

- Evidence-based practice (EBP) helps clinicians keep up with emerging evidence, practices, and technologies.

- The Johns Hopkins Evidence-Based Practice (JHEBP) Model for Nursing and Healthcare Professionals provides a structured and systematic way for clinicians to effectively use current scientific and experiential evidence to determine best practices and provide safe, high-quality care.

- Numerous healthcare organizations encourage the use and prioritization of EBP.

- EBP can be used during resource-limited times such as with the COVID-19 pandemic. Clinicians may need to think creatively and expand their skill sets.

- Artificial intelligence (AI) can potentially enhance the EBP process by speeding up the process or replacing many of the human tasks. In the future, AI may complete entire EBP projects in seconds.

- EBP teams can address health equity locally by considering diversity, equity, and inclusion from the start of the EBP project.

INTRODUCTION

As far back as 2003, the Institute of Medicine (IOM), now the National Academy of Medicine (NAM), published a set of five core competencies required of each health professional. This is not an exhaustive list but represents the competencies common among various health professionals and the most important to advancing healthcare. These competencies included providing patient-centered care, working in interdisciplinary teams, applying quality improvement, utilizing informatics, and employing *evidence-based practice* (EBP; IOM, 2003). Today, EBP remains a significant core competency for nurses and other healthcare providers, who have considerable influence on healthcare decisions and the quality and safety of care. EBP allows clinicians and interprofessional teams to keep up with the rapidly changing environment.

INFORMATION EXPLOSION

The world is experiencing an information and technology explosion. Unfortunately, in healthcare, the growth of knowledge outpaces the application to practice. The process of incorporating new knowledge into clinical practice is often considerably delayed. Curry (2018) reports that it may take up to 15 years to approve new drugs. The average time for the uptake of research into actual practice is 15 years (Balas & Boren, 2000; Khan et al., 2021). New knowledge has grown exponentially. Early in the 20th century, many healthcare professionals had but a few, hard-to-access journals available to them. Today, the healthcare database MEDLINE indexes 5,200 journals (National Library of Medicine, 2024) with more than 31 million references. The Cumulative Index to Nursing and Allied Health Literature (CINAHL) indexes more than 5,600 journals and includes over 4.1 million records (EBSCO Publishing, 2024). Resources for clinicians on EBP are available through the addition of free and fee-for-service applications that provide evidence-based practices, clinical practice guidelines, and standards of care at one's fingertips. The key to these and other resources is knowing and understanding which applications are resource-rich with peer-reviewed data and provide decision-making support clinicians can rely on.

Accessibility of information on the web also has increased consumer expectations of participating in treatment decisions. Patients with chronic health problems have accumulated considerable expertise in self-management, increasing the pressure on providers to be up to date with the best evidence for care. The EBP process is one of the best strategies enabling healthcare providers to stay abreast of new practices and technology amid this continuing information explosion.

EBP DEFINED

EBP is a problem-solving approach to clinical decision-making that integrates the best available scientific evidence with the best available experiential (patient and practitioner) evidence and encourages critical thinking in the judicious application of such evidence to the care of individual patients, a patient population, or a system (Dang et al., 2022). The challenge for healthcare providers is to use such evidence to implement the best interventions to improve patient outcomes. The Johns Hopkins Evidence-Based Practice (JHEBP) Model for Nursing and Healthcare Professionals provides a structured and systematic way for clinicians to effectively use current scientific and experiential evidence to determine best practices and provide safe, high-quality care.

EBP can support and inform clinical, administrative, and educational decision-making. Combining evidence from various sources—including research, quality improvement, clinical expertise, and expert opinion—ensures that clinical decisions are based on all available information. EBP enhances *efficacy* (the ability to reach a desired result under ideal circumstances); *efficiency* (the achievement of a desired result with minimal expense, time, and effort); and *effectiveness* (the ability to produce a desired result in the "real world"; Burches & Burches, 2020). Additionally, the EBP process weighs risk, benefit, and cost against a backdrop of patient preferences and organizational considerations. This evidence-based decision-making encourages healthcare providers to question practice and determine which interventions are ready to be implemented or de-implemented in clinical practice, administration, or education. EBP can lead to:

- Optimal outcomes
- Reductions in unnecessary variations in care
- Standardization of care
- Equivalent care at lower cost and/or in less time
- Improved patient satisfaction
- Increased clinician satisfaction and autonomy
- Higher health-related quality of life

THE PAST

EBP in healthcare is not conceptually new. It is grounded in the assumption that patient care should be informed and guided by scientific evidence, clinical experience, and patient preferences to ultimately improve patient, provider, and system outcomes but also to address the need for cost-effective practice, availability of information, consumer knowledge, and treatment options (Melnyk & Fineout-Overholt, 2023; O'Brien et al., 2023).

From a nursing perspective, Florence Nightingale pioneered the concept of using research evidence to dictate care. She documented her experimental evidence and published it in her book *Notes on Nursing: What It Is, and What It Is Not* (1859). Though recently under scrutiny for her views on race and colonialism (Bates & Greenwood, 2022), Nightingale's work remains an early example of using evidence in practice. She used her data and evidence to influence patient care, positively impacting patient outcomes long before any formal knowledge of EBP (Mackey & Bassendowsky, 2017). In the 1920s, Mary McMillan worked to bring a scientific basis to the practice of physical therapy and to standardize the practice (American Physical Therapy Association, 2023). The EBP movement gained momentum in 1972, when Archibald L. Cochrane, a British medical researcher, criticized the health profession for administering treatments not supported by evidence but rather by unfounded assumptions, individual assessment, and choice (Cochrane, 1972; Mackey & Bassendowsky, 2017). By the 1980s, the term *evidence-based medicine* was being used at McMaster University Medical School in Canada. Positive reception given to systematic reviews of care during pregnancy and childbirth prompted the British National Health Service in 1992 to approve funding for a "Cochrane Centre" to facilitate the preparation of systematic reviews of randomized controlled trials of healthcare, eventually leading to the establishment of the Cochrane Collaboration in 1993 (Cochrane Collaboration, 2016). Cochrane continues to provide systematic reviews about the effectiveness of healthcare and sound scientific evidence for providing effective treatment regimens. David Sackett, widely considered the father of evidence-based medicine, and colleagues expanded Cochrane's definition in the mid-1990s to include individual patient preferences, values, and beliefs (Sackett et al., 1996). It was then that evidence-based medicine changed its name to evidence-based practice and was subsequently adopted by other healthcare professions to be used in their respective specialized fields (Mackey & Bassendowsky, 2017). In 1996, Alan Pearson founded the Joanna Briggs Research Institute (now JBI) to link research with practice, thus impacting global health outcomes and providing evidence to inform clinical decision-making (JBI, 2020). Concurrent with the rapid development of EBP in the mid-1990s, the first detailed description of EBP and nursing in primary care was published in 1996; less than 10 years later, an entire journal dedicated to EBP, *Worldviews on Evidence-Based Nursing*, was published.

Experts from the IOM, now NAM, recommended expanding the use of EBP in healthcare across disciplines to inform best practices, ultimately supporting the quadruple aim of improving population health outcomes, reducing the cost of care, enhancing the patient's experience (inclusive of quality and safety), and improving clinician satisfaction, experience, and well-being (Bodenheimer & Sinsky, 2014; Stevens, 2013). More recently, the fifth aim of "health equity" was added (Nundy et al., 2022). The following reports by IOM/NAM have urged healthcare professionals to prioritize EBP:

- *Crossing the Quality Chasm* (IOM, 2001) called for the healthcare system to adopt six aims for improvement and 10 principles for redesign. The report recommended that healthcare decision-making be evidence-based to ensure that patients receive care based on the best scientific evidence available and that the evidence is transparent to patients and their families to assist them in making informed decisions.

- The second report, *Health Professions Education: A Bridge to Quality* (IOM, 2003), described five key competencies for health professionals: delivering patient-centered care, working as part of interprofessional teams, focusing on quality improvement, using information technology, and practicing evidence-based medicine.

- The third report, *Roundtable on Evidence-Based Medicine* (IOM, 2007), brought medical researchers and clinicians together to set a goal that by the year 2020, 90% of clinical decisions would be supported by accurate, timely, and up-to-date clinical information and will reflect the best available evidence—a goal that, unfortunately, healthcare professionals did not meet.

- The fourth report, *The Future of Nursing: Leading Change, Advancing Health* (IOM, 2011), urged that schools of nursing ensure that nurses achieve competency in leadership, health policy, systems improvement, teamwork and collaboration, and research and EBP.

- The most recent report, *The Future of Nursing 2020–2030: Charting a Path to Achieve Health Equity* (National Academies of Sciences, Engineering, and Medicine [NASEM], 2021), addresses the focus on social disparities in healthcare and nurses' unique position to help address equitable health and healthcare systems for all while taking costs, new technology, and patient- and family-centered care into account.

THE PRESENT

Given these rapid developments over the last 50 years, where does EBP stand now?

EBP has experienced tremendous growth in the past few decades. The increased emphasis on EBP can be attributed to two main factors. First, as mentioned previously, knowledge development is outpacing our ability to put findings into practice, driving the need for a systematic way of evaluating evidence. Second, the development of EBP has been further driven by a desire to improve outcomes, pressure from consumers for more accountability, and regulatory requirements by accreditation bodies.

As a result, many healthcare organizations have created strategic initiatives for EBP. Current national pay-for-performance initiatives, both voluntary and mandatory, provide reimbursement to hospitals and practitioners for implementing healthcare practices supported with evidence. Consumer pressure and increased patient expectations place an even greater emphasis on this need for true EBP. In an often-cited study, McGlynn et al. (2003) reported that Americans receive only about 50% of the healthcare recommended by evidence. For example, there is currently an increased focus on maternal health, a crisis with rising but preventable deaths of women in the US in recent years. According to the Centers for Disease Control and Prevention (2021, 2022), approximately 1,200 women died in 2021 (numbers may be somewhat skewed due to the COVID-19 pandemic) from pregnancy-related causes, and an estimated four in five deaths could have been prevented by addressing gaps in hospital-level system factors, social determinants of health, and EBP (Bovbjerg et al., 2022).

The International Council of Nurses (ICN), as well as the American Nurses Association (ANA), recommend the use of EBP and promote its use in nursing to disseminate findings, use those findings for advocacy, and build partnerships and capacity (ANA, 2023; ICN, 2012, 2023). In addition, the development of best-practice guidelines by nursing organizations has led to expanded access and availability (Mackey & Bassendowsky, 2017). For example, the Registered Nurses' Association of Ontario (RNAO) in Canada has published over 50 best-practice guidelines on their website in nine categories that are accessible to anybody (RNAO, 2024). Additionally, other disciplines have developed evidence-based guidelines specific to their practices. The American Occupational Therapy Association (AOTA) maintains resources and guidelines for EBP, including evidence infographics and evidence-informed interventions (AOTA, 2024). The American Association for Respiratory Care (AARC) provides evidence-based clinical guidelines for various practices (AARC, 2023).

Despite this trend, many healthcare clinicians in the US and the world still practice care grounded in traditions, operating in "comfort zones" rather than applying the best evidence into practice (Lehane et al., 2019; Melnyk et al., 2018). Saunders and Vehviläinen-Julkunen (2016) suggest that nurses generally value and believe in the EBP process yet point to a lack of knowledge and skills as factors for not using the approach. Barriers related to giving nurses dedicated time to learn about the components of EBP, providing them with time and resources to apply the entire EBP process to an identified problem, and organizational leadership support of EBP are key issues that need to be addressed if we want to improve the uptake of EBP at organizations (Kerr & Rainey, 2021; Melnyk & Fineout-Overholt, 2023). Lastly, the need for rapid translation of evidence into practice during the COVID-19 pandemic suggests an even greater imperative to build infrastructure that not only supports EBP but also infuses it into practice environments.

THE FUTURE: EMERGING TRENDS

COVID-19

The COVID-19 pandemic, which started in late 2019 in Wuhan, China, was an incredibly difficult time for healthcare providers and highlighted areas of strength and weakness in our healthcare system. An area of strength was the healthcare team's readiness to do what was needed. However, there was minimal and often conflicting evidence on how patients infected with COVID-19 should be treated and how healthcare providers should protect themselves against infection. While nurses were trying to base their care on the evidence available to them (Rudman et al., 2023), important questions related to EBP were raised: "What if there is no evidence to review? What if the resources and interventions that we know are best practices are not available? What if the credible authorities' guidelines contradict the best evidence?" (Rudman et al., 2023; Yingling, 2020). For the healthcare team to practice competently, the team had to find what evidence was available and adapt and adopt information appropriate to the situation at hand. This highlights how imperative critical thinking and EBP skills are as competencies for the healthcare professional. According to Rudman et al. (2023), nurses used EBP during COVID-19 to guide practice and make decisions in their activities with about the same frequency as they did before COVID-19, which speaks to how quickly the COVID-19 information was assessed, reviewed, and made available for the interdisciplinary teams on the front lines and in the boardroom.

Still, lack of time and resources, high patient load, and other factors present barriers to EBP. Given the most recent experiences related to the COVID-19 pandemic, there is a need for guidelines on how to adapt EBP models when scarcity of materials and time is a major factor when practicing nursing (Yingling, 2020). Additionally, gaps between rapidly evolving evidence and complex and time-consuming policymaking, as evidenced during the COVID-19 pandemic, lead to delays in evidence-based care (Tussing et al., 2023). One practical example that applied the EBP process during resource-limited times while focusing on positive patient outcomes is the "Choosing Wisely" initiative (Pramesh et al., 2021). Despite being a physician-patient intervention, it addresses questions related to avoiding unnecessary medical interventions in times of scarcity that could be adapted by other healthcare specialties and in different environments. To facilitate EBP projects and research endeavors during the pandemic, remote teleconferencing platforms such as Zoom and Webex evolved. Now, widely available internet platforms for research data collection, such as REDCap and Microsoft Teams, have created mechanisms for sharing information and collaboration that were less common before the pandemic (Britt, 2021; Gralton et al., 2020). Using these new technology platforms, however, requires different expertise and skills, which will require adaptation of the process used to conduct research and EBP in the past (Fowler, 2023).

Artificial Intelligence

In 2007, the Institute of Medicine Roundtable on Evidence-Based Medicine projected that "by the year 2020, ninety percent of clinical decisions will be supported by accurate, timely, and up-to-date clinical information, and will reflect the best available evidence" (App. D, para. 1). However, achieving this target remains challenging, even in 2024. A new and evolving technology, artificial intelligence (AI), can support efforts to increase the use of evidence-based practices.

AI, according to the University of Illinois Chicago College of Engineering (2024), "represents a branch of computer science that aims to create machines capable of performing tasks that typically require human intelligence" (para. 1). AI is entering healthcare practice and education in a variety of mechanisms. The Organisation for Economic Co-operation and Development (2023) suggests that "different AI systems vary in their levels of autonomy and adaptiveness after deployment" (p. 3). AI uses large amounts of training data to develop patterns of algorithm responses, including reinforcement learning components provided by human feedback (Zhavoronkov, 2023). Large language models (LLMs) such as ChatGPT have been made available to the public in the recent past. They can answer questions, summarize, and paraphrase text in a matter of seconds in a quality that is equal to or even better than what a human being could have produced (Clusmann et al., 2023).

As technologies develop, AI could both support the EBP process and replace the need for EBP. In terms of supporting the process, AI has the potential to:

- Analyze large volumes of data from various sources, completing an evidence search, screening, and appraisal

- Apply "few-shot learning," a technique that requires only a limited amount of training data to generate EBP questions (Peng et al., 2023)

- Transform complex clinical jargon into plain language to increase engagement and empowerment, which is particularly useful for clinicians as consumers of research evidence (Peng et al., 2023)

- Speed up the efficiency with which we integrate new knowledge into practice by developing implementation plans

- Evaluate the implementation and measure outcomes and analyze data

- Provide "living systematic reviews" by automatically updating clinical evidence as soon as new information becomes available (NASEM, 2019)

In terms of replacing EBP, AI may be able to complete the entire EBP process with a simple prompt or query. In the future, EBP teams could provide the AI system with an EBP question and wait as the system produces best-evidence recommendations within seconds. Teams would presumably still need to determine the fit, feasibility, and acceptability for their organization, but even those considerations may eventually be part of the AI knowledge bank.

While the promises of AI are intriguing and potentially game-changing, clinicians must proceed with caution. Current available AI technology is not where it would need to be to truly impact EBP. For example, as Zhavononkov (2023) reports, programs like ChatGPT were not trained on the entire body of available healthcare literature or tested or trained by expert clinicians. Currently, these systems exclude relevant information and generate inaccurate outputs, missing important components when synthesizing evidence such as the distinction between short-term and long-term outcomes (Peng et al., 2023). Moreover, these systems are trained on data and models created by humans who may impart their own implicit or explicit biases (Adams et al., 2024). As such, AI-generated content may perpetuate healthcare inequalities by continuing to underrepresent certain populations or push forward biases. Additionally, more recent data available after the training point are not incorporated in the latest evidence but might be more accurate (Adams et al., 2024; Zhavononkov, 2023). Until real-time updating or training can be achieved, evidence identified by LLMs should be compared with manually extracted reviews by human reviewers, and regardless of the technological advances with AI, EBP teams must remain well-versed in the EBP process.

Health Equity

In 2021, NASEM published their much-anticipated report *The Future of Nursing 2020–2030*. While the report was specific to nursing, the concepts are relevant to all healthcare providers. The report expands its previous focus to include a road map to "applying evidence linking health and health care equity to health outcomes for individuals, families, and communities, populations, as well as further building out evidence-based models" (p. xv). One year after this publication, Nundy and colleagues (2022) proposed to include health equity in the quadruple aim of healthcare improvement, thus creating a quintuple aim.

Health equity as defined by the World Health Organization (2024) is "the absence of unfair, avoidable or remediable differences among groups of people, whether those groups are defined socially, economically, demographically, or geographically or by other dimensions of inequality (e.g., sex, gender, ethnicity, disability, or sexual orientation)" (para. 1). In the United States and worldwide, the complex interactions between individual social determinants of health and structural multisystem factors such as access to care and racialized health inequities remain challenges in addressing health disparities and population health outcomes (Still et al., 2023). As has been previously reported, the US spends more on healthcare than any other comparable high-income country but has higher mortality rates, worse outcomes, highest poverty rates, and greatest income inequality (NASEM, 2021; Tikkanen & Abrams, 2020). Sadly, in the US, the COVID-19 pandemic highlighted these existing health disparities, resulting in high mortality rates in underserved and marginalized communities (NASEM, 2021). Despite this, only 58% of healthcare organizations consider health equity one of their top three priorities (Ratersdorf et al., 2022).

To address health equity, the focus of research and thus EBP has shifted in recent years to include population health-focused interventions. Because nurses and other healthcare providers are some of the most trusted professionals in the US, their expertise and involvement in many aspects of healthcare could be leveraged to address disparities and promote health equity for all (Gallup, 2024). Building partnerships with communities by including them in research activities, aligning mutual priorities, and collaborating with policy experts will help nurse researchers address these persistent problems (Still et al., 2023). Implementation science could be used to scale evidence-based practices as well as educational strategies and public policies (Hassmiller & Wakefield, 2022). However, for these strategies to succeed, healthcare leaders must provide practitioners with the needed resources, such as dedicated time and leadership support to conduct evidence-based interventions, engage with communities, collect data, and publish the findings (Nundy et al., 2022).

EBP teams can address health equity at the local level as well. From the start of the project, teams should consider diversity, equity, and inclusion (DEI). They may start by creating an EBP team of diverse backgrounds and experiences. When exploring and developing the problem, the team should ask, "Does the problem impact one group more than another?" or, "Are we looking at this from all diverse perspectives?" EBP questions should incorporate DEI. Does the EBP question capture all those affected, or is the team eliminating important groups? During the search and screening process, teams should be aware of populations left out of the literature and recognize who may be underrepresented in the evidence. While appraising the evidence, teams should note who participated in the study—that is, what populations, age groups, etc., were represented in the sample. Recommendations should be developed to be inclusive and ensure that best practices reach everyone. Healthcare inequality is a large global problem. However, ensuring that DEI considerations are part of local EBP projects is a step in the right direction.

SUMMARY

This chapter defines EBP and discusses the evolution that led to the focus on using evidence-based practices to guide decision-making. EBP creates a culture of critical thinking and ongoing learning and is the foundation for an environment where evidence supports clinical, operational, and educational decisions. EBP is an explicit process that facilitates decision-making to support effective, efficient, and equitable patient-centered care. Recent global challenges such as COVID-19 highlighted the need for clinicians to be well-versed in rapidly accessing and appraising available evidence for practice or adapting in the absence of evidence. Despite many advances in EBP and access to evidence, healthcare professionals continue to practice by tradition, and barriers to EBP still exist. Emerging technologies such as AI promise to make EBP more accessible or replace it altogether. However, even those advances would still require clinicians knowledgeable in the EBP process to verify AI findings. Healthcare equality can be addressed through EBP and should be a regular consideration starting at the local level.

REFERENCES

Adams, L., Fontaine, E., Lin, E., Crowell, T., Chung, V. C. H., & Gonzalez, A. A. (Eds.). (2024, April 8). Artificial intelligence in health, health care and biomedical science: An AI code of conduct principles and commitments discussion draft. *NAM Perspectives*. National Academy of Medicine. https://doi.org/10.31478/202403a

American Association for Respiratory Care. (2023). *Clinical practice guidelines*. https://www.aarc.org/resource/clinical-practice-guidelines/

American Nurses Association. (2023, June 1). *What is evidence-based practice in nursing?* https://www.nursingworld.org/content-hub/resources/workplace/evidence-based-practice-in-nursing/

American Occupational Therapy Association. (2024). *Evidence-based practice and knowledge translation*. https://www.aota.org/practice/practice-essentials/evidencebased-practiceknowledge-translation

American Physical Therapy Association. (2023). *100 milestones of physical therapy*. https://timeline.apta.org/

Balas, E. A., & Boren, S. A. (2000). Managing clinical knowledge for health care improvement. *Yearbook of Medical Informatics, 1*, 65–70.

Bates, R., & Greenwood, A. (2022). Could Nightingale get cancelled? The rise, endurance, and possible fall of Florence Nightingale in British historical culture since 1854. *Women's History Review, 31*(7), 1080–1106. https://doi.org/10.1080/09612025.2022.2045110

Bodenheimer, T., & Sinsky, C. (2014). From triple to quadruple aim: Care of the patient requires care of the provider. *Annals of Family Medicine, 12*(6), 573–576.

Bovbjerg, M., Tucker, C. M., & Pillai, S. (2022). Current resources for evidence-based practice. *Journal of Obstetric, Gynecologic, and Neonatal Nursing, 51*(2), 225–237. https://doi.org/10.1016/j.jogn.2022.01.005

Britt, K. C. (2021, January). Meeting the nursing research world in the time of COVID-19. *Clinical Nursing Research, 30*(1), 3–4. https://doi.org/10.1177/1054773820984642

Burches, E., & Burches, M. (2020). Efficacy, effectiveness and efficiency in health care: The need for an agreement to clarify its meaning. *International Archives of Public Health & Community Medicine, 4*(1). doi.org/10.23937/2643-4512/1710035

Centers for Disease Control and Prevention. (2021). *Maternal mortality rates in the United States, 2021*. https://www.cdc.gov/nchs/data/hestat/maternal-mortality/2021/maternal-mortality-rates-2021.htm

Centers for Disease Control and Prevention. (2022, Sept. 19). *Four in 5 pregnancy-related deaths in the U.S. are preventable*. https://www.cdc.gov/media/releases/2022/p0919-pregnancy-related-deaths.html

Clusmann, J., Kolbinger, F. R., Muti, H. S., Carrero, Z. I., Eckardt, J.-N., Laleh, N. G., Loffler, C. M. L., Schwarzkopf, S.-C., Unger, M., Veldhuizen, G. P., Wagner, S. J., & Kather, J. N. (2023). The future landscape of large language models in medicine. *Communications Medicine, 3*(141). https://doi.org/10.1038/s43856-023-00370-1

Cochrane, A. L. (1972). *Effectiveness and efficiency: Random reflections on health services*. Nuffield Provincial Hospitals Trust.

Cochrane Collaboration. (2016). *About us*. http://www.cochrane.org/about-us

Curry, S. H. (2018). Translational science: Past, present, and future. *BioTechniques, 44*(Suppl. 2). https://doi.org/10.2144/000112749

Dang, D., Dearholt, S., Bissett, K., Ascenzi, J., & Whalen, M. (2022). *Johns Hopkins evidence-based practice for nurses and healthcare professionals: Model and guidelines* (4th ed.). Sigma Theta Tau International.

EBSCO Publishing. (2024). *CINAHL database*. https://www.ebsco.com/products/research-databases/cinahl-database#:~:text=CINAHL%20indexes%20the%20top%20nursing,companion%20to%20the%20CINAHL%20index

Fowler, S. B. (2023). Sustainability of nursing research during the pandemic: Reflections and directions. *Research in Nursing and Health, 46*(2), 188–189.

Gallup. (2024). *Ethics ratings of nearly all professions down in U.S.* https://news.gallup.com/poll/608903/ethics-ratings-nearly-professions-down.aspx

Gralton, K. S., Korom, N., Kavanaugh, K., Wenne, S., & Norr, K. (2020). COVID-19: Impact for pediatric research, evidence-based practice and quality processes and projects. *Journal of Pediatric Nursing, 55*, 264–265. https://doi.org/10.1016/j.pedn.2020.08.009

Hassmiller, S. B., & Wakefield, M. K. (2022). The future of nursing 2020–2030: Charting a path to achieve health equity. *Nursing Outlook, 70*(6), S1–S9. https://doi.org/10.1016/j.outlook.2022.05.013

Institute of Medicine. (2001). *Crossing the quality chasm: A new health system for the 21st century*. National Academies Press. https://www.ncbi.nlm.nih.gov/books/NBK222274/

Institute of Medicine. (2011). *The future of nursing: Leading change, advancing health*. National Academies Press.

Institute of Medicine. (2003). *Health professions education: A bridge to quality*. National Academies Press. https://doi.org/10.17226/10681

Institute of Medicine Roundtable on Evidence-Based Medicine, Olsen, L. A., Aisner, D., & McGinnis, J. M. (Eds.). (2007). *The learning healthcare system: Workshop summary*. Appendix D. National Academies Press. https://www.ncbi.nlm.nih.gov/books/NBK53486/

International Council of Nurses. (2012, May). *Closing the gap: From evidence to action*. https://www.nursingworld.org/~4aff6a/globalassets/practiceandpolicy/innovation--evidence/ind-kit-2012-for-nnas.pdf

International Council of Nurses. (2023). *International Nurses Day 2023 report: Our nurses, our future*. https://www.icn.ch/sites/default/files/2023-07/ICN_IND_2023_Report_EN.pdf

JBI. (2020). *About JBI*. https://jbi.global/about-jbi

Kerr, H., & Rainey, D. (2021). Addressing the current challenges of adopting evidence-based practice in nursing. *British Journal of Nursing, 30*(16), 970–974. https://doi.org/10.12968/bjon.2021.30.16.970

Khan, S., Chambers, D., & Neta, G. (2021). Revisiting time to translation: Implementation of evidence-based practices (EBPs) in cancer control. *Cancer Causes & Control, 32*(3), 221–230. https://doi.org/10.1007/s10552-020-01376-z

Lehane, E., Leahy-Warren, P., O'Riordan, C., Savage, E., Drennan, J., O'Tuathaigh, C., O'Connor, M., Corrigan, M., Burke, F., Hayes, M., Lynch, H., Sahm, L., Heffernan, E., O'Keeffe, E., Blake, C., Horgan, F., & Hegarty, J. (2019). Evidence-based practice education for healthcare professions: An expert view. *BMJ Evidence-Based Medicine, 24*(3), 103–108. https://doi.org/10.1136/bmjebm-2018-111019

Mackey, A., & Bassendowski, S. (2017). The history of evidence-based practice in nursing education and practice. *Journal of Professional Nursing, 33*(1), 51–55. https://doi.org/10.1016/j.profnurs.2016.05.009

McGlynn, E. A., Asch, S. M., Adams, J., Keesey, J., Hicks, J., DeCristofaro, A., & Kerr, E. A. (2003). The quality of health care delivered to adults in the United States. *New England Journal of Medicine, 348*(26), 2635–2645. https://doi.org/10.1056/nejmsa022615

Melnyk, B. M., & Fineout-Overholt, E. (2023). *Evidence-based practice in nursing and healthcare: A guide to best practice* (5th ed.). Wolters Kluwer.

Melnyk, B. M., Gallagher-Ford, L., Zellefrow, C., Tucker, S., Thomas, B., Sinnott, L. T., & Tan, A. (2018). The first U.S. study on nurses' evidence-based practice competencies indicates major deficits that threaten healthcare quality, safety, and patient outcomes. *Worldviews on Evidence-Based Nursing, 15*(1), 16–25. https://doi.org/10.1111/wvn.12269

National Academies of Sciences, Engineering, and Medicine. (2019). *Artificial intelligence in health care: The hope, the hype, the promise, the peril*. https://doi.org/10.17226/227111

National Academies of Sciences, Engineering, and Medicine. (2021). *The future of nursing 2020–2030: Charting a path to achieve health equity*. National Academies Press. https://doi.org/10.17226/25982

National Library of Medicine. (2024). *MEDLINE overview*. https://www.nlm.nih.gov/medline/medline_overview.html#:~:text=MEDLINE%20is%20the%20National%20Library,with%20a%20concentration%20on%20biomedicine

Nundy, S., Cooper, L. A., & Mate, K. S. (2022). The quintuple aim for health care improvement. A new imperative to advance health equity. *JAMA, 327*(6), 521–522.

O'Brien, T., Hood, A., King, T. S., & Brinkman, B. (2023). Nurturing a spirit of inquiry: Fundamentals of evidence-based practice in nursing. *Nephrology Nursing Journal, 50*(6), 509–511.

Organisation for Economic Co-operation & Development. (2023). *Recommendation of the Council on Artificial Intelligence*. https://legalinstruments.oecd.org/en/instruments/OECD-LEGAL-0449#mainText

Peng, Y., Rousseau, J. F., Shortliffe, E. H., & Weng, C. (2023, May). AI-generated text may have a role in evidence-based medicine. *Nature Medicine, 29*, 1593–1594. https://doi.org/10.1038/s41591-023-02366-9

Pramesh, C. S., Babu, G. R., Basu, J., Bushan, I., Booth, C. M., Chinnaswamy, G., Guleria, R., Kalantri, S. P., Kang, G., Mohan, P., Mor, N., Pai, M., Prakash, M., Rupali, P., Sampathkumar, P., Sengar, M., Sullivan, R., & Ranganathan, P. (2021, July). Choosing wisely for COVID-19: Ten evidence-based recommendations for patients and physicians. *Nature Medicine, 27*, 1324–1327. https://doi.org/10.1038/s41591-021-01439-x

Raderstorf, T., Bisognano, M., & Trinter, K. (2022). How to leverage innovation models to achieve health equity: Build. Measure. Share. *Nursing Outlook, 70*(6), S88–95. https://doi.org/10.1016/j.outlook.2022.05.009

Registered Nurses' Association of Ontario. (2024). *Best practice guidelines*. https://rnao.ca/bpg/guidelines

Rudman, A., Boström, A.-M., Wallin, L., Gustavsson, P., & Ehrenberg, A. (2023). The use of the evidence-based practice process by experienced nurses to inform and transform clinical practice during the COVID-19 pandemic: A longitudinal national cohort study. *Worldviews on Evidence-Based Nursing, 21*(1), 14–22. https://DOI.org/10.1111/wvn.12692

Sackett, D. L., Rosenberg, W. M., Gray, J. A., Haynes, R. B., & Richardson, W. S. (1996). Evidence based medicine: What it is and what it isn't. *BMJ, 312*(7023), 71–72. https://doi.org/10.1136/bmj.312.7023.71

Saunders, H., & Vehviläinen-Julkunen, K. (2016, April). The state of readiness for evidence-based practice among nurses: An integrative review. *International Journal of Nursing Studies, 56*, 128–140. https://doi.org/10.1016/j.ijnurstu.2015.10.018

Stevens, K. (2013). The impact of evidence-based practice in nursing and the next big ideas. *The Online Journal of Issues in Nursing, 18*(2). https://doi.org/10.3912/OJIN.Vol18No02Man04

Still, C. H., Flores, D. D., & Santa Maria, D. (2023). Advancing health equity through nursing research. *Nursing Outlook, 71*(6), 102049. https://doi.org/10.1016/j.outlook.2023.102049

Tikkanen, R., & Abrams, M. K. (2020, Jan. 30). *U.S. health care from a global perspective, 2019: Higher spending, worse outcomes?* The Commonwealth Fund. https://doi.org/10.26099/7avy-fc29

Tussing, T. E., Welch, J. C., & Loversidge, J. M. (2023). Using evidence to influence health and organizational policy. In B. Melnyk & E. Fineout-Overholt (Eds.), *Evidence-based practice in nursing & healthcare: A guide to best practice* (5th ed., Ch. 20). Wolters Kluwer.

University of Illinois Chicago. (May 2024). *What is (AI) artificial intelligence?* https://meng.uic.edu/news-stories/ai-artificial-intelligence-what-is-the-definition-of-ai-and-how-does-ai-work/

World Health Organization. (2024). *Health equity.* https://www.who.int/health-topics/health-equity#tab=tab_1

Yingling, J. K. (2020). Rationing evidence-based nursing practice: Considering a resource-based approach. *The Online Journal of Issues in Nursing*, 26(1). https://doi.org/10.3912/OJIN.Vol26No01PPT62

Zhavoronkov, A. (2023, Feb. 7). Caution with AI-generated content in biomedicine. *Nature Medicine*, 29, 532. https://doi.org/10.1038/d41591-023-00014-w

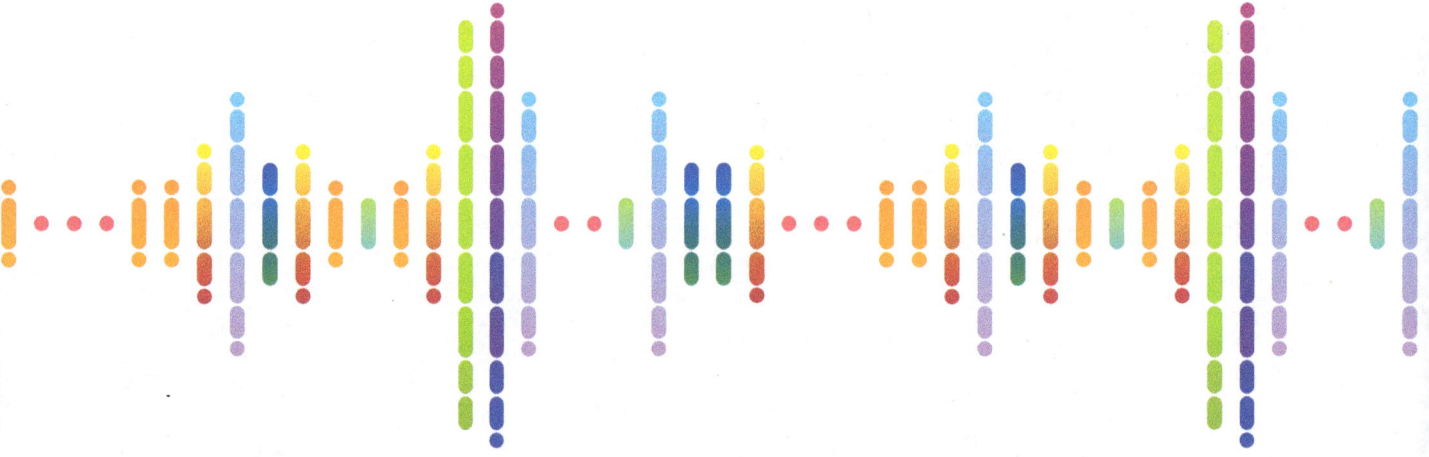

OBJECTIVES

- Differentiate between the three forms of inquiry: quality improvement (QI), research, and evidence-based practice (EBP)

- Describe the revised Johns Hopkins Evidence-Based Practice (JHEBP) Model for Nurses and Healthcare Professionals

- Introduce frontline HCPs and leaders to the PET process (**P**ractice Question, **E**vidence, and **T**ranslation)

- Identify ongoing considerations important to the success of the EBP project

2

THE JOHNS HOPKINS EVIDENCE-BASED PRACTICE (JHEBP) MODEL FOR NURSES AND HEALTHCARE PROFESSIONALS (HCPs) PROCESS OVERVIEW

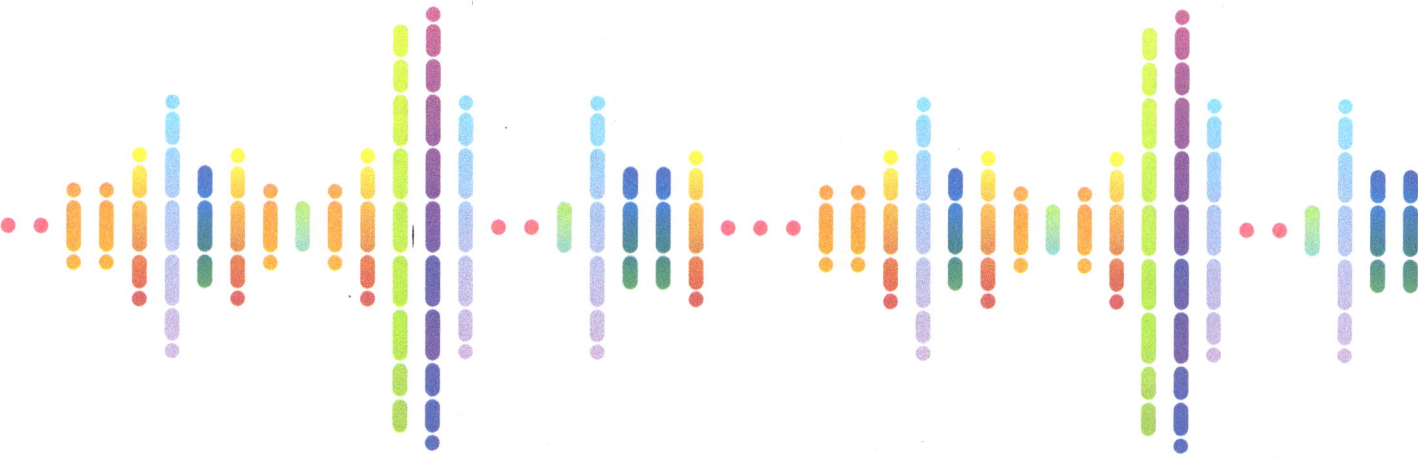

KEY POINTS

This chapter summarizes all the steps in the JHEBP model. The JHEBP Project Steps and Overview (Appendix A) mirrors this overview.

- QI, research, and EBP are the three forms of inquiry common to healthcare.

- The JHEBP model is built on the concepts of inquiry, practice, and learning.

- Critical thinking and clinical reasoning are essential components of the model.

- The EBP process can be influenced by both internal and external factors.

- The JHEBP model uses the PET process: Practice Question, Evidence, and Translation.

- The JHEBP model consists of 16 steps with associated tools to guide the EBP process.

INTRODUCTION

Evidence-based practice (EBP) is a core competency for all healthcare professionals (HCPs) in all practice settings (Saunders et al., 2019). Using an evidence-based approach to care and practice decision-making is not only an expectation in all practice settings but also a requirement established by professional standards, regulatory agencies, health insurers, and purchasers of healthcare insurance. EBP is an important component of high-reliability organizations. It is a process that can enable organizations to meet the quadruple healthcare aim to enhance patient care, improve population health, reduce healthcare costs, and increase the well-being of healthcare staff (Migliore et al., 2020).

In 2009, the Institute of Medicine (IOM) set an ambitious goal that 90% of clinical decisions would be evidence-based by 2020. Although HCPs are increasingly adopting EBP in practice, we have not met this grand challenge. However, licensed healthcare staff have the potential to make a major impact on improving patient outcomes through the appraisal and translation of evidence (American Association of Colleges of Nursing [AACN], 2020; IOM, 2011; Wilson et al., 2015). This requires leaders in academia and service settings to align their learning and practice environments to promote evidence-based healthcare, cultivate a spirit of continuous inquiry, and translate the highest-quality evidence into practice. Using a model for EBP within an organization fosters end-user adoption of evidence, enables users to speak a common language, standardizes processes, improves care and care outcomes, and embeds this practice into the organization's fabric.

DIFFERENTIATING BETWEEN QUALITY IMPROVEMENT, RESEARCH, AND EBP

Before an in-depth discussion of the JHEBP model, it is important to consider EBP in the context of the three forms of inquiry. Differentiating between research, QI, and EBP can be challenging. Although QI, research, and EBP use distinctly different processes, commonalities among these concepts include teamwork, critical thinking, and a commitment to improving care. The methods used and outcomes sought differ for each inquiry type (see Table 2.1).

TABLE 2.1 Differentiating Between the Three Forms of Nursing Inquiry

	QUALITY IMPROVEMENT	RESEARCH	EVIDENCE-BASED PRACTICE
Starting point	A gap in performance of practice, process, or system	A gap in knowledge or evidence	A gap in knowledge of the best available evidence
Method	Plan-Do-Study-Act (PDSA), Six Sigma, Lean principles	Scientific process	Practice Question, Evidence, Translation (PET) process
Outcome	Produces evidence for application at the local level (unit, department, organization)	Generates new knowledge for broad application	Synthesizes the best evidence for adoption in practice

Quality improvement is a process to improve healthcare services, systems, and processes at the local level (e.g., unit, department, organization) to ameliorate outcomes (Jones, 2019). QI generally includes measuring a particular outcome, making changes to improve practice, and monitoring performance. QI may uncover a practice problem that initiates an EBP project. Some examples of QI initiatives are lowering catheter-associated urinary tract infections, reducing wait times in the emergency department, decreasing falls among patients, reducing surgical site infections, improving patient satisfaction, increasing pneumococcal and influenza immunization rates, and decreasing restraint use.

Research is a systematic investigation designed to develop, uncover, create, or contribute to new knowledge that can be generalized for broader applications (US Department of Health and Human Services, 2018). It is often undertaken when no evidence or weak, conflicting, or incomplete evidence is returned during the search phase of an EBP project. Research requires approval by an institutional review board because the intent is to generalize knowledge beyond the usual care of the patient or setting. Research can impose additional risks or burdens not experienced in usual care, and the subject has the ethical right to decide whether they want to participate. Some examples of research are to create new evidence to compare pain management protocols on the experience of pain for ventilated patients, or to evaluate two methods of communication (daily rounds conducted with clinicians only versus huddles incorporating patients and families) to compare satisfaction with patient engagement in decision-making for end-of-life care.

Evidence-based practice projects are undertaken when clinicians raise a concern or question important to practice that existing literature addresses. The EBP process starts with identifying a practice problem and reviewing the data or experience related to the problem; creating a specific question based on the identified problem; searching, retrieving, and reviewing the best available evidence; appraising the retrieved evidence; synthesizing the results; creating and implementing a translation to practice plan; and evaluating results and lessons learned.

While these three forms of inquiry are distinct, they are linked when determining a course of action based on the nature of the question or problem raised by healthcare providers. For example, an interdisciplinary team raised the issue of increased infection rates in orthopedic patients with traction pins. Initially, efforts to decrease rates began as a QI project reinforcing protocol adherence. However, on examining the current practice using the PDSA method, the team discovered variations in pin care among the nurses and found a knowledge gap related to best practices. The team then undertook an EBP project to find the best evidence on pin care. Finding no evidence in their search, they initiated a research study to generate new knowledge on the most effective pin care cleaning protocol for minimizing infection. Figure 2.1 outlines this process.

ESSENTIAL COMPONENTS OF THE JHEBP MODEL FOR NURSES AND HCPs: INQUIRY, PRACTICE, AND LEARNING

The JHEBP Model for Nurses and HCPs (see Figure 2.2) is composed of three interrelated components—inquiry, practice, and learning—that take place in the context of interprofessional collaborative practice.

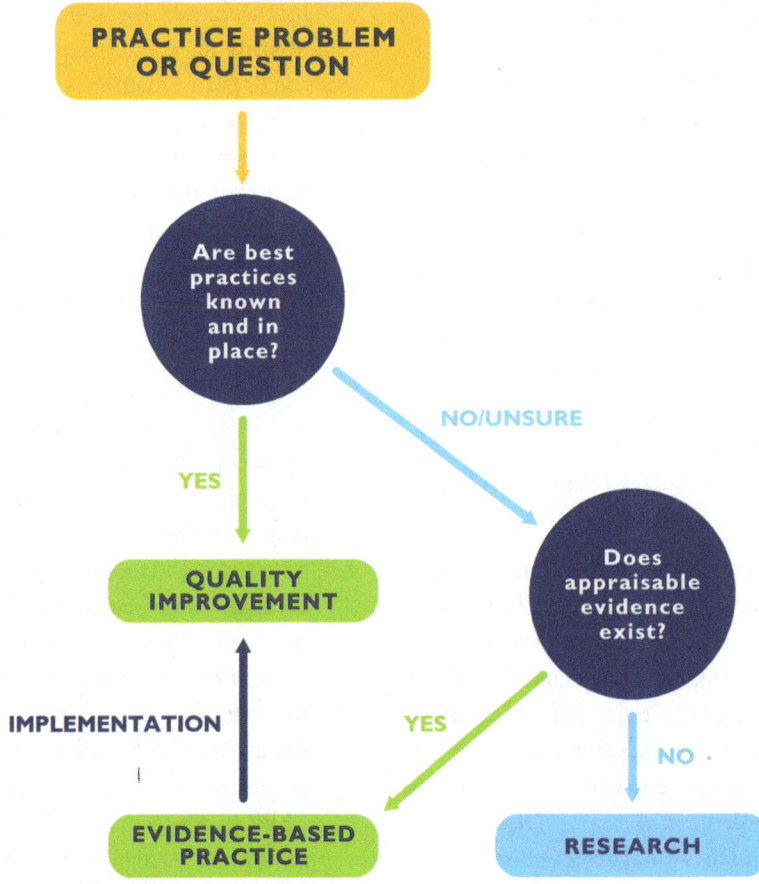

FIGURE 2.1 Three forms of inquiry and practice problems.

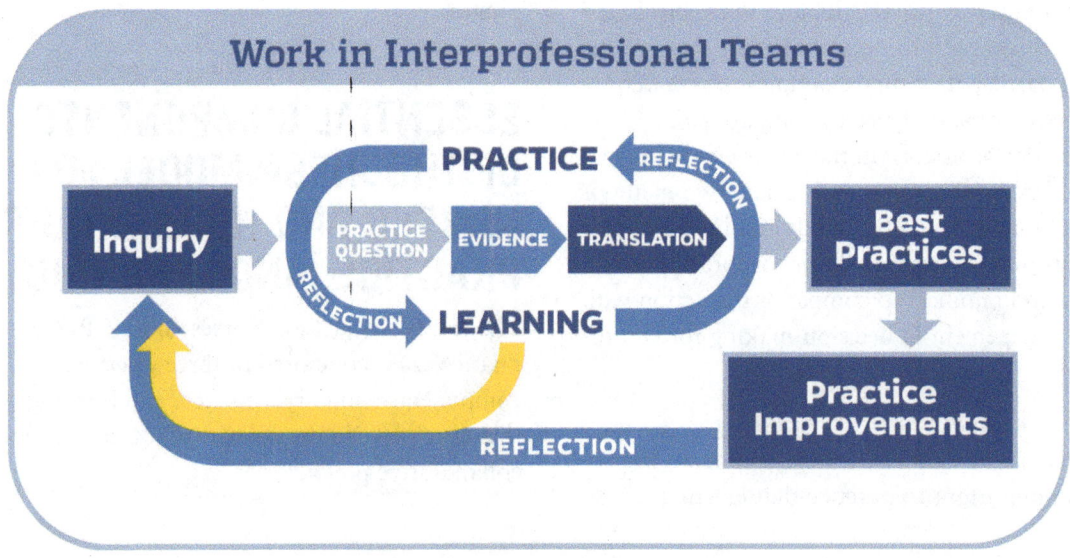

FIGURE 2.2 The JHEBP Model for Nurses and HCPs (2022).
© *Johns Hopkins Health System*

Inquiry

Inquiry is the initial component that launches the EBP process. The concept of *inquiry*, a foundation for healthcare practice, encompasses a focused effort to question, examine, and collect information about a problem, an issue, or a concern generally identified through observation, assessment, and personal experience within the clinical setting. Curiosity and inquiry can foster meaningful learning experiences by prompting individuals to look for learning opportunities to know more. The National League for Nursing (NLN, 2014) describes a spirit of inquiry as:

> a persistent sense of curiosity that informs both learning and practice. A nurse infused by a spirit of inquiry will raise questions, challenge traditional and existing practices, and seek creative approaches to problem-solving . . . A spirit of inquiry . . . engenders innovative thinking and extends possibilities for discovering novel solutions in both predictable and unpredictable situations. (NLN, 2014, para. 1)

Within the practice setting, inquisitiveness and curiosity about the best evidence to guide clinical decision-making are what drives EBP (Melnyk et al., 2009). Practice questions commonly arise from HCPs as they provide everyday care to their patients. These questions may include whether the best evidence is being used or if the care provided is safe, effective, timely, accessible, cost-effective, and/or of high quality. Organizations that foster a culture of inquiry are more likely to have staff that will embrace and actively participate in EBP activities (Migliore et al., 2020). When HCPs, individually and collectively, commit to inquiry and apply new knowledge and best evidence in practice, two outcomes are more likely—high-quality outcomes and a culture that promotes inquiry.

Practice

Practice, one component of all HCPs' activity, reflects the translation of what clinicians know into what they do. It is the who, what, when, where, why, and how that address the range of activities that define the care a patient receives (American Nurses Association [ANA], 2010, 2015).

All HCPs are bound by and held to standards established by their respective professional organizations. For example, the ANA (2015) has identified six standards of nursing practice (scope) based on the nursing process and 11 standards of professional performance. In addition to the ANA, professional nursing specialty organizations establish standards of care for specific patient populations. Collectively, these standards define nurses' scope of practice, set expectations for evaluating performance, and guide the care provided to patients and families. Similarly, other HCP organizations establish practice standards for a variety of care providers such as the American College of Clinical Pharmacy's Standards of Practice for Clinical Pharmacists (2014) and the American Association of Respiratory Care's Respiratory Care Scope of Practice (2018). These standards provide broad expectations for practice in all settings where healthcare is delivered and are translated into organization-specific standards such as policies, protocols, and procedures.

According to the IOM *Health Professions Education* report (2003), regardless of their discipline, all HCPs should have a core set of competencies that include the ability to use EBP, work in interdisciplinary teams, apply QI methods, utilize informatics, and provide patient-centered care (see Figure 2.3). These competencies are achieved using consistent communication skills, obtaining knowledge and skills, and using clinical reasoning and reflection routinely in the practice setting.

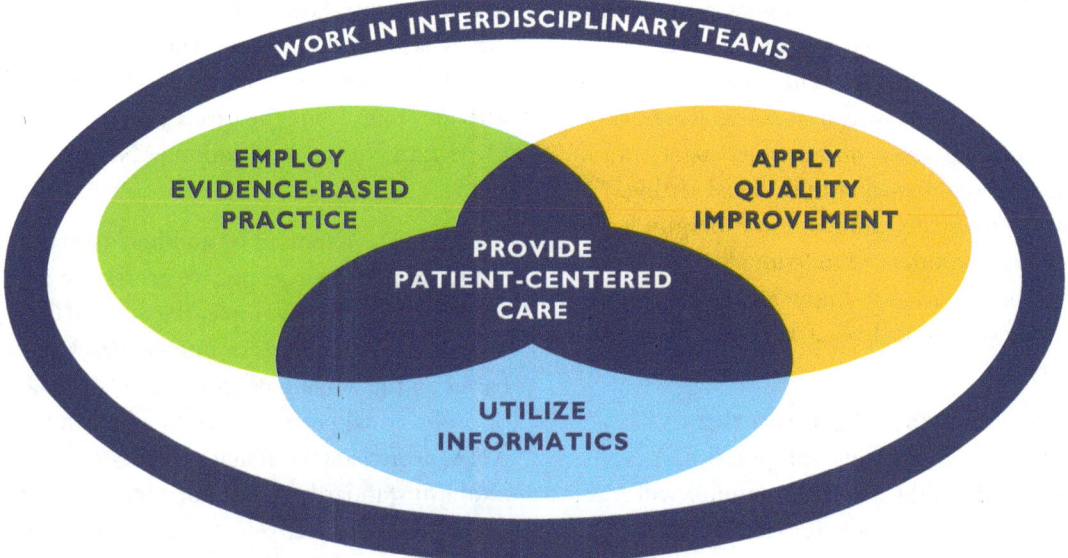

FIGURE 2.3 Relationship among core competencies for health professionals.

The *Health Professions Education* report's core competencies support the use of interprofessional team collaboration in which a variety of diverse professionals share their observations and knowledge through communication and collaboration. Both EBP and research initiatives have become more interprofessional, and interdisciplinary teams have been shown to enhance quality outcomes through the integration of professional perspectives, lower costs, and improved interactions among team members, thereby promoting patient safety and reducing medical errors (Aein et al., 2020; Bohnenkamp et al., 2014; IOM, 2003). Working in interprofessional teams allows all team members to contribute their expertise to achieve the best possible outcomes for patients and fosters role appreciation and job satisfaction between team members (Bohnenkamp et al., 2014). Practice change and improvement will also be more accepted within the organization and by all disciplines when it is based on evidence evaluated through an interprofessional EBP process. An organization's ability to create opportunities for HCPs as part of an interprofessional team, develop EBP questions, evaluate evidence, promote critical thinking, make practice changes, and promote professional development is no longer optional.

The use of an evidence-based approach in developing clinical practice standards and guidelines is also an expectation of regulatory agencies such as the Joint Commission (Joint Commission International, 2016) and certifying bodies such as the American Nurses Credentialing Center [ANCC], which reviews organizations for Magnet® certification (ANCC, 2011). For example, healthcare organizations are standardizing practices based on evidence to reduce variations in care and practice to improve patient safety and quality while reducing healthcare costs (James, 2018; Warren et al., 2016).

Learning

According to Braungart et al. (2014), *learning* is "a relatively permanent change in mental processes, emotional functioning, skill, and/or behavior as a result of experience" (p. 64). Learning incorporates the active process of observing, interacting with phenomena, and engaging with others (Teaching Excellence in Adult Literacy, 2011). It builds on prior knowledge and often occurs in a complex social environment in which knowledge is built by engaged members. Learning requires the learner to be motivated because it often uses significant mental energy and involves persistence. Learning allows the learner to adopt new knowledge by applying it in practice, resulting in behavior change (Lancaster, 2016). In addition to behavioral changes, learning can also lead to changes in how participants think about themselves, their world, and others, which is referred to as *transformational learning* (Teaching Excellence in Adult Literacy, 2011). In this type of learning, critical reflection is used to examine issues or beliefs by assessing the evidence and arguments and being open to differing points of view and new information (Western Governors University, 2020). Ultimately, learning is what the learner hears and understands (Holmen, 2014).

A *learning culture* is a culture of inquiry that inspires staff to increase their knowledge and develop new skills (Linders, 2014; McCormick, 2016) and one that supports a growth mindset—the belief that a person can acquire new skills and knowledge over time (*Psychology Today*, 2021). Staff with a growth mindset tend to actively seek out challenges and believe their true potential can be achieved through effort. Learning cultures also improve employee engagement, increase employee satisfaction, promote creativity, and encourage problem-solving (McCormick, 2016; Nabong, 2015). Both individual learning and a culture of learning are necessary to build practice expertise and maintain staff competency. Education is different from learning in that *education* imparts knowledge through teaching at a point in time, often in a formal setting. Education makes knowledge available. According to Prabhat (2011), education is largely considered formal and shapes resources from the top down. Formalized education starts with an institution that offers accreditation and then provides resources to meet that expressed goal. In contrast, learning begins with individuals and communities. The desire to learn, a natural desire, is considered informal learning and is based on the interests of individuals or groups that access resources in pursuit of that interest.

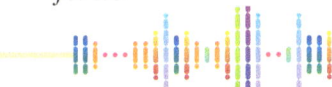

"Education is what people do to you. Learning is what you do for yourself."
–Joi Ito

Ongoing learning is necessary to remain current with new knowledge, technologies, skills, and clinical competencies. Learning also serves to inform practice, which leads to changes in care standards that drive improvements in patient outcomes. Because the field of healthcare is becoming increasingly more complex and technical, no single individual can know everything about how best to provide safe and effective care, and no single degree can provide the knowledge needed to span an entire career. It is, therefore, an essential expectation that healthcare clinicians participate in lifelong learning and continued competency development (IOM, 2011).

Lifelong learning is not only individual learning but also interprofessional, collaborative, and team-oriented learning. For example, joint learning experiences between nursing, medical, and pharmacy students facilitate a better understanding of roles and responsibilities, make communication more effective, aid in conflict resolution, and foster shared decision-making. They can also improve collaboration and the ability to work more effectively on interprofessional EBP teams. Interprofessional education and learning experiences foster collaboration, improve services, and prepare teams to solve problems using an EBP approach that exceeds the capacity of any single professional (Aein et al., 2020; IOM, 2011).

DESCRIPTION: THE JHEBP MODEL

The JHEBP model is an inquiry-based learning framework in which individuals or interprofessional teams actively control their own learning to gain new knowledge and to update existing knowledge (Jong, 2006; Pedaste et al., 2015). This approach emphasizes the learner's role in the process instead of a teacher telling learners what they need to know. Learners or teams are encouraged to explore, ask questions, and share ideas (Grade Power Learning, 2018). The inquiry-learning process often starts with the investigation of a specific topic or problem to determine what currently is known and where there are gaps in knowledge. This phase may be followed by the development of an inquiry question or hypothesis leading to a plan to address the question through observation, the collection of evidence, experimentation, and/or data analysis (Jong, 2006; Pedaste et al., 2015). Based on the findings, conclusions are drawn and communicated. Future phases may include applying knowledge to new situations followed by evaluation. *Reflection*, which involves describing, critiquing, evaluating, and discussing, is an integral part of all phases of the inquiry-learning model. Reflection by learners leads to deeper learning and the ability to internalize complex knowledge (Kori et al., 2014).

Examples of reflective questions might include:

- What do we need to know about a particular problem?
- How can we find the information that we need?
- Are the resources used reliable?
- What were the barriers in the process?
- What could be done differently next time to improve the process?

An inquiry-learning framework has its foundation in the work of earlier theorists such as Dewey and Piaget, whose learning philosophies were based on the belief that experience provides the best process for acquiring knowledge (Barrow, 2006; Zaphir, 2019). Learners are encouraged to be self-directed based on personal experiences and participate in group collaboration and peer grading or review. A second learning philosophy—*connectivism*—evolving from the development and rapid growth of digital technology (Duke et al., 2013) includes concepts such as self-directed social learning, content sharing, and group collaboration. Technology allows learners to access a large array of concepts networked by information sets. The core skill then for the learner is to be able to identify connections between information sources and maintain those connections to facilitate continual learning because data is constantly changing and updating (Duke et al., 2013).

Inquiry is the starting point for the JHEBP model (refer to Figure 2.1). An individual or a team, sparked by a genuine spirit of curiosity, seeks to clarify practice concerns by reflecting on such questions as whether current practices are based on the best evidence for a specific problem or a particular patient population, or perhaps considering whether there is a more efficient and cost-effective way of achieving a particular outcome. The PET (Practice Question, Evidence, and Translation) process shown in the EBP model provides a systematic approach for developing a practice question, finding the best evidence, and translating the best evidence into practice. As the individual or team moves through the PET process, they are continually learning by gaining new knowledge, improving skills in collaboration, and gaining insights. These insights generate new EBP questions for future investigation at any time throughout the EBP process. The model also depicts that practice improvements are often clinical, learning, or operational and are based on the translation of best evidence into practice. The ongoing cycle of inquiry, practice, and learning, and identifying best evidence and implementing practice improvements makes the JHEBP model a dynamic and interactive process for making practice changes that impact system, staff, and patient outcomes. As depicted in the model, reflection by the team based on their discipline perspective and experiences serves to deepen learning through intentional discourse and articulation of important lessons learned throughout the entire EBP process (Di Stefano et al., 2014).

Critical Thinking, Clinical Reasoning, and Evidence-Based Practice

The ability of the EBP team to apply elements of critical thinking and clinical reasoning to the EBP process is vital to the success of any EBP project because it ensures that outcomes are based on sound evidence (Canada, 2016; Finn, 2011; Kim et al., 2018; Profetto-McGrath, 2005). *Critical thinking* is the process of questioning, analysis, synthesis, interpretation, inference, reasoning, intuition, application, and creativity (AACN, 2008). It is a means of imposing intellectual standards in the approach to any subject in a non-discipline-specific way (Victor-Chmil, 2013). Clinical reasoning employs critical thinking in the cognitive process used by HCPs when examining a patient care concern (Victor-Chmil, 2013). Critical thinkers bring various skills to the EBP team that help effectively support the EBP process. They see problems from differing perspectives, use a variety of investigative approaches, and generate many ideas before developing a plan of action (Murawski, 2014). They see problems as challenges, rely on evidence to make judgments, are interested in what others have to say, think before acting, and engage in active listening.

When critical thinking skills are applied to the EBP process, a team is more apt to examine problems carefully, clarify assumptions and biases, and identify any missing information (Herr, 2007). The team uses critical thinking when appraising the evidence, and the quantity and consistency of the evidence, and then combines these findings to determine the best-evidence recommendations, a process referred to as *synthesis*. Critical thinking fosters the use of logic to evaluate arguments, gather facts, weigh the evidence, and arrive at conclusions.

Based on this sound process, the EBP team uses clinical reasoning to think beyond traditional patient care routines and protocols and engage in critical analysis of current healthcare practices to determine the relevance of the evidence as it applies to a specific clinical situation (Profetto-McGrath, 2005; Victor-Chmil, 2013). For example, consider how clinical reasoning skills might be used by an EBP team looking at how hourly rounding impacts fall rates and patient satisfaction with nurse responsiveness. In developing the EBP question, the team employs clinical reasoning when questioning if they have a full understanding of the current practices on the nursing units impacted by the project and what additional information might be needed. The team may consider if they have gathered all available data that substantiates the problem (e.g., current fall rates, falls with injuries, and Health Consumer Assessment of Healthcare Providers and Systems

[HCAHPS] scores). The team may also examine differences between different levels of care (e.g., critical, acute, or behavioral care). The team must also determine whether the recommendations for translation are a good fit for the clinical area and impacted groups, are feasible to implement in the identified areas, and are deemed acceptable within the organization.

Factors Influencing the JHEBP Model

The JHEBP model is an open system with interrelated components. Because it is an open system, inquiry, learning, and practice are influenced by not only evidence but also factors external and internal to the organization. *External factors* can include accreditation bodies, legislation, quality measures, regulations, and standards. Accreditation bodies (e.g., the Joint Commission, Commission on Accreditation of Rehabilitation Facilities) require an organization to achieve and maintain high standards of practice and quality. Legislative and regulatory bodies (local, state, and federal) enact laws and regulations designed to protect the public and promote access to safe, quality healthcare services. Failure to adhere to these laws and regulations has adverse effects on an organization, most often financial. Examples of regulatory agencies are the Centers for Medicare & Medicaid Services, Food and Drug Administration, and state boards of nursing. State boards of nursing regulate nursing practice and enforce the Nurse Practice Act, which serves to protect the public. Quality measures (outcome and performance data) and professional standards serve as yardsticks for evaluating current practices and identifying areas for improvement or change. The ANCC, through its Magnet Recognition Program®, developed criteria to assess the quality of nursing and nursing excellence in organizations. Additionally, many external groups, such as healthcare networks, special interest groups/organizations, vendors, patients and their families, the community, and third-party payors exert influence on healthcare organizations.

Internal factors include organizational culture, values, and beliefs; practice environment (e.g., leadership, resource allocation, patient services, organizational mission and priorities, availability of technology, library support, and time to conduct EBP activities); equipment and supplies; staffing; and organizational standards. Enacting EBP within an organization requires:

- A culture that believes EBP will lead to optimal patient outcomes

- A culture that supports interprofessional collaboration

- Strong and visible leadership support at all levels with the necessary resources (human, technological, and financial) to sustain the process

- Clear expectations that incorporate EBP into standards and job descriptions

- Availability of EBP mentors such as unit-based EBP champions, advanced practice clinicians, and those with practice doctorates in nursing, pharmacy, and physical therapy, as well as other organizational experts in the EBP process to serve as coaches and role models

Partnerships and interprofessional collaboration are crucial for the implementation of EBP initiatives that align with a healthcare organization's mission, goals, and strategic priorities (Moch et al., 2015). Mentors with knowledge of the patient population and the context of internal and external factors are essential for the successful implementation and sustainability of EBP.

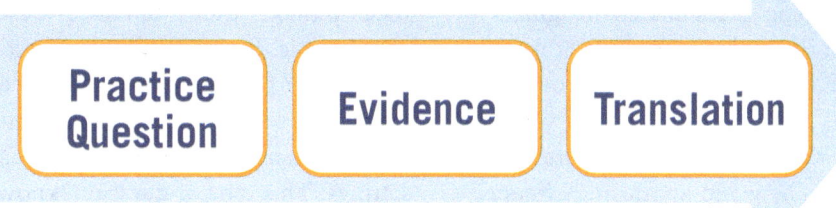

FIGURE 2.4 JHEBP PET process.
© Johns Hopkins Health System

JHEBP PET PROCESS: PRACTICE QUESTION, EVIDENCE, AND TRANSLATION

The JHEBP process occurs in three phases and can be described as Practice Question, Evidence, and Translation (PET; see Figure 2.4). The 16-step process (see Appendix A) begins with exploring and describing the practice problem, issue, or concern. This step is critical because the problem statement drives the remaining steps in the process. Based on the problem statement, the EBP team develops a practice question, refines it, and searches for, appraises, and synthesizes the evidence. Based on this synthesis, the team decides whether the evidence supports a change in practice. If it does, evidence translation begins and the practice change is planned, implemented, and evaluated. The final step in translation is to enact the sustainability plan and monitor ongoing outcomes. Throughout these steps, there are ongoing considerations: EBP teams must maintain the project plan, involve impacted groups (formerly referred to as stakeholders), monitor alignment with organizational priorities, and disseminate findings.

Practice Question

The first phase of the process (Steps 1–3) includes developing a problem statement and writing an answerable EBP question. An interprofessional team examines a practice concern, develops and refines an EBP question, and determines its scope. Refer to the EBP Project Steps and Overview (Appendix A) frequently throughout the process to direct the team's work. To gauge progress, teams may decide to use the project Gantt chart, an additional resource found online at Hopkins.org/resources. Appendix A highlights the following steps.

Step 1: Explore and Describe the Problem To define a problem accurately, the EBP team invests time to identify the gap between the current practice and the desired practice—in other words, between what the team sees and experiences and what they want to see and experience. This is accomplished by stating the problem in different ways and soliciting feedback from nonmembers to see whether there is agreement on the problem statement. Teams should gather information, both narrative and numerical, to identify why the current practice is a problem. To do this, team members might observe the practice and listen to how actual users describe the problem in comparison to anticipated practice changes. The time devoted to probing issues and challenging assumptions about the problem, looking at it from multiple angles, and obtaining feedback from as many sources as possible is always time well spent. Incorrectly identifying the problem results in wasted effort searching and appraising evidence that, in the end, does not provide the insight that allows the team to achieve the desired outcomes. The Question Development Tool (Appendix B) walks teams through aspects of the exploration process.

Step 2: Develop the Problem Statement The culmination of exploring, refining, and describing the problem should be a robust yet succinct problem statement. A good problem statement describes the gap between the current state and the desired state. Ideally, it provides all necessary information about the problem such as where it occurs, who is affected, how it impacts, and why it is important. One or two sentences may be all that is needed to create a high-impact problem statement (see the Question Development Tool, Appendix B).

Step 3: Write the EBP Question With a clear problem statement, the EBP team develops and refines the clinical, learning, or operational EBP question (see the Question Development Tool, Appendix B). Keeping the EBP question narrowly focused makes the search for evidence specific and manageable. For example, the question "What are the best practices for providing discharge teaching?" is extremely wide-ranging and could encompass many interventions and all practice settings. This type of question, known as a *broad question* (previously known as a background question), is often used when the team knows little about the area of concern or is interested in identifying best practices. In contrast, a more focused question is, "According to the evidence, in the critical care setting, what is the impact of using the teach-back method, as compared to traditional teaching for discharge education, on readmission rates?" This type of question, known as an *intervention question* (previously, foreground), is generally used by more experienced teams with specialized knowledge to compare interventions or make decisions. In general, intervention questions are narrow and allow the search for evidence to be more precise and focused.

To build an EBP question, teams should consider three or four elements: the population, setting, topic/intervention, and outcomes. See Table 2.2 for an example. The structure provided below replaces the traditional PICO format. More information on these changes can be found in Chapter 4.

TABLE 2.2 Components of an EBP Question

	BROAD	INTERVENTION
Population	Adult patients	Adult patients
Setting	General medical units	General medical units
Topic (broad question) or intervention (intervention question)	MRSA transmission	Handwashing with soap and water Alcohol-based hand cleanser
Outcomes (intervention only)		Rates of hospital-acquired MRSA

Using a simple format, the Question Development Tool (Appendix B) guides the team to write either a broad or an intervention EBP question. For example, using the concepts from Table 2.2, a broad EBP question may look like this:

Among adult medicine patients, what are the best practices regarding preventing MRSA transmission?

An intervention question may be:

According to the evidence, among adult medicine patients, what is the impact of handwashing with soap and water as compared to alcohol-based cleansers on the rates of hospital-acquired MRSA?

Evidence

The second phase (Steps 4–10) of the PET process addresses the search for, screening, appraisal, and synthesis of the evidence. Based on these results, the team makes best-evidence recommendations regarding practice changes.

Before proceeding further with the EBP process, the team should determine if EBP is the correct approach and what kind of search needs to be conducted. The EBP Project Steps and Overview (Appendix A) contains a decision tree to guide this process. The algorithm helps teams determine if EBP is the best option and the type of evidence search required. For example, if a best-evidence search reveals a high-quality, recent clinical practice guideline (CPG), the EBP team determines whether the CPG is sufficient to address the EBP problem or whether an exhaustive evidence search is warranted. Alternatively, if the search indicates a lack of evidence related to the problem, consideration should be given to whether conducting a research study would be the most effective way of addressing the problem. Only when the preliminary scan of the literature indicates that it is likely that sufficient evidence is available should the team move forward with the EBP project (see Appendix A). Using the decision tree can save valuable time for teams and should not be overlooked.

Step 4: Conduct Best-Evidence Search and Appraisal To begin this phase, teams should conduct a best-evidence search specifically for recent *pre-appraised* evidence. The EBP team should search first for CPGs followed by literature reviews with a systematic approach (LRSAs) and finally, evidence summaries (see Chapters 6 and 7). Any pre-appraised evidence uncovered should be reviewed for suitability and adequacy (see Chapter 8). The Searching and Screening Tool (Appendix C) provides direction.

Step 5: Conduct Targeted Search or Exhaustive Search and Screening Here the team has two potential paths, also guided by the Searching and Screening Tool (Appendix C):

1. **Targeted search:** After finding an adequate review or guideline that addresses all aspects of the EBP question, the EBP team searches for any additional evidence published since the original review was conducted (see Chapter 7). If this focused search does not yield further evidence or support the original synthesis, the team does not need to perform a full evidence review and can proceed to the translation phase of the PET process. If newer evidence contradicts the original evidence, the team would need to convene impacted groups and determine which recommendations to adopt and move into translation (see Chapters 8 and 9).

2. **Exhaustive search and screening:** If no recent pre-appraised evidence exists, what exists does not address all aspects of the question, or what exists is not of high quality, the team conducts an exhaustive search (Chapter 7). Enlisting the assistance of a health information specialist (librarian) is highly recommended. Such assistance saves time and ensures a comprehensive and relevant search. All results should

undergo a systematic screening process to minimize bias. If an exhaustive search fails to identify appraisable evidence, the EBP project cannot proceed. The team should discuss alternatives such as waiting for more evidence to be published or conducting a research study.

Step 6: Appraise the Evidence Provided sufficient evidence exists, the team appraises the evidence to 1) determine the level of support for decision-making, and 2) assess the quality. The JHEBP model no longer uses a traditional evidence hierarchy. The JHEBP model now recognizes four types of decision-making support: independent, strong, moderate, and limited. Table 2.3 provides a snapshot of these levels of support and associated study designs along with examples. See Chapter 6 for more details.

The Appraisal Tool Selection Algorithm (Appendix D) guides the team in determining 1) the level of decision-making support, and 2) which appraisal tools to use. Specific action items will vary for each type of evidence and are discussed. Teams will use the Pre-appraised Evidence Appraisal Tool (Appendix E1) for CPGs, LRSAs, and evidence summaries. Single studies are appraised using the appropriate section of the Single Study Evidence Appraisal Tool (Appendix E2). Anecdotal evidence, such as expert opinions or case studies, are appraised using the Anecdotal Evidence Appraisal Tool (Appendix E3). Each tool includes a set of questions to determine the adequacy of each piece of evidence. See Chapter 8 for more details.

Based on this assessment, each piece of evidence is either included or excluded. Previously, teams using the JHEBP model would rate evidence quality using a letter value, A, B, or C. Team members spent valuable time trying to discern between A or B quality evidence, often landing on A– or B+. This granularity was unnecessary and did not impact the decision to draw recommendations from the evidence. To eliminate some of that granularity, the JHEBP model eliminated the letter grading and now suggests that, based on a thorough appraisal, evidence is either good enough to be included in the next steps or not.

TABLE 2.3 Levels of Support for Decision-Making and Associated Designs

TYPE OF EVIDENCE	LEVEL OF SUPPORT FOR DECISION-MAKING	DESIGN	EXAMPLE
Pre-appraised	Independent	N/A	CPG
Single studies with a formal study design	Strong	Controlled trials with or without randomization	Randomized control trial (RCT)
	Moderate	Interventional studies without control or randomization and observational designs	Descriptive correlational study or a qualitative focus-group study
Anecdotal	Limited	N/A	Expert opinion or case study

Step 7: Summarize the Evidence At this step, the EBP team has identified and evaluated the literature either through a best-evidence and targeted search or an exhaustive search. The type of search and subsequent evidence collection from Steps 4, 5, and 6 will determine which tool the EBP team uses to complete the summary process. Best-evidence searches with pre-appraised evidence and supplementary literature use the Best-Evidence Summary Tool (Appendix G1). Exhaustive searches that have gathered pre-appraised evidence that doesn't fully answer the EBP question, single studies, and anecdotal evidence will use the Individual Evidence Summary Tool (Appendix G2). Regardless of the tool, the purpose and process are essentially the same.

The team completes this step by filling in the table on the tool using the prompts provided in the headers. The appraisal tools from Step 6 provide a single-row table with identical headers to assist with collecting and compiling the information in real time. A detailed set of instructions and guidance on what data to include in each box can be found on each tool. See Chapter 9 for a more detailed discussion.

Step 8: Organize the Data Organization or preparation of the collated data involves sorting the information into various groups, clusters, or visual representations to aid the team in interpretation. This step can occur during or after the data summary process to help the team understand the evidence for the next step, synthesis. Teams should always group and analyze evidence by the level of support for decision-making (independent, strong, moderate, or limited). Additionally, the team may also decide to divide the evidence into more meaningful sub-categories such as populations or interventions. While this is most important when preparing the Individual Evidence Summary Tool (Appendix G2) for synthesis, depending on the amount of additional evidence gathered from their supplementary targeted search, the EBP team may also want to organize their reports of single studies (Section II of the Best-Evidence Summary Tool; Appendix G1) to facilitate analysis.

Step 9: Synthesize the Findings Once summarizing is completed, the team turns to synthesis. In this step, the EBP team applies critical thinking skills to deliberate and thoughtfully evaluate the body of evidence and come to an agreement on new insights, understandings, and perspectives. Synthesis contains all the elements of summary, with greater context and connection, and is the opportunity to turn information into knowledge. EBP projects that used an exhaustive search and have gathered literature on the Individual Evidence Summary Tool (Appendix G2) will complete this step by filling out Section I of the Summary, Synthesis, & Best-Evidence Recommendations Tool (Appendix H). Of note, like the organizing step, information gathered from a targeted search to supplement *pre-appraised* evidence may need to be synthesized to facilitate the next step, best-evidence recommendations. Teams can do so by annotating their entries in the Best-Evidence Summary Tool (Appendix G1). Chapter 9 provides a complete overview of the synthesis process.

Step 10: Record Best-Evidence Recommendations Best-evidence recommendations are succinct statements, drawn from synthesized evidence, that answer the practice question. The team completes this step by filling out Section II of Appendix H. Many EBP questions will include multiple best-evidence recommendations with varying levels of certainty. Characterizing the individual recommendations, not the overall evidence, aids in determining specific best practices as well as interventions that do not have the requisite evidence to support moving forward with practice change. Recommendations can be put in one of four groups based on their characteristics. They include:

High certainty recommendations: Robust, well-documented, consistent, and persuasive evidence, based mostly on evidence that provides strong support for decision-making

Reasonable certainty recommendations: Good, mostly compelling, consistent evidence, based mostly on evidence that provides moderate to strong support for decision-making

Reasonable-to-low certainty recommendations: Good but conflicting evidence and inconsistent results, based mostly on evidence that provides moderate support for decision-making

Low certainty recommendations: Little to no evidence; information is minimal, inconsistent, and/or based mostly on evidence that provides limited support for decision-making

Practice change can be based on recommendations with high and reasonable certainty. Recommendations with reasonable-to-low and low certainty do not provide adequate support for practice change. Keep in mind that an EBP team may recommend stopping or de-implementing a practice if there is high or reasonable certainty that it is *not* effective or if there is low certainty it *is* effective.

The process for identifying best-evidence recommendations varies by the type of evidence the team is using and is discussed in Chapter 9.

Translation

In the third phase (Steps 11–16) of the PET process, the EBP team determines the risk, feasibility, fit, and acceptability of the best-evidence recommendations within the target setting. If the assessment for feasibility, fit, and acceptability is positive, the team proceeds with creating an action plan, secures support and resources, implements and evaluates the change, and communicates the results to appropriate individuals both internal and external to the organization.

Step 11: Assess the Risk, Fit, Feasibility, and Acceptability of Best-Evidence Recommendations Translation of evidence may introduce safety risks to patients, staff, or the environment. A risk assessment focuses on identifying, analyzing, and discussing safety vulnerabilities that a potential change may create for the organization. In contrast, various risks are inherent to healthcare, such as clinical, financial, reputational, or technological. This step of the translation process focuses on safety risk identification. Determination of fit includes the team's perceived relevance or compatibility of the change with the user's workflow for the given practice setting, provider, or consumer, and/or perceived relevance of the change to address a particular issue or problem. When considering feasibility, the team determines the extent to which a change (system process improvement, innovation, or practice change) can be successfully implemented within a given organization or practice setting. Lastly, acceptability is the team's perception regarding the extent to which impacted groups and organizational leadership perceive a change to be agreeable, palatable, and satisfactory for the organization.

Step 12: Identify Practice Setting-Specific Recommendations   After completing Step 11 with the best-evidence recommendations, the team develops practice setting-specific recommendations. These are the recommendations the team decides can be implemented at that point in time.

Even with high-certainty recommendations, EBP teams may find it difficult to implement practice changes in some cases. For example, an EBP team examined the best strategy for ensuring appropriate enteral tube placement after initial tube insertion. The evidence indicated that X-ray was the only 100% accurate method for identifying tube location. The EBP team recommended that a post-insertion X-ray be added to the enteral tube protocol. Despite their presenting the evidence to clinical leadership and other impacted groups in the organization, the team's recommendation was not accepted within the organization. Concerns were raised by organizational leadership about the additional costs and adverse effects that may be incurred by patients (acceptability). Other concerns related to delays in workflow (fit) and the availability of staff to perform the additional X-rays (feasibility). Risk management data showed a lack of documented incidents related to inappropriate enteral tube placement. As a result, after weighing the risks and benefits, the organization decided that making this change was not a good fit at that time. The team records the practice setting-specific recommendations on the Translation Tool (Appendix I).

Step 13: Identify an Implementation Framework   According to Milat and Li (2017), there are 41 different frameworks and models to translate research evidence into policy and practice. Implementation frameworks or models apply to many fields, such as health services research, public health, guideline development, and preventive medicine (Milat & Li, 2017). While many choices exist, and the EBP team's specific problem and setting can inform their selection, Chapter 11 reviews the Johns Hopkins Quality and Safety Research Group Translating Evidence Into Practice (TRIP) Model. See Chapter 11 for a list of implementation frameworks and their best use.

Step 14: Create an Implementation/Action Plan   In this step, the team develops a plan to implement the practice change(s). The plan may include, but is not limited to:

- Development of (or change to) a standard (policy, protocol, guideline, or procedure), a critical pathway, or a system or process related to the EBP question

- Development of a detailed timeline assigning team members to the tasks needed to implement the change (including the evaluation process and reporting of results)

- Solicitation of feedback from organizational leaders, bedside clinicians, and other impacted groups

Essentially, the team must consider the who, what, when, where, how, and why when developing an action plan for the proposed change. The Implementation and Action Planning (A3) Tool (see Appendix J) provides a guide for the EBP team to develop the action plan.

Step 15: Implement   Implementation is one of the final steps of the EBP process and is essential to bring the best evidence to the bedside. To ensure not only success but also sustainability, the EBP team should be deliberate in the planning and execution of their intervention or innovation (White et al., 2024). Chapter 11 provides an overview of action-planning tools that will help teams achieve success.

An essential piece of implementation is identifying appropriate metrics. Measures of success should be related to the goals and the problem identified. For example:

- Use process measures, such as compliance to EBP, attendance to education, and so on (80% compliance to infection prevention bundle).

- Use patient/population outcomes, such as improvement in infection rates, length of stay, etc. Be specific— demonstrate improvement comparison from pre-implementation to post-implementation (reduction of infection by 25% or reduction of infection rate from 10.0 to 7.5 per 1,000 patient days).

- Use timelines on when the metrics will be achieved (example: a month from implementation).

Although the team desires positive outcomes, unexpected outcomes often provide learning opportunities, and the team should examine why these occurred. This examination may indicate the need to alter the practice change or the implementation process, followed by reevaluation.

One way to evaluate outcomes, particularly for uncomplicated, small tests of change, is through the QI process. The PDSA QI cycle is a tested way to determine whether a practice change has met the desired outcomes/improvements (Institute for Healthcare Improvement, 2020). When using the PDSA cycle, the team begins by planning the change, implementing it, observing the results, and then acting on what is learned. The process can help teams determine whether the change brought about improvement; how much improvement can be expected; whether the change will work in the actual environment of interest; and the costs, social impact, and side effects of the change. It can also serve to minimize resistance to the change.

Step 16: Monitor Sustainability and Identify Next Steps Enduring and expanding a project allows the implementation to thrive after a project team closes. Sustainability is essential to maintain the quality of healthcare. Additional strategies to sustain the project include incorporating the project into organizational policy, new employee onboarding, and electronic medical records. An accountable person or department may monitor data and practice compliance periodically beyond the project period. Considerations include:

- Any new barriers and facilitators that may have surfaced

- Additional resources (e.g., people, training, equipment) that may be required

- Any additional outcomes or metrics that are needed to fully evaluate ongoing success

Chapter 11 describes sustainability planning in more detail. Additionally, the Implementation and Action Planning (A3) Tool (Appendix J) provides a section for sustainability planning.

In terms of next steps, EBP team members review the process and findings and consider whether any lessons have emerged that should be shared or whether additional steps need to be taken. These lessons or steps may include a new question that has emerged from the process, the need to do more research on the topic, additional training that may be required, suggestions for new tools, the writing of an article on the process or outcome, or the preparation of an oral or poster presentation at a professional conference. Chapter 12 provides information about dissemination, including podium and poster presentations.

ONGOING CONSIDERATIONS

In addition to the 16 steps of the PET process, the JHEBP model identifies several ongoing considerations. Some of these considerations were once distinct steps in the process. However, years of using the model in practice revealed that they did not fit well within the linear steps, either taking place at multiple unrelated steps or encompassing the entire process. Instead of depicting actionable items at distinct points in the process, the considerations represent areas requiring ongoing attention. Their removal as actionable steps should not convey any less importance. Rather, teams should pay close attention to these considerations as they move through the PET process.

Maintain Project Plan, Including Timeline and Responsibilities

Identifying a leader for the EBP project facilitates the process, accountabilities, and responsibilities and keeps the project moving forward. The ideal leader is knowledgeable about EBP and has experience and a proven track record in leading interprofessional teams. It is also helpful if this individual knows the structure and strategies for implementing change within the organization. See Appendix I and Hopkins.org/resources for project planning and timeline tools.

The leader takes initial responsibility for setting up the first EBP team meeting and involves members in the following activities:

- Reserving a room with adequate space conducive to group work and discussion
- Asking team members to bring their calendars so that subsequent meetings can be scheduled
- Ensuring that a team member is assigned to record discussion points and group decisions
- Establishing a project plan and timeline for the project
- Keeping track of important items (e.g., copies of the EBP tools, literature searches, materials, and resources)
- Providing a place to keep project files

See Chapter 5 for more information on the team.

Teams and Impacted Groups

It is important for the EBP team to identify early the appropriate individuals and impacted groups who should be involved in and kept informed during the EBP project. An *impacted group* is a person, group, or department in an organization that has an interest in, or a concern about, the topic or project under consideration (Agency for Healthcare Research and Quality, 2023). Impacted groups may include a variety of clinical and nonclinical staff, departmental and organizational leaders, patients and families, regulators, insurers, or policymakers. Keeping key groups informed is instrumental to successful change. The team also considers whether the EBP question is specific to a unit, service, or department or involves multiple departments. If it is the latter, representatives from all areas involved need to be recruited for the EBP team. The team regularly communicates with key leaders in the affected departments on the team's progress. If the problem affects multiple disciplines (e.g., nursing, medicine, pharmacy, respiratory therapy), these disciplines need to be a part of the team. The Impacted Groups Analysis and Communication Resource guides group identification and can be accessed online at Hopkins.org/resources. See Chapter 5 for more on teams and impacted groups.

Monitor Alignment With Organizational Priorities

Once the EBP teams have sufficiently defined the problem and crafted a searchable EBP question, they must ask if the problem meets the organization's strategic priorities. Problems and projects that do not match the organization's priorities and focus may receive little support or traction. If facing a project not aligned with strategic priorities, teams should consider alternatives to conducting the EBP project. Perhaps there is another avenue to resolve the issue or a different aspect of the problem that would align with the strategic priorities. While this consideration occurs at a specific point in the process, it should be considered throughout the project. Teams may consider if best-practice recommendations align with strategic priorities or if adaptation is required. See Chapter 4 and the EBP Project Steps and Overview (Appendix A) for more information.

Communication and Dissemination

Communication is not limited to one or two points in time or a distinct step in the process. It is, however, no less important. Communication is vital and ongoing. Teams must communicate throughout the project, from the earliest stages through implementation. A communication plan may help facilitate the sharing of information. It should address:

- The goals of the communication
- Target audiences
- Available communication media
- Preferred frequency

Key messages and methods of communication should align with the audience:

- **Audience:** Think about the project recommendations. Identify the end-users—who is your audience? Revisit the Impacted Groups Analysis and Communication Resource (Hopkins.org/resources) to confirm who may be impacted and the key messages they need to receive. What do you want the target audience(s) to hear, know, and understand?

- **Key messages:** Messages should be clear, succinct, personalized to the audience, benefit-focused, actionable, and repeated three to six different times and ways.

- **Method:** Communication can occur on many levels using varying strategies.

    - Internal dissemination methods can include newsletters, internal websites, private social media groups, journal clubs, grand rounds, staff meetings, toolkits, podcasts, and lunch-and-learns.

    - External dissemination can be in the form of conference posters and podium presentations, peer-reviewed articles, opinion pieces, letters to the editor, book chapters, interviews, or social media (blogs, X [formerly Twitter], YouTube; see Chapter 12 for more information).

- **Timing:** When will your message have the most impact? Consider the audience and time communication when the content may be most relevant to them and their priorities. Also, keep in mind events such as holidays and the academic calendar, which can distract audiences' attention.

Sharing and disseminating the results, both favorable and unfavorable, may generate additional practice or research questions. Valuable feedback obtained can overcome barriers to implementation or help develop strategies to improve unfavorable results. The Impacted Groups Analysis and Communication Resource (Hopkins.org/resources) guides the EBP team in identifying the audience(s), key message points, and methods to communicate the team's findings, recommendations, and practice changes.

SUMMARY

This chapter introduces the revised JHEBP model and the 16 steps of the PET process, designed as an intentional and systematic approach to EBP that requires support and commitment at the individual, team, and organizational levels. HCPs with varied experience and educational preparation have successfully used this process with coaching, mentorship, and organizational support (Dearholt & Dang, 2012).

REFERENCES

Aein, F., Hosseini, R., Naseh, L., Safdari, F., & Banaian, S. (2020). The effect of problem-solving-based interprofessional learning on critical thinking and satisfaction with learning of nursing and midwifery students. *Journal of Education and Health Promotion*, 9(109). https://doi.org/10.4103/jehp.jehp_640_19

Agency for Healthcare Research and Quality. (2023, July). *Patient-centeredness, diversity, and stakeholder engagement*. https://www.ahrq.gov/pcor/strategic-framework/stakeholder-engagement.html

American Association of Colleges of Nursing. (2008). *The essentials of baccalaureate education for professional nursing practice*. http://www.aacnnursing.org/portals/42/publications/baccessentials08.pdf

American Association of Colleges of Nursing. (2020). *Nursing workforce fact sheet*. https://www.aacnnursing.org/News-Information/Fact-Sheets/Nursing-Fact-Sheet

American Association of Respiratory Care. (2018). *Respiratory care scope of practice*. https://www.aarc.org/wp-content/uploads/2017/03/statement-of-scope-of-practice.pdf

American College of Clinical Pharmacy. (2014, August). Standards of practice for clinical pharmacists. *Pharmacotherapy*, 34(8), 794–797. https://doi.org/10.1002/phar.1438

American Nurses Association. (2010). *Nursing: Scope and standards of practice*. Author.

American Nurses Association. (2015). *Nursing: Scope and standards of practice* (3rd ed.). Author.

American Nurses Credentialing Center. (2011). *Magnet model – Creating a Magnet culture*. https://www.nursingworld.org/organizational-programs/magnet/magnet-model/

Barrow, L. H. (2006). A brief history of inquiry: From Dewey to standards. *Journal of Science Teacher Education, 17*(3), 265–278. https://www.jstor.org/stable/43156392

Bohnenkamp, S., Pelton, N., Rishel, C. J., & Kurtin, S. (2014). Implementing evidence-based practice using an interprofessional team approach. *Oncology Nursing Forum, 41*(4), 434–437. https://doi.org/10.1188/14.ONF.434-437

Braungart, M., Braungart, R. G., & Gramet, P. R. (2014). Applying learning theories to healthcare practice. In S. B. Bastable (Ed.), *Nurse as educator, principles of teaching and learning for nursing practice* (pp. 64–110). Jones & Bartlett Learning.

Canada, A. N. (2016). Probing the relationship between evidence-based practice implementation models and critical thinking in applied nursing practice. *The Journal of Continuing Education in Nursing, 47*(4), 161–168. https://doi.org/10.3928/00220124-20160322-05

Dearholt, S. L., & Dang, D. (2012). *Johns Hopkins nursing evidence-based practice: Model and guidelines* (2nd ed.). Sigma Theta Tau International.

Di Stefano, G., Gino, F., Pisano, G., & Staats, B. (2014, April 11). Learning by thinking: How reflection improves performance. *Harvard Business School Working Knowledge*. https://hbswk.hbs.edu/item/learning-by-thinking-how-reflection-improves-performance

Duke, B., Harper, G., & Johnston, M. (2013). Connectivism as a digital age learning theory. *The International HETL Review, Special Issue*. https://www.hetl.org/wp-content/uploads/2013/09/HETLReview2013SpecialIssueArticle1.pdf

Finn, P. (2011). Critical thinking: Knowledge and skills for evidence-based practice. *Language, Speech, and Hearing Services in Schools, 42*, 69–72.

Grade Power Learning. (2018, April 3). *What is inquiry-based learning (and how is it effective)?* https://gradepowerlearning.com/resources/enrichment/what-is-inquiry-based-learning/

Herr, N. (2007). *Critical thinking*. https://www.csun.edu/science/ref/reasoning/critical_thinking/index.html

Holmen, M. (2014, Aug. 6). *Education vs learning— What exactly is the difference?* EdTechReview. http://edtechreview.in/trends-insights/insights/1417-education-vs-learning-what-exactly-is-the-difference?utm_content=buffer4e5b8&utm_medium=social&utm_source=twitter.com&utm_campaign=buffer#.U-NdPce3yG4.twitter

Institute for Healthcare Improvement. (2020). *Model for improvement: Testing changes.* https://www.ihi.org/how-improve-model-improvement-testing-changes

Institute of Medicine. (2003). *Health professions education: A bridge to quality.* National Academies Press. https://www.ncbi.nlm.nih.gov/books/NBK221528/

Institute of Medicine. (2009). *Roundtable on evidence-based medicine.* National Academies Press. https://www.ncbi.nlm.nih.gov/books/NBK52847

Institute of Medicine. (2011). *The future of nursing: Leading change, advancing health.* National Academies Press. https://www.ncbi.nlm.nih.gov/books/NBK209880/

James, T. (2018). *The science of health care improvement: Overcoming unintended variation.* Harvard Medical School. https://www.soa.org/globalassets/assets/files/e-business/pd/events/2019/health-meeting/pd-2019-06-health-session-063.pdf

Joint Commission International. (2016). *Clinical practice guidelines: Closing the gap between theory and practice.* https://www.hhmglobal.com/images/stories/pdf/white6.pdf?phpMyAdmin=0BSDHG8m4NpoYHjERcBikX0RWyb

Jones, B., Vaux, E., & Olsson-Brown, A. (2019). How to get started in quality improvement. *BMJ, 364.* doi:10.1136/bmj.k5437

Jong, T. (2006). Technological advances in inquiry learning. *Science, 312*(5773), 532–533.

Kim, S. S., Kim, E. J., Lim, J. Y., Kim, G. M., & Baek, H. C. (2018). Korean nursing students' acquisition of evidence-based practice and critical thinking skills. *Journal of Nursing Education, 57*(1), 21–27. https://doi.org/10.3928/01484834-20180102-05

Kori, K., Maeots, M., & Pedaste, M. (2014). Guided reflection to support quality of reflection and inquiry in web-based learning. *Procedia: Social and Behavioral Sciences, 112,* 242–251. https://www.sciencedirect.com/science/article/pii/S1877042814011781

Lancaster, J. (2016). Changing health behavior using health education with individuals, families, and groups. In M. Stanhope & J. Lancaster (Eds.), *Public health nursing* (pp. 355–376). Elsevier Mosby.

Linders, B. (2014, July 24). *Nurturing a culture for continuous learning.* InfoQ. https://www.infoq.com/news/2014/07/nurture-culture-learning

McCormick, H. (2016). *Seven steps to creating a lasting learning culture.* University of North Carolina.

Melnyk, B. M., Fineout-Overholt, E., Stillwell, S. B., & Williamson, K. M. (2009). Igniting a spirit of inquiry: An essential foundation for evidence-based practice. *American Journal of Nursing, 109*(11), 49–52.

Migliore, L., Chouinard, H., & Woodlee, R. (2020). Clinical research and practice collaborative: An evidence-based nursing clinical inquiry expansion. *Military Medicine, 185*(2), 35–42. https://doi.org/10.1093/milmed/usz447

Milat, A. J., & Li, B. (2017). Narrative review of frameworks for translating research evidence into policy and practice. *Public Health Research & Practice, 27*(1), 2711704. https://doi.org/10.17061/phrp2711704

Moch, S. D., Quinn-Lee, L., Gallegos, C., & Sortedahl, C. K. (2015). Navigating evidence-based practice projects: The faculty role. *Nursing Education Perspectives, 36*(2), 128–130. https://doi.org/10.5480/12-1014.1

Murawski, L. M. (2014). Critical thinking in the classroom . . . and beyond. *Journal of Learning in Higher Education, 10*(1), 25–30.

Nabong, T. (2015, April 7). *Creating a learning culture for the improvement of your organization.* Training Industry. https://trainingindustry.com/articles/professional-development/creating-a-learning-culture-for-the-improvement-of-your-organization/

National League for Nursing. (2014). *Practical/vocational nursing program outcome: Spirit of inquiry.* https://www.nln.org/docs/default-source/uploadedfiles/default-document-library/spirit-of-inquiry-final.pdf

Pedaste, M., Maeots, M., Siiman, L. A., Jong, T., Van Riesen, S., Kamp, E. T., Manoli, C. C., Zacharia, Z. C., & Tsourlidaki, E. (2015). Phases of inquiry-based learning: Definitions and the inquiry cycle. *Educational Research Review, 14*(2015), 47–61. https://doi.org/10.1016/j.edurev.2015.02.003

Prabhat, S. (2011, July 28). *Difference between education and learning.* Difference Between. http://www.differencebetween.net/miscellaneous/difference-between-education-and-learning

Profetto-McGrath, J. (2005). Critical thinking and evidence-based practice. *Journal of Professional Nursing, 21*(6), 364–371. https://doi.org/10.1016/j.profnurs.2005.10.002

Psychology Today. (2021). *Growth mindset: What is a growth mindset?* https://www.psychologytoday.com/us/basics/growth-mindset

Saunders, H., Gallagher-Ford, L., Kvist, T., & Vehvilainen-Julkunen, K. (2019). Practicing healthcare professionals' evidence-based practice competencies: An overview of systematic reviews. *Worldviews on Evidence-Based Nursing, 16*(3), 176–185. https://doi.org/10.1111/wvn.12363

Teaching Excellence in Adult Literacy. (2011). *Adult learning theories.* https://lincs.ed.gov/sites/default/files/11_%20TEAL_Adult_Learning_Theory.pdf

Victor-Chmil, J. (2013). Critical thinking versus clinical reasoning versus clinical judgment: Differential diagnosis. *Nurse Educator, 38*(1), 34–36. https://doi.org/10.1097/NNE.0b013e318276dfbe

US Department of Health and Human Services. (2018). *Code of Federal Regulations, Title 45 Public Welfare, Part 46 Protection of Human Subjects.* https://www.hhs.gov/ohrp/regulations-and-policy/regulations/45-cfr-46/index.html

Warren, J. I., McLaughlin, M., Bardsley, J., Eich, J., Esche, C. A., Kropkowski, L., & Risch, S. (2016). The strengths and challenges of implementing EBP in healthcare systems. *Worldviews on Evidence-Based Nursing, 13*(1), 15–24.

Western Governors University. (2020, July 17). *What is the transformative learning theory.* WGU Blog. https://www.wgu.edu/blog/what-transformative-learning-theory2007.html

White, K. M., Dudley-Brown, S., & Terhaar, M. F. (Eds.). (2024). *Translation of evidence into nursing and healthcare.* Springer.

Wilson, M., Sleutel, M., Newcomb, P., Behan, D., Walsh, J., Wells, J. N., & Baldwin, K. M. (2015). Empowering nurses with evidence-based practice environments: Surveying Magnet, Pathway to Excellence, and non-Magnet facilities in one healthcare system. *Worldviews on Evidence-Based Nursing, 12*(1), 12–21. https://doi.org/10.1111/wvn.12077

Zaphir, L. (2019, Dec. 12). Knowledge is a process of discovery: How constructivism change education. *The Conversation*. https://theconversation.com/knowledge-is-a-process-of-discovery-how-constructivism-changed-education-126585

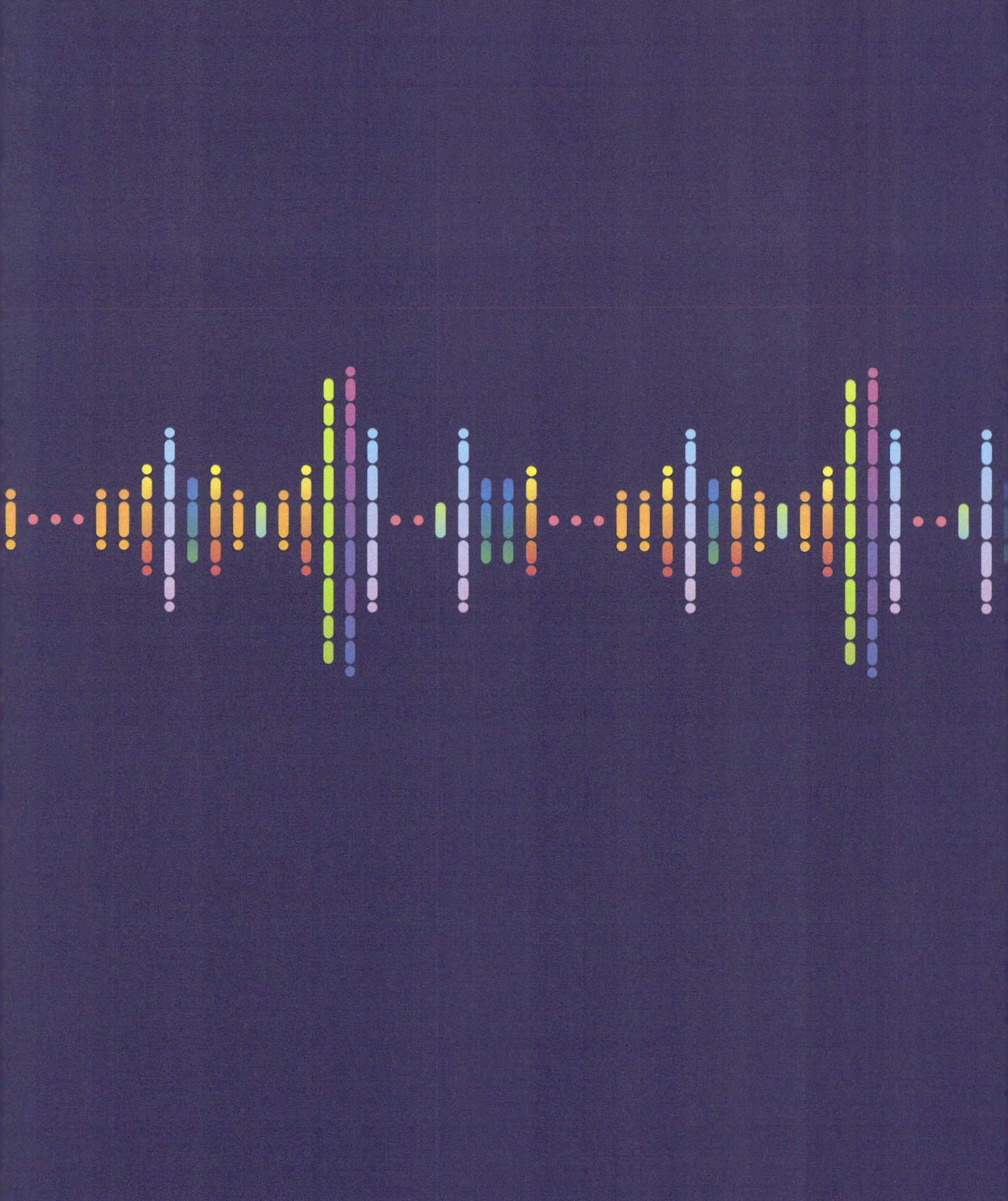

PART II
PRACTICE QUESTION, EVIDENCE, TRANSLATION (PET)

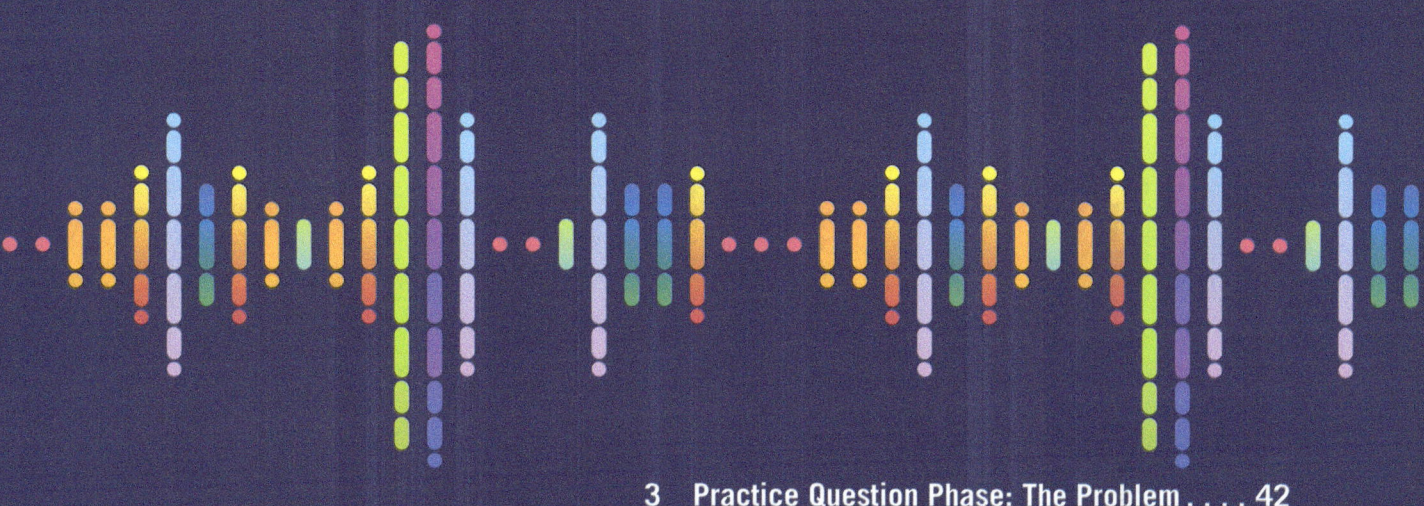

3	Practice Question Phase: The Problem	42
4	Practice Question Phase: The EBP Question	54
5	The Interprofessional Team	64
	Overview of the Evidence Phase	76
6	Evidence Phase: Introduction to Evidence	78
7	Evidence Phase: The Evidence Search and Screening	92
8	Evidence Phase: Appraising the Evidence	118
9	Evidence Phase: Summary, Synthesis, and Best-Evidence Recommendations	132
10	Translation Phase: Translation	146
11	Translation Phase: Implementation	156
12	Ongoing Considerations: Communication and Dissemination	170

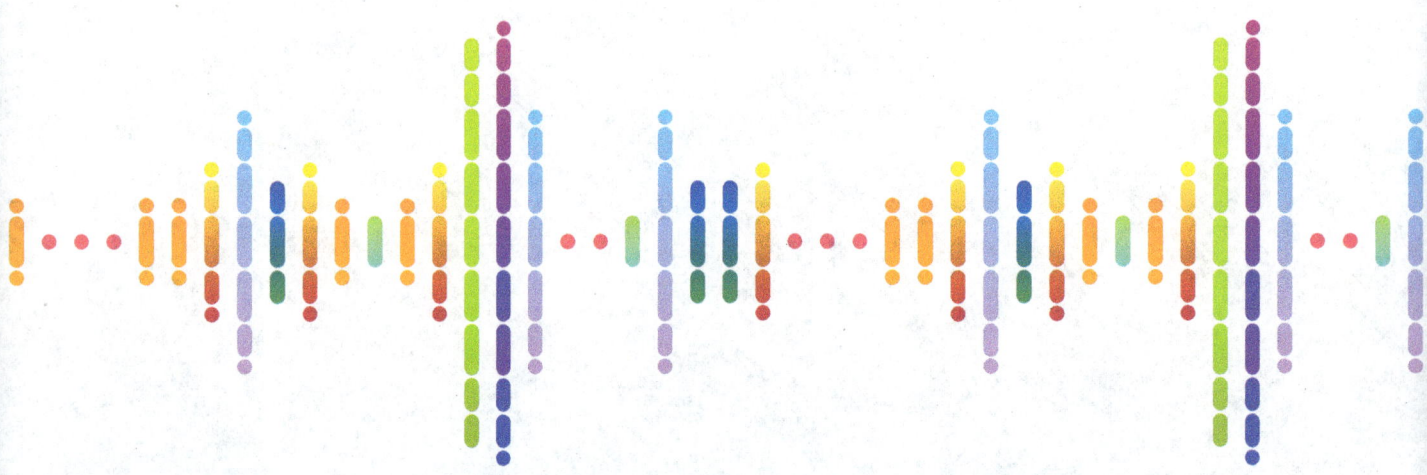

OBJECTIVES

- Describe ways in which an EBP team may realize there is a problem that needs to be addressed

- Discuss strategies for exploring problems to ensure that the root of the issue is being addressed

- Explore techniques for developing a problem statement

3

PRACTICE QUESTION PHASE: THE PROBLEM

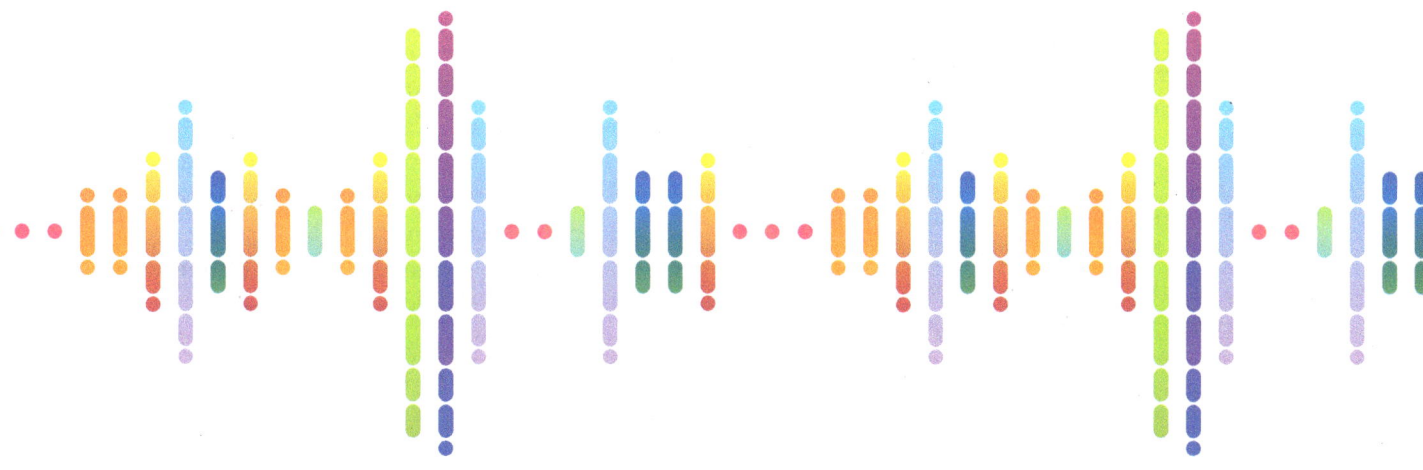

KEY POINTS

The practice question phase contains three steps. This chapter reviews the first and second (see Box 3.1). The Johns Hopkins Evidence-Based Practice (JHEBP) Question Development Tool (Appendix B) facilitates this phase.

- Failing to fully describe and define the problem can lead to ineffective solutions.

- Teams should avoid starting with a solution in mind, focusing on the symptoms of the problem, and jumping on the first problem identified.

- Spending time exploring the problem with techniques such as a root cause analysis will help identify the true problem.

- Inaccurate or poorly defined problem statements may lead to wasted time, resources, and potential dead ends in the EBP process.

> **BOX 3.1** STEPS IN THE PRACTICE QUESTION PHASE: THE P IN THE PET PROCESS
>
> 1. **Explore and describe the problem**
> 2. **Develop the problem statement**
> 3. **Write the EBP question**

INTRODUCTION

The practice question phase is the first phase of the PET process. Evidence-based practice (EBP) projects are born out of questions, curiosities, problems, or other issues that require further investigation. Exploring and establishing the problem lays the foundation for the project's trajectory and ensures that efforts are focused on addressing not only the correct problem but also problems that are well-suited to the EBP process.

EXPLORE THE PROBLEM

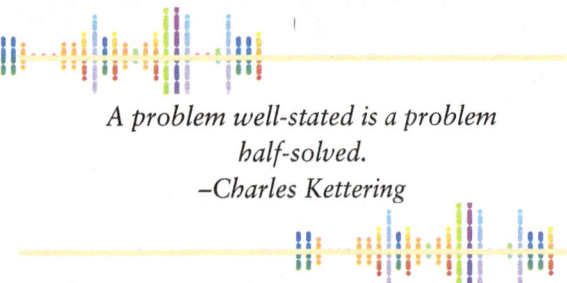

A problem well-stated is a problem half-solved.
–Charles Kettering

Merriam-Webster (n.d.) defines a *problem* as "a question raised for inquiry, consideration, or solution" and "an intricate unsettled question." While the word may have many negative connotations (e.g., the problem with illicit drug use), use of the word *problem* in the context of developing an EBP question is not meant to be wholly negative but rather to represent any topic of interest. For example, a problem may be a knowledge gap around how best to implement a new employee rewards program.

EBP projects are often sparked by curious healthcare clinicians seeking to understand the evidence supporting current practice. Clinicians may ask, "Why are we doing this procedure this way?" or, "What is the evidence that supports this intervention?" This spirit of inquiry, coupled with a culture that supports and encourages questioning, is essential for EBP to thrive within an organization (Melnyk & Fineout-Overholt, 2023).

Problems can be approached by the type of trigger that indicates there is an issue that requires further investigation: problem-focused or knowledge-focused triggers (Titler et al., 1994, 2001). *Problem-focused triggers* are identified by staff during routine monitoring of quality, risk, financial, or benchmarking data or adverse events. *Knowledge-focused triggers* are identified by reading published reports or learning new information at conferences or professional meetings (see Table 3.1). Finally, problems may be recognized because of an identified knowledge gap. *Knowledge gaps* represent the difference between the current state (clinical practice, patient care, etc.) and the ideal state. These triggers may be identified through firsthand experience, active observation, or secondhand experiences (e.g., patient, colleague, client, or business).

DESCRIBE THE PROBLEM

Once the team has identified an issue or concern, the next—and arguably one of the most important—step is to clarify and describe the problem. This includes identifying the local problem, which may be a bulleted list or phrases describing what is happening. Teams can use several strategies to help define problems. For example, phrasing the problem statement in terms of the knowledge gap rather than the solution, or asking clarifying questions (e.g., where, why, when, how), allows the team to probe deeper into the nature or root cause of the problem. Table 3.2 provides specific strategies for defining the problem with examples. Time spent defining the problem clearly and concisely will facilitate the construction of a good EBP question. Failing to fully define the problem may lead to a problem statement that doesn't truly reflect the issue at hand and may lead to the wrong solution.

TABLE 3.1 Sources of Evidence-Based Practice Problems

TRIGGER	SOURCES
Problem-focused	Financial concerns
	Evidence for current practice questioned
	Quality concern (efficiency, effectiveness, timeliness, equity, patient-centeredness)
	Safety or risk management concerns
	Unsatisfactory patient, staff, or organizational outcomes
	Variations in practice compared with external organizations
	Variations in practice within the setting
Knowledge-focused	New sources of evidence
	Changes in standards or guidelines
	New philosophies of care
	New information provided by organizational standards committees

TABLE 3.2 Strategies for Defining the EBP Problem

STRATEGY	RATIONALE	EXAMPLES
Describe in precise terms the perceived gap between what one sees and what one wants to see.	Allows the team to assess the current state and envision a future state in which broken components are fixed, risks are prevented, new evidence is accepted, and missing elements are provided	Patient satisfaction with pain management is low. This falls short of national benchmarks and a unit goal of 85%.

continues

TABLE 3.2 Strategies for Defining the EBP Problem (cont.)

STRATEGY	RATIONALE	EXAMPLES
Examine the problem critically without making assumptions to ensure that the final statement defines the specific problem.	Gives the team time to gather information, observe, listen, and probe to ensure a true understanding of the problem	Patients are not following the prescribed pain management regimen. Patients expressed confusion regarding the regimen to follow after discharge, citing that the paperwork was too complicated.
State the problem differently.	Helps gain clarity by using different verbs	40% of patients discharged post total knee replacement complain that they were not able to manage their pain. 40% of patients discharged post total knee replacement reported low patient satisfaction scores related to pain management after discharge.
Ask clarifying questions.	Helps the team get to the specific problem by using question words such as when, what, and how	When are these patients experiencing pain? What are their precipitating factors? How often are patients taking their pain medications?
Challenge assumptions.	Helps the team avoid conjecture and question everyday processes and practices that are taken for granted	Are patients filling their pain medication prescriptions and taking pain medication in the way it was prescribed?
Expand and contract the problem.	Helps the team understand whether the problem is part of a larger problem or is made up of many smaller problems	Expanded problem: Is dissatisfaction with post-discharge pain management part of general dissatisfaction with the hospital stay? Contracted problem: Are there unit- or patient-level factors contributing to the issue?
Refrain from blaming the problem on external forces or focusing attention on the wrong aspect of the problem.	Keeps the team focused on processes and systems as the team moves to define the EBP question	Avoid attributing blame such as: The patients are noncompliant with the prescribed pain medication therapy. The nurses did not educate the patient properly about the importance of taking pain medications as prescribed.

Though very important, identifying and clarifying the problem(s) is not always easy. Often, teams can be derailed by a few common mistakes. Understanding these potential pitfalls and developing strategies to overcome them is vital.

Pitfall 1: Approaching With a Solution in Mind

Well-intentioned teams or individuals may already know what they think or want the solution to the problem to be. They may inadvertently insert the solution into the problem statement and ultimately the EBP question. When clarifying the problem, it is important not to infer the cause of the problem. Consider a nurse manager faced with an increase in falls in the bathrooms on their unit. The manager recently heard of another unit with a different patient population that is using patient observers to prevent falls. The manager approaches the EBP team with this problem statement—*We need to understand how to implement patient observers to reduce falls*—and directs them to conduct an EBP project. The EBP team develops this into an EBP question, gathers and appraises evidence, develops an implementation plan, and begins a pilot of patient observers. The team quickly realizes that implementation of patient observers is not improving their fall rates. What went wrong? They explored the *solution* (patient observers, which may not have been supported by the best evidence in the context of all available solutions) and not the *cause* of the problem (staff lack knowledge of best practices to prevent falls in bathrooms).

Pitfall 2: Focusing on the Symptoms of the Problem

EBP teams may sometimes mistake symptoms for the actual problem. *Symptoms* are the outward signs that a problem exists and are often low-hanging fruit—easy to see and seemingly easy to solve. However, resolving a symptom serves as a band-aid and does not remedy the true problem. Additionally, solving one symptom inevitably brings forth others. Imagine a patient has low blood pressure (BP), prompting the team to give fluids. The fluids cause respiratory distress, so the team increases their fluid output, in turn causing their potassium to drop. The team can continue chasing the symptoms but never fix the underlying cause of the low BP, which is an infection. Chasing symptoms without a clear picture of the problem can lead to frustration and demotivation. Table 3.3 provides examples of symptoms disguised as problems.

TABLE 3.3 Symptoms Disguised as Problems

SYMPTOM	ACTUAL PROBLEM
Patients with total knee replacement were not satisfied after discharge.	40% of patients discharged post total knee replacement weren't receiving adequate pain control.
Patients are not meeting their mobility goals in an intensive care unit.	The culture in the ICU is to keep patients in restraints, on ECMO, or mechanical ventilation in bed.
Staff in the emergency department are facing burnout.	Following numerous behavioral emergencies in the emergency department, staff felt unsupported and unprepared to manage these types of events.

Pitfall 3: Accepting the First Problem Identified

Just as focusing on symptoms can lead teams astray, stopping at the first problem identified by the team may also lead to inappropriate and/or ineffective solutions. For example, a team investigating nasogastric tube dislodgement may immediately identify the problem as patients pulling the tubes out. They could build an EBP project looking for the best ways to prevent patients from pulling the tubes. However, exploring other potential problems may reveal a knowledge gap related to securing the tubing or a defect in the products used for securing the tubes. Each problem would lead to different solutions, and not every solution would be appropriate or effective.

Solutions

Approaching With an Open Mind EBP teams should be suspicious when presented with a problem statement that includes a solution. Recognizing this helps the EBP team to take a step back, look at the problem to address, and move forward in the spirit of inquiry. Instead, the EBP team can review patient fall trends on the unit, observe that most are happening in the bathroom, and ask the EBP question, "What are the best practices to prevent patient falls when toileting patients?" Patient observers may be one solution, but there may be several better solutions identified in the evidence. Problem statements reflecting an openness to possible causes of the problem allow teams to see those other, potentially more effective solutions.

Focusing on the Actual Problem One strategy to identify the actual problem is to conduct a *root cause analysis* (RCA). An RCA is a process for identifying the causes of problems to implement solutions (Centers for Medicare & Medicaid Services, n.d.). There are many tools, techniques, and approaches to conducting an RCA, but the general process is as follows (Reid & Smyth-Renshaw, 2012):

1. Identify if there is a problem.
2. Collect and analyze data surrounding the problem.
3. Determine possible causative factors.
4. Identify the root cause(s).
5. Recommend and implement solutions.

An RCA uses a systematic approach to investigate issues and contributory factors that led to an incident (Haxby, 2018). RCAs are performed among a multidisciplinary team to confirm the sequence of preceding factors before an event, to complete an analysis of these factors to identify errors, and to determine implementation measures to prevent and eliminate these errors to prevent a repeat of the adverse event (PSNet, 2019). Table 3.4 outlines several useful examples.

Each of these root cause analysis or problem identification techniques has different goals and may provide different insights about the problem. Teams should select the method best suited for their team, problem, resources, and experience. While helpful in avoiding accepting the first problem identified, problem identification tools can be used to avoid many of the pitfalls previously mentioned.

TABLE 3.4 Techniques for Conducting a Root Cause Analysis

TECHNIQUE	DESCRIPTION	AIM
Brainstorming	A technique for generating ideas and information about a particular subject or topic	Particularly useful in generating information about problems, causes, solutions, and barriers to implementation
The Five Whys	Asking "why" five times to get to the root of the problem	Useful when defining the problem or identifying if more data or analysis is needed
Mind Mapping	A diagram that visually organizes information as it relates to or radiates from a central theme or concept	Helpful in brainstorming a problem or organizing and planning tasks
Ishikawa Fishbone Diagram	A visual display that explores problems using categories such as man, machine, methods, materials, and environment	Robust method for conducting root cause analysis, generating causes
Affinity Diagram	A visual display organizing large amounts of information into categories for further reflection	Useful after brainstorming to summarize the information
Relation Diagram	A visual display of various issues and ideas and their relationship to one another using arrows to and from the concepts	Useful when exploring complex cause-and-effect relationships

(Nickols, 2021)

Asking Why to Get More Answers To improve processes at Toyota manufacturing plants, Taiichi Ohno (1988) created a now classic exercise called the *Five Whys*. This exploration involves asking "why" five times when confronted with a problem. The goal is to uncover the true root of the problem and correct it. While named the *Five Whys*, this process may take as few as three or more than 10 questions. The questioning continues until the team is satisfied and the real problem has been identified. The Five Whys process is one technique under the umbrella of an RCA and can be applied to developing problem statements.

Consider this example: An occupational therapist (OT) is working with a client to better understand a recent weight gain (symptom). During the interview and assessment, the client admits to a lack of movement or physical activity (problem). The OT provides education related to the importance of healthy behaviors including movement (solution) to decrease weight gain. The client returns for a six-month follow-up and has gained more weight and is moving less than before. The OT reevaluates and this time asks more questions, as outlined in Figure 3.1. Each time a potential problem is identified, the OT probes further by asking "why," such as, "Why

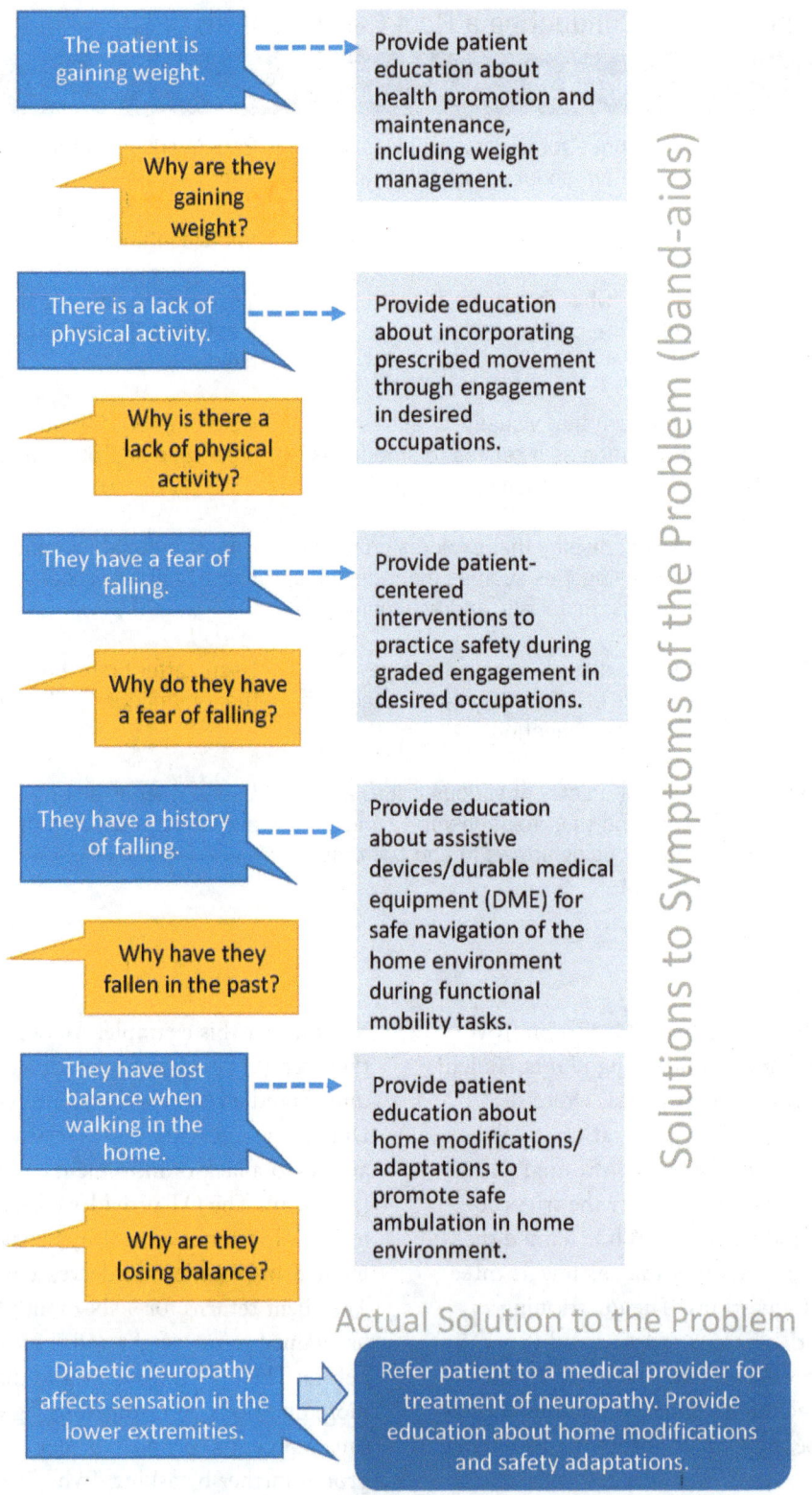

FIGURE 3.1 Using the Five Whys in practice.
(A. Cecil, personal communication, October 10, 2023)

are you not moving around?" The process can stop at any stage of questioning, and solutions can be implemented. However, until the root problem is identified, the solutions are only temporary fixes at best. As depicted, the current problem becomes a symptom as "why" questions are asked. The final problem may then become the focus of the problem statement and the team's efforts.

Using the Five Whys method can be difficult and may not work well in complex situations (Markovitz, 2020). Teams may also consider using a Fishbone or Ishikawa diagram (Ishikawa, 1990), process map, mind-mapping exercises, or other brainstorming techniques to further clarify the problem.

DEVELOP THE PROBLEM STATEMENT

After a thorough exploration and definition of the problem, the EBP team must craft a problem statement. A well-developed problem statement sets the stage for effective solutions that truly address the issue at hand and ensures that team members and impacted groups have a clear understanding of the foundation of the project. Inaccurate or poorly defined problem statements may lead to wasted time, resources, and potential dead ends in the EBP process. Proceeding without a clear problem statement may result in:

- EBP projects that do not address the true problem or are limited by a predetermined solution

- Literature searches that are too broad and lead the team to review more evidence than is needed to answer the question or too narrow to produce useful evidence

- Missing evidence that is important to answer the question

- Team frustration with the ineffectiveness of the EBP process

The EBP team uses the Question Development Tool (Appendix B) to guide this process. To assist in crafting the problem statement, EBP teams should consider the following:

- What is the local problem (defined and clarified from the previous steps)?

- Why is the problem important and relevant? What would happen if it were not addressed? This is vital information to convey to impacted groups and leadership.

- What is the current practice in the EBP team's setting? Understanding what is currently happening allows the team to further highlight the problem and need for the EBP project.

- What data from the EBP team's setting indicates there is a problem? Getting buy-in often involves data. Impacted groups want to know the magnitude of the problem and its effect on operations.

The result of identifying, clarifying, and defining the problem in the previous step should be a succinct (one or two concise sentences) and robust (strongly constructed) problem statement. Articulating a well-developed problem statement provides a comprehensive understanding of the population of interest (e.g., patients, families, staff, and their characteristics), the topic (e.g., medication administration, falls, wound care), and how the population is affected (e.g., morbidity, mortality, satisfaction). Precise descriptions clarify the scope and magnitude of the problem related to the outcome of interest. Problem statements do not include solutions or plans for solving the problem.

ADAPTING THE PROBLEM STATEMENT FOR DIFFERENT AUDIENCES

Once a problem statement has been developed, it can be adapted to accommodate different audiences. For example, consider the problem statement as the elevator pitch or quick, impactful statement of key points meant to introduce an idea or persuade someone to action. The statement must convey all the pertinent information in a concise statement or two. While crafting the problem statement, the team should consider the audience. What is important to them? What would they need to hear or understand to support your project? The goal is to encourage buy-in. The answers to these questions may differ if the team considers delivering the elevator pitch to hospital leadership or bedside staff. What each group values or needs may differ, and statements may need to be slightly reworded to accommodate that. Ultimately, teams need to craft a problem statement that conveys a sense of urgency to encourage the audience to react.

SUMMARY

Exploring and defining the practice problem is an important phase in the PET process. Lack of a well-developed practice problem may lead to answering the wrong EBP question. Asking questions, challenging assumptions, exploring the data, or performing an RCA may help home in on the specific area to address. Exploring the problem enables the interprofessional team to reflect, gather information, observe current practice, listen to clinicians, visualize how the process can be different or improved, and probe the description—together fostering a shared understanding and better reflecting the true nature of an issue. Understanding the problem allows the EBP team to develop an accurate and succinct problem statement. Statements should reflect the intended audience and convey a sense of urgency to spur an action.

A well-developed problem statement leads to an answerable EBP question that will be developed in the next step. The potential for problems to generate practice questions is limitless. Time spent refining the problem and articulating a problem statement is invaluable.

REFERENCES

Centers for Medicare & Medicaid Services. (n.d.). *Guidance for performing root cause analysis (RCA) with performance improvement projects (PIPs)*. https://www.cms.gov/medicare/provider-enrollment-and-certification/qapi/downloads/guidanceforrca.pdf

Haxby, E., & Shuldham, C. (2018). How to undertake a root cause analysis investigation to improve patient safety. *Nursing Standard, 32*(20), 41–46. https://doi.org/10.7748/ns.2018.e10859

Ishikawa, K. (1990). *Introduction to quality control*. 3A Corporation.

Markovitz, D. (2020). *The conclusion trap: Four steps to better decisions*. D&L Publications.

Melnyk, B., & Fineout-Overholt, E. (2023). *Evidence-based practice in nursing and healthcare: A guide to best practice* (5th ed.). Wolters Kluwer.

Merriam-Webster. (n.d.). Problem. In *Merriam-Webster.com dictionary*. https://www.merriam-webster.com/dictionary/problem

Nickols, F. (2021, May 28). *Problem-solving tools*. https://www.nickols.us/24PSTools.pdf

Ohno, T. (1988). *Toyota production system: Beyond large-scale production*. Productivity Press.

PSNet. (2019, Sept. 7). *Root cause analysis*. https://psnet.ahrq.gov/primer/root-cause-analysis

Reid, I., & Smyth-Renshaw, J. (2012). Exploring the fundamentals of root cause analysis: Are we asking the right questions in defining the problem? *Quality and Reliability Engineering International, 28*(5), 535–545.

Titler, M. G., Kleiber, C., Steelman, V., Goode, C., Rakel, B., Barry-Walker, J., Small, S., & Buckwalter, K. (1994). Infusing research into practice to promote quality care. *Nursing Research, 43*(5), 307–313.

Titler, M. G., Kleiber, C., Steelman, V. J., Rakel, B. A., Budreau, G., Everett, L. Q., Buckwalter, K. C., Tripp-Reimer, T., & Goode, C. J. (2001). The Iowa model of evidence-based practice to promote quality care. *Critical Care Nursing Clinics of North America, 13*(4), 497–509.

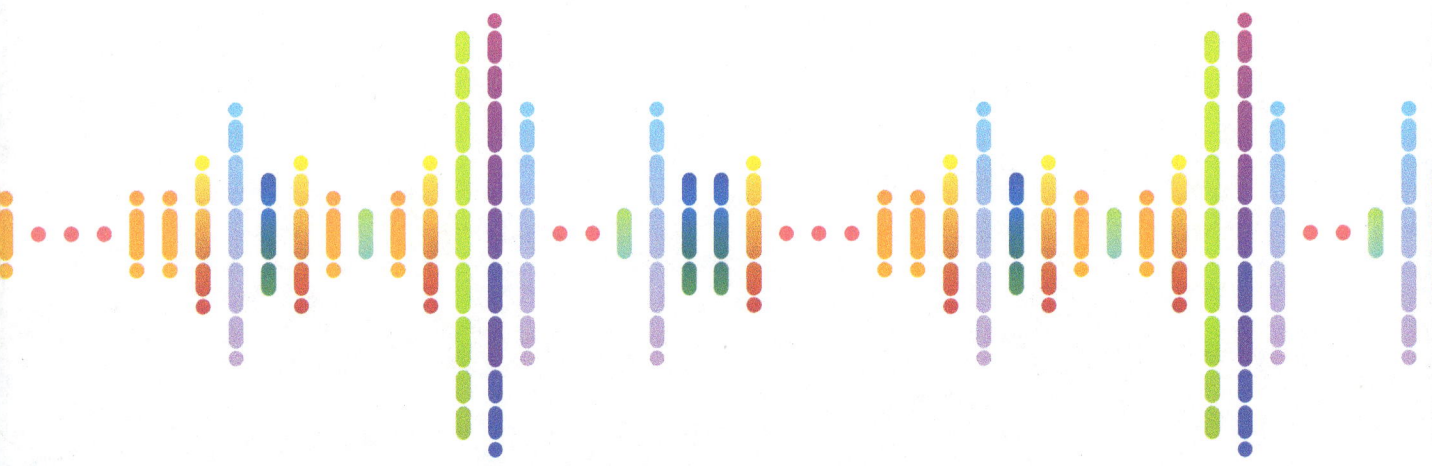

OBJECTIVES

- Establish the purpose of a well-written EBP question

- Describe past and current approaches to creating EBP questions

- Review the new Johns Hopkins Evidence-Based Practice (JHEBP) model approach to EBP questions, including types of questions and strategies to build them

4
PRACTICE QUESTION PHASE: THE EBP QUESTION

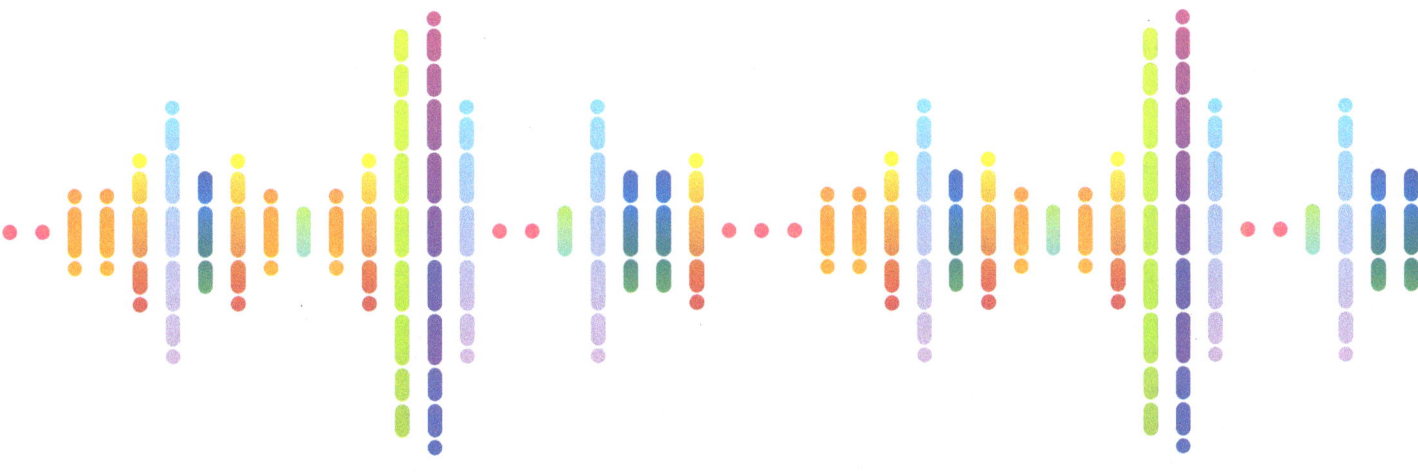

KEY POINTS

The practice question phase contains three steps. This chapter covers the final step (see Box 4.1). The Johns Hopkins Evidence-Based Practice (JHEBP) Question Development Tool (Appendix B) facilitates this step.

- In many instances, the PICO question—Patient/Population/Problem, Intervention, Comparison, and Outcome—has become synonymous with the EBP question, with teams using "PICO question" and "EBP question" interchangeably. However, PICO guides searches. It doesn't support question development as well.

- Searchable questions are concise and focused, possibly limited to two to three main ideas.

- Broad (formerly background) EBP questions cast a wide net and provide a good starting point.

- Intervention (formerly foreground) EBP questions provide more precise knowledge to drive decision-making.

- Before embarking on a full EBP project, teams should examine the project's potential alignment with organizational priorities, impact on outcomes, and ability to be implemented in the current climate.

> **BOX 4.1   STEPS IN THE PRACTICE QUESTION PHASE: THE P IN THE PET PROCESS**
>
> 1. Explore and describe the problem
> 2. Develop the problem statement
> 3. **Write the EBP question**

INTRODUCTION

Having explored and defined the problem and developed the problem statement, the evidence-based practice (EBP) team generates an answerable EBP question to address their area or topic of interest. This helps the team understand the specific information that needs to be gathered and is used to generate a search strategy to identify evidence in the next phase—evidence. The thoughtful development of a well-structured EBP question is vital because the question drives the strategies the team will use to search for evidence. A well-defined and answerable EBP question may reduce time spent searching and increase the likelihood of finding relevant evidence. There are different types and structures of EBP questions depending on the project's starting point and objectives. This chapter provides guidance on which structures work best for a given situation.

PREVIOUS APPROACHES TO EBP QUESTIONS

Types of EBP Questions

When developing the original JHEBP model in 2005, in addition to the nursing literature, nurse leaders looked to the foundational evidence-based medicine work of Dr. David Sackett and others. A prevailing approach then was the use of background and foreground questions. According to Sackett et al. (2000), a background question is employed when clinicians have limited expertise in an area. It includes a question word (what, where, how, etc.) and a clinical term (test, treatment, or an aspect of medical care). It served to identify the incidence and prevalence of a disease, condition, or topic. As knowledge is gained, clinicians develop foreground questions that seek specific information to inform decision-making and contain four components: patient/population/problem, intervention, comparison, and outcomes of clinical importance, now commonly known as the *PICO question* (Straus et al., 2019). Historically, background questions were not intended to be used as EBP questions but rather provided fundamental information, often found in textbooks, to formulate a foreground question (Fineout-Overholt & Johnson, 2023).

Since its inception, the JHEBP model has treated background questions differently. According to the model, a background question is broad and produces a wide range of evidence for review. EBP teams use background questions to identify and understand what is known when the team has little knowledge, experience, or expertise in the area. For example, to better understand pain management for people with a history of substance abuse, a background question is: "What are the best interventions to manage pain for adult patients with a history of substance abuse enrolled in outpatient rehabilitation?" This question would produce an array of evidence—for example, pharmacology, alternative therapies, behavioral contracting, or biases in prescribing and administering pain medication. Evidence identified for background questions often provides many results with diverse interventions. Teams could then break the problem into an appropriate number of background or foreground questions, creating questions that relate to each of the components identified during the initial evidence review. Often informed by background questions, foreground questions produce a refined, limited body of evidence specific to the EBP question. Foreground questions yield specific knowledge that informs decisions or actions and are generally used to compare two or more specific interventions. These questions typically align with the PICO (Population, Intervention, Comparison, Outcome) approach.

However, as the JHEBP model has evolved, the use of the words *background* and *foreground* to describe types of EBP questions may no longer be ideal. First, using the term *background* for a question to determine best practices and not simply looking at incidence and prevalence has caused confusion. When directed to start with a background question, teams may only search for incidence and prevalence, as would be expected in a true background question/search. The team may then move prematurely into a more specific foreground question without full awareness of all the variables or potential interventions. Secondly, referring to EBP questions as background questions indicates that there needs to be another step—something must follow the background question. As mentioned, background questions could lead to more background questions or foreground questions. However, most often, teams implement findings of background questions.

Building the EBP Question: The PICO Approach

In 1995, Richardson and colleagues published a now widely used format for constructing an answerable EBP question referred to as PICO—Patient/Population/Problem, Intervention, Comparison, and Outcome. The PICO format is broadly accepted as the standard for defining clinical questions for EBP and facilitating evidence retrieval by identifying key search terms (Cooke, 2012; Eriksen, 2018; Kloda, 2020; McKenzie et al., 2019; Schiavenato, 2021). Historically, PICO was intended to be utilized in clinical medicine and research, not EBP (Cullen et al., 2023; Schiavenato, 2021). In many instances, PICO has become synonymous with the EBP question, with teams using "PICO question" and "EBP question" interchangeably. However, the search strategy and the EBP question are not interchangeable.

For example, not all elements of an EBP question should be included in the search, and all search terms need not be a part of the EBP question. Using PICO to structure the EBP question and develop the search strategy has added unnecessary complexity. For example, EBP teams spend much time and energy figuring out which parts of their problem or question belong in the "intervention" category. First, it does not matter where various components end up if the appropriate terms are selected for the search strategy. Second, filling all the PICO components often results in prematurely selecting an intervention without a full review of the evidence (Cullen et al., 2023; Milner, 2024). Third, EBP teams leave the "C" blank, as it does not pertain to background questions, and they often omit the "O" when formulating the question. Using only half of the acronym proves confusing (Whalen, 2024). Not all types of EBP questions are suitable for PICO. It works well for foreground questions or questions targeting specific interventions. However, it is not well-suited for background questions where interventions are unknown. In addition to PICO, there are many other question development structures. A rapid review conducted in 2023 exploring structures for formulating questions found 38 question formulation frameworks providing a structure for almost any type of question asked (Booth et al., 2023).

THE UPDATED EBP QUESTION

After reviewing the recent literature, talking with users of the JHEBP model, and working through countless scenarios, a decision was made to update the approach to building EBP questions. This includes moving away from the terms *background* and *foreground*, as they are not well-suited to many projects undertaken by teams using the JHEBP model, and de-emphasizing the PICO structure in the EBP process. Components of PICO could still be considered as guidance for search strategies, but there is greater freedom to the structure of the EBP question (Bramer et al., 2018). Evidence points to improved search results for evidence when utilizing a less restrictive approach, especially when searching for qualitative evidence (Booth et al., 2000; Ericksen, 2018; Kloda, 2020; Schiavenato, 2021). More on search structure and strategy follows in Chapter 7.

Building New Types of EBP Questions

The updated JHEBP model will no longer utilize background or foreground questions for EBP question development. Instead, this model will guide the reader in formulating a broad EBP question or an intervention EBP question (see Figure 4.1). While this change in terminology may not functionally change the way a team approaches a question, moving away from outdated terms and better meeting the needs of the users of the JHEBP model demonstrates continued use of evidence and provider preference to update practice, even within EBP itself. Additionally, instead of trying to frame questions in PICO format, this new approach provides EBP teams with fill-in-the-blank sentence structures and suggested terms to build a question, rather than match areas of the problem to a prescribed letter.

> **NOTE**
>
> **SEARCHABLE QUESTIONS**
>
> - Are concise and focused to facilitate a more efficient search
> - May be limited to two to three main concepts
> - Often address who, what, when, where, why, and how of the problem or issue at hand
> - Can be created with question frameworks
> - Are neither too broad or vague nor too specific

Broad EBP Questions   *Broad* is defined as wide in range or amount; widely applicable or applied (Merriam-Webster, n.d.). Like the JHEBP model's previous background questions, broad questions cast a wide net, looking for all the evidence on the topic. Broad EBP questions are a good place to start when the interprofessional team lacks extensive knowledge of the topic at hand. Broad questions have a very simple structure aligning the topic, population, and setting.

> **EXAMPLE**
>
> **CONSTRUCTING A BROAD EBP QUESTION**
>
> In/among (population and/or setting), what are the best (practices/strategies/interventions) for/regarding (topic)?
>
> *In elderly patients on a psychiatric unit, what are the best practices for safe wandering?*

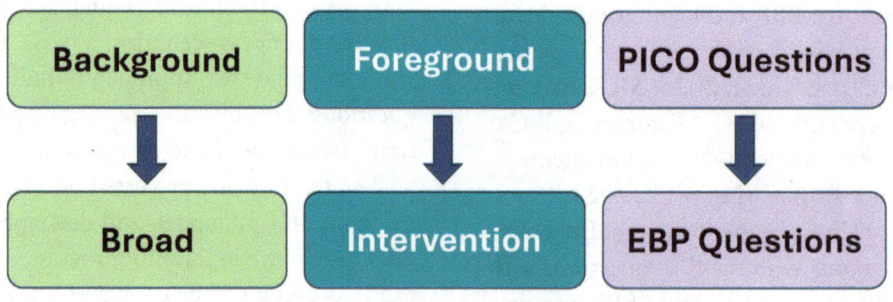

FIGURE 4.1   Changes to question terminology.

As an aid to formulating the practice question, consider the:

- Population—types of patients, clients, healthcare providers, people; consider attributes such as age, gender, symptoms, diagnosis, or roles
- Setting—place, environment
- Topic—problem, issue

Notice that the broad question structure does not include a specific intervention. Doing so at this stage in the EBP process is premature. Teams do not yet have a solid understanding of all available interventions for a particular topic. Therefore, asking them to select an intervention only leads to selecting what they think will work best and working backward to find evidence to support that practice (Cullen et al., 2023). Additionally, it is important to use the plural form of the noun—i.e., practices, interventions, strategies. This expands the expectations from one possible solution to many and primes the team to explore all options.

Assuming appropriate evidence is available, there are a few possible outcomes of a broad question. First, the evidence gleaned from a broad question can be developed into a practice change without creating further questions. For example, to implement best practices for pressure injury prevention in the intensive care unit (ICU), the EBP team posed this question: Among adults in the ICU, what are best practices regarding pressure ulcer prevention? The question yielded high-certainty recommendations in support of several interventions implemented as a bundle. The team identified gaps in the current practice and implemented components of the bundle that were lacking.

Alternatively, evidence gathered from a broad question can lead to additional broad questions.

For example, to design a physical therapist preceptor program in a community hospital, the EBP team posed this broad question: "Among physical therapist preceptors in a community hospital, what are best practices regarding training programs?" This question yielded much evidence that seemed to fall into three distinct categories: initial training/orientation, competencies, and ongoing support. From this evidence review, the team developed three more targeted and manageable broad questions:

- Among physical therapist preceptors in a community hospital, what are best practices regarding program orientation?
- Among physical therapist preceptors in a community hospital, what are best practices regarding essential competencies?
- Among physical therapist preceptors in a community hospital, what are best practices regarding ongoing support programs?

Finally, evidence gathered from broad questions may lead to a second type of question—the intervention question.

Intervention EBP Questions *Intervention* EBP questions provide more precise knowledge to inform decisions or actions. As discussed above, based on their knowledge of the subject matter, or after reviewing the wide range of evidence from a broad question, the team may select one (or more) specific intervention to review in further detail. This selection may be based on identified gaps in practice (i.e., the team identified interventions that were not already a part of their routine care), feasibility (i.e., the team identified recommendations that could easily be put into practice), or interventions with greater support for practice change (i.e., high certainty recommendations).

These focused questions follow the structure of broad questions, with the addition of an outcome and the use of a specific intervention instead of a general topic. It may be helpful for the stem of the question to begin, "According to the evidence, …". This serves two purposes: 1) to dissuade teams from starting with a focused question before reviewing the evidence, and 2) to differentiate the intervention EBP question from a research question.

> **NOTE**
> **EXPERIENCE MATTERS**
> Teams with little experience with a topic or condition will have more broad best-practice questions, whereas teams with more experience with the subject matter will generally have more intervention best-practice questions. Often, EBP teams benefit from a thorough understanding of all the best practices for an issue before diving into the more specific interventions. As their understanding and experience with the topic or issue expand, they move into more focused intervention best-practice questions (see Figure 4.2).

To build an intervention question, identify the:

- Population: types of patients, clients, healthcare providers, and people; consider attributes such as age, gender, symptoms, or diagnosis
- Setting: place or environment
- Intervention(s): treatment, intervention, or process
- Outcome: measures that indicate the effect of the intervention in achieving the desired change, improvement, or outcome

For example, an EBP team begins with a broad question asking, "Among children receiving injections in the outpatient setting, what are the best practices regarding anxiety management?" This question may yield evidence for various interventions, such as using virtual reality as a distraction, education, or gradual exposure. Virtual reality surfaces as the intervention with the highest certainty recommendations. To investigate this further, they formulate an intervention EBP question to address that gap: "According to the evidence, among pediatric patients receiving injections in the outpatient setting, what is the effect of virtual reality on levels of anxiety?" Intervention questions can also compare two interventions—for example, "According to the evidence, among pediatric patients receiving injections in the outpatient setting, what is the effect of virtual reality vs. gradual exposure on levels of anxiety?"

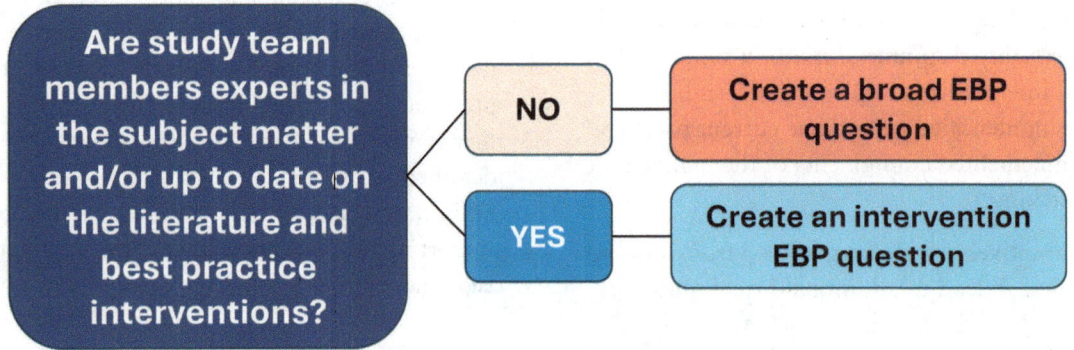

FIGURE 4.2 Team experience level and type of EBP question.

> **EXAMPLE**
>
> **SINGLE INTERVENTION EBP QUESTION**
>
> According to the evidence, in/among (population and/or setting), what is the impact of (intervention) on (outcome)?
>
> According to the evidence, in the pediatric ICU, what is the impact of changing electrodes daily on the amount of nuisance alarms?
>
> **COMPARISON INTERVENTION EBP QUESTION**
>
> According to the evidence, in/among (population and/or setting), what is the impact of (intervention) compared to (intervention) on (outcome)?
>
> According to the evidence, in post-operative adult patients, what is the impact of coughing, deep breathing, and early ambulation compared to incentive spirometry on post-operative atelectasis rates?

EBP teams may find evidence or have other compelling reasons (such as a directive from their leadership) that an intervention should be put into place but need more information on how to best implement it. This can lead to a broad EBP question that includes a specific intervention framed as best practices for implementation. In other words, not does it work but how to make it work. For example, an EBP team may be told an organizational priority is the implementation of a virtual nursing program. They need more information not about whether it will be successful but how to make it successful. Their broad EBP question would be, "In the intensive care unit, what are best practices for implementing virtual nursing?"

ADDITIONAL CONSIDERATIONS

EBP is a powerful, problem-solving approach; however, it does not work in all situations. Teams should assess if the problem lends itself to the EBP process. First, is there existing literature on the topic? EBP projects are undertaken when clinicians raise a concern or question important to practice that *existing* literature addresses. For example, a clinician inquiring about the best positioning for patients with COVID-19-related respiratory complications could find more than 300 references with a quick search. However, at the beginning of the pandemic, there would not have been any information or evidence to answer an EBP question. At the start of the pandemic, no research had been conducted on the novel virus, so best practices could not be established. If no evidence exists, teams may need to consider conducting a research study. Refer to Chapter 2 for more information on the three forms of inquiry.

Another important area for the EBP team to consider before fully beginning an EBP project is whether the problem or focus aligns with the organization's priorities. These may be strategic, financial, reputational, or value-based. Due to the time and resources needed to change practice, all efforts should align with the organization's current focus to ensure financial and leadership support. Keep in mind that some problems have multiple implications. For example, decreasing hospital-acquired infection rates leads to better patient outcomes, improved patient satisfaction, and cost savings due to the non-reimbursable cost associated with this quality indicator. Before embarking on an EBP project and committing the necessary time and resources, consider the following questions:

- Would the resulting practice changes from this project improve clinical or staff outcomes, unit structures or processes, or patient or staff satisfaction or engagement?
- Would the practice changes reduce the cost of care?
- Can potential practice changes be implemented given the practice setting's current culture, practices, and organizational structure?

Teams should consider holding off on an EBP project if the identified problem does not align with organizational priorities, would not improve outcomes, or could not be reasonably implemented in the practice setting. The topic may be better supported later with a change in climate or shifting priorities.

In addition to considering whether the problem and EBP question match organizational priorities, EBP teams should conduct a preliminary search for evidence. This search should include both internal and external resources. First, teams should do an inventory of projects undertaken in their organization. Perhaps others have addressed similar problems. Teams can save valuable time by exploring and learning from previous work.

SUMMARY

The goal of the P phase in the PET process is a well-framed question to guide the next phase of the EBP process, the E (evidence) phase, successfully and efficiently. This chapter provides a new approach to building an answerable EBP question. EBP teams may choose a broad or an intervention best-practice question. The EBP team does not need to create a broad best practice-question before creating an intervention best-practice question, but starting with a broad best practice-question will ensure a high-quality intervention best-practice question that is reflective of currently available information. For EBP teams that are unfamiliar with the subject matter or are unsure about a process or alternative interventions, it's recommended to start with a broad best-practice question. Additionally, teams should take time to determine if an EBP project is necessary or appropriate for a particular issue. Understanding the organizational strategic values and priorities is one aspect of this decision. Projects matched to the organization's strategic goals may be better supported in time and resources. Time spent developing the searchable question and determining the need for the project will be time well spent in the long run.

REFERENCES

Booth, A., O'Rourke, A. J., & Ford, N. J. (2000). Structuring the pre-search reference interview: A useful technique for handling clinical questions. *Bulletin of the Medical Library Association, 88*(3), 239.

Booth, A., Noyes, J., Flemming, K., Moore, G., Tuncalp, O., & Shakibazadeh, E. (2023). Rapid review of existing question formulation frameworks. *BMJ Global Health, 4*, 001107.

Bramer, W. M., De Jonge, G. B., Rethlefsen, M. L., Mast, F., & Kleijnen, J. (2018). A systematic approach to searching: An efficient and complete method to develop literature searches. *Journal of the Medical Library Association, 106*(4), 531541. https://doi.org/10.5195/jmla.2018.283

Cooke, A., Smith, D., & Booth, A. (2012). Beyond PICO: The SPIDER tool for qualitative evidence synthesis. *Qualitative Health Research, 22*(10), 1435–1443. https://doi.org/10.1177/1049732312452938

Cullen, L., Hanrahan, K., Tucker, S., Edmonds, S. W., & Laures, E. (2023). The problem with the PICO question: Shiny object syndrome and the PURPOSE statement solution. *Journal of PeriAnesthesia Nursing, 38*(3), 516–518.

Eriksen, M. B., & Frandsen, T. F. (2018). The impact of patient, intervention, comparison, outcome (PICO) as a search strategy tool on literature search quality: A systematic review. *Journal of the Medical Library Association, 106*(4), 420–431. https://doi.org/10.5195/jmla.2018.345

Fineout-Overholt, E., & Johnson, S. J. (2023). Asking compelling clinical questions. In B. Melnyk & E. Fineout-Overholt (Eds.), *Evidence-based practice in nursing & healthcare* (5th ed., pp. 37–61). Wolters Kluwer.

Kloda, L. A., Boruff, J. T., & Cavalcante, A. S. (2020). A comparison of patient, intervention, comparison, outcome (PICO) to a new, alternative clinical question framework for search skills, search results, and self-efficacy: A randomized controlled trial. *Journal of the Medical Library Association, 108*(2), 185–194. https://doi.org/10.5195/jmla.2020.739

McKenzie, J. E., Brennan, S. E., Ryan, R. E., Thomson, H. J., Johnston, R. V., & Thomas J. (2019). Defining the criteria for including studies and how they will be grouped for the synthesis. In J. P. T. Higgins, J. Thomas, J. Chandler, M. Cumpston, T. Li, M. J. Page, & V. A. Welch (Eds.), *Cochrane handbook for systematic reviews of interventions* (Version 6.0, Chapter 3). https://training.cochrane.org/handbook/archive/v6/chapter-03

Merriam-Webster. (n.d.). Broad. In *Merriam-Webster.com dictionary*. https://www.merriam-webster.com/dictionary/broad

Milner, K. A., Hays, D., Farus-Brown, S., Zonsius, M. C., Saska, E., & Fineout-Overholt, E. (2024). National evaluation of DNP students' use of the PICOT method for formulating clinical questions. *Worldviews on Evidence-Based Nursing, 21*(2), 216–222. https://doi.org/10.1111/wvn.12709

Richardson, W. S., Wilson, M. C., Nishikawa, J., & Hayward, R. S. (1995). The well-built clinical question: A key to evidence-based decisions. *ACP Journal Club, 123*(3), A12–A13.

Sackett, D. L., Straus, S. E., Richardson, W. S., Rosenberg, W., & Haynes, R. B. (2000). *Evidence-based medicine: How to practice and teach EBM*. Churchill.

Schiavenato, M., & Chu, F. (2021). PICO: What it is and what it is not. *Nurse Education in Practice, 56,* 103194. https://doi.org/10.1016/j.nepr.2021.103194

Straus, S. E., Glasziou, P., Richardson, W. S., & Haynes, R. B. (2019). *Evidence-based medicine: How to practice and teach EBM* (5th ed.). Elsevier Health Sciences.

Whalen, M. (2024, Aug. 21). Reducing decision-making: A simple solution to making evidence-based practice more accessible to all. *Worldviews on Evidence-Based Nursing*. https://doi.org/10.1111/wvn.12740

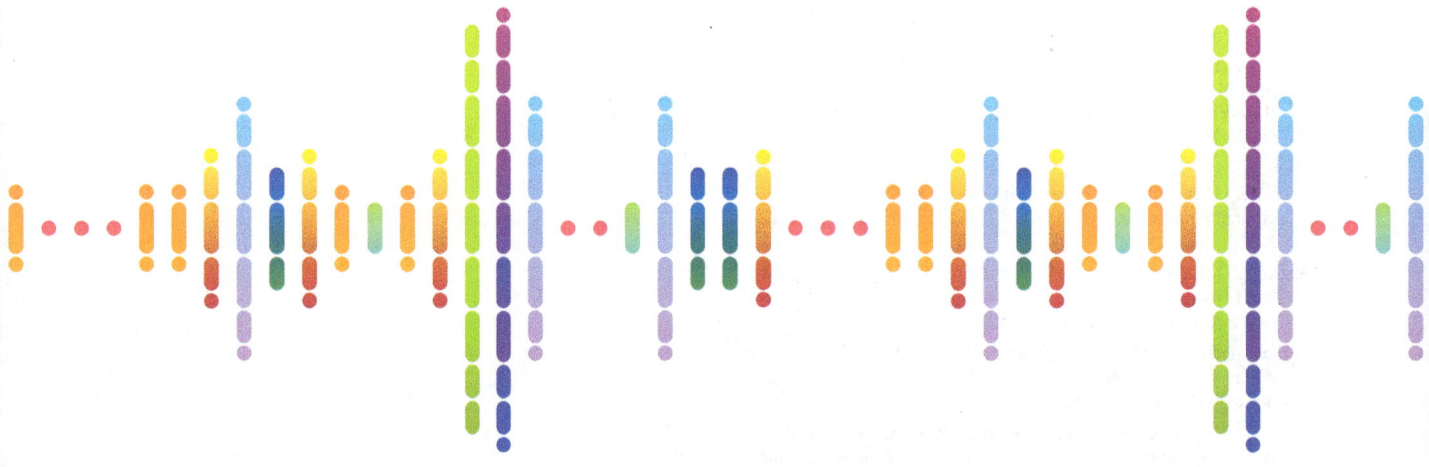

OBJECTIVES

- Describe the formation of the interprofessional team
- Discuss important characteristics of core team members
- Identify strategies for success

5
THE INTERPROFESSIONAL TEAM

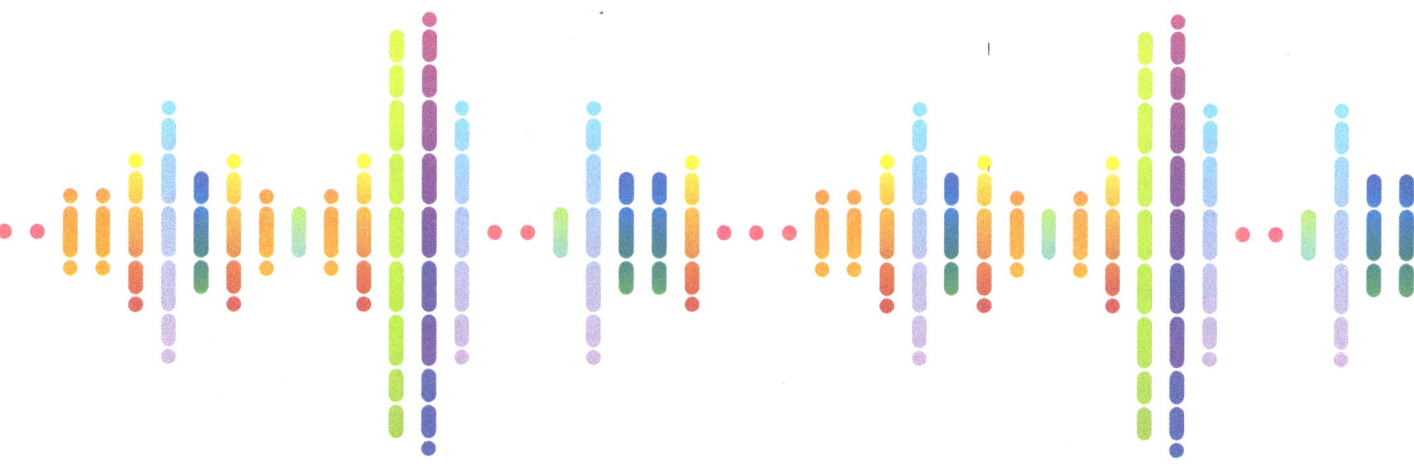

KEY POINTS

- It is critical to build an interprofessional team to collaborate with when embarking on an EBP project.

- When building core EBP team members and the team leader, consider their expertise, influence, character traits, behavior traits, and team dynamics.

- Consider impacted groups that may influence or be influenced by the EBP project. Impacted groups can include patients, families, managers, and policymakers.

- Impacted groups can broaden the team's perspective, enhance the project's impact, and make the audience feel inclusive and considerate of all perspectives.

- Recognizing and appreciating contributions within the team enhances belonging and commitment to the project.

- Successful teams tend to have a clear vision and direction.

INTRODUCTION

This chapter is intended for health professionals interested in or involved in EBP projects who want to learn how to collaborate with other disciplines to achieve better patient care and outcomes. The chapter provides examples, tables, and figures to illustrate and facilitate the application of the concepts and methods discussed. It also includes references for further reading and exploration of the topic.

Evidence-based practice (EBP) requires collaboration among health professionals who bring their diverse and specialized knowledge, skills, and methods to the project. This chapter guides the team on how to form and manage an effective interprofessional EBP team. It empowers them with the knowledge and tools to translate evidence into practice and overcome the challenges and barriers that may arise along the way.

THE EBP TEAM

In 2003, the Institute of Medicine (IOM) suggested five "core competencies that all health clinicians should have, no matter their discipline, to meet the needs of the 21st-century health care system" (pp. 45–46):

- Care for patients' needs
- Collaborate across disciplines
- Use EBP
- Improve quality
- Use informatics

Since then, the best evidence shows that interprofessional teams produce better patient care with improved outcomes than healthcare professionals who work alone (IOM, 2003).

In 2014, the Robert Wood Johnson Foundation conducted a study investigating best practices for interprofessional teams in the real world (CFAR Inc. et al., 2015). The study found that effective interprofessional teams:

- Encourage the active involvement of each discipline in patient care. All disciplines work together, fully engaging patients and those who support them. Team leadership changes based on patient needs.
- Respect patient- and family-centered goals and values, provide a way for continuous communication among caregivers, and maximize participation in clinical decision-making within and across disciplines. Teams value the disciplinary contributions of all professionals (p. 1).

These findings are relevant to creating interprofessional EBP teams with members from different disciplines who bring their diverse and specialized knowledge, skills, and methods. Throughout the project, team members integrate their observations, areas of expertise, and decision-making to coordinate, collaborate, and translate evidence into practice.

Action Item 1: Choose Team Members

At the outset of an EBP project, the people beginning the initiative must build the right interprofessional team. This will help ensure diverse views, strong cooperation, and solid suggestions. While a detailed analysis of who will be affected by or is interested in the project is needed, the initiators should first form a core EBP team with some of these impacted individuals. A core EBP team should have enough members to cover the topic well but not too many to slow things down—ideally six to eight people.

Expertise The EBP team members should have different skills depending on the problem's focus and scope. They should know about the EBP problem and who is affected by any potential change. For example, nurses, pharmacists, and oncologists could work on a question about managing nausea in chemotherapy patients, as this may involve prescribing, formulating, dispensing, and administering medications. A question about the early mobilization of ICU patients could involve nursing, respiratory therapy, intensive care physicians, and physical and occupational therapy, as this may involve writing mobility orders, assessing patient capacities, assisting patients in meeting goals, and coordinating care.

Level of Influence It is also essential to consider how influential or supportive a team member will be. Leaders, formal or informal, should be included on the team. Formal leaders have defined roles and power based on their position or title. Informal leaders have influence based on their clinical expertise and experience. Formal leaders can help with securing resources and funding or eliminating barriers. Informal leaders can help with change and adaptation among colleagues. An effective core EBP team should include both formal and informal leaders. Descriptions of informal leaders are displayed in Figure 5.1 (Morena et al., 2022).

Character Traits Along with their expertise and level of influence, the character traits of crucial EBP team members are helpful to think about. One way to do this is to use the Ten Faces of Innovation (Kelly & Littman, 2005) framework, which suggests that people have different roles, such as learning, organizing, and building roles. Learning roles tend to be receptive to new ideas and practice sincere and respectful inquiry. Organizing roles can be skillful at finding and overcoming obstacles to progress and are good at staying on track. Building roles can use the work done by others and promote it to others on the local and system level.

Behavior Traits It is also essential to consider how different EBP team members may help or hinder change. Rogers' Theory of Diffusion of Innovation (2003) describes five categories of adopters who can speed up or slow down the adoption of improvements or changes in practice. Inviting individuals considered late majority or laggards to join the EBP team lets them be part of the process and learn about the project gradually. This strategy may encourage the late majority and laggard members to adopt evidence recommendations more quickly, supporting their successful implementation into the practice environment.

Opinion Leaders
- Part of local peer group
- Have a wide sphere of influence
- Trusted to judge fit between innovation and unit norms
- Viewed as respected and trustworthy sources of information

Change Champions
- Respected members of local group setting (clinic, care unit)
- Expert clinicians with positive relations with other professionals
- Encourage peers to adopt innovation; are persistent and passionate about innovation

FIGURE 5.1 Characteristics of informal leaders *(Morena et al., 2022).*

Behavioral categories are:

- **Innovators:** Risk-takers who want to create change. This is 2.5% of all people.
- **Early adopters:** Adventurous, trendy, influential, and respected by others. They are 13.5% of the population.
- **Early majority:** Also influential but more practical and careful to avoid risk. The early majority is 34% of the population.
- **Late majority:** More wary or doubtful and can be swayed by laggards. This is 34% of all people.
- **Laggards:** Distrustful, preferring the current situation over change. They are 16% of the population.

Figure 5.2 shows a pediatric intensive care unit (PICU) that completed an EBP project on telenursing to support new nurses. The core EBP team knew they needed to choose more members wisely based on their early adopter role from Rogers' theory. They assigned early adopter roles based on experience with those staff members on other projects and everyday work.

Team Dynamics Understanding team dynamics is also crucial for effective teamwork. Google and MIT researchers identified five critical factors of productive teams in Project Aristotle (Google re:Work, 2024). They are:

1. **Psychological safety:** Team members can take risks and share their vulnerability in a supportive environment.
2. **Mutual trust:** Team members are reliable, clear about their roles and responsibilities, and trust each other to finish work on time.
3. **Structure and clarity:** Team members know the team goals and agree on specific and achievable plans to achieve them.
4. **Meaning:** Team members value the project or their role on the team.
5. **Impact:** The team can see that their work matters and contributes to the project's impact on the unit or organization.

All the above factors should be considered when forming the ideal core EBP team. Having team members with as many qualities as possible will help the team perform well and succeed in the project. This will help to balance the team. The team may be ineffective if the membership has an unbalanced ratio of laggards to early adopters. Keep in mind that some team members may have more than one quality. For example, a

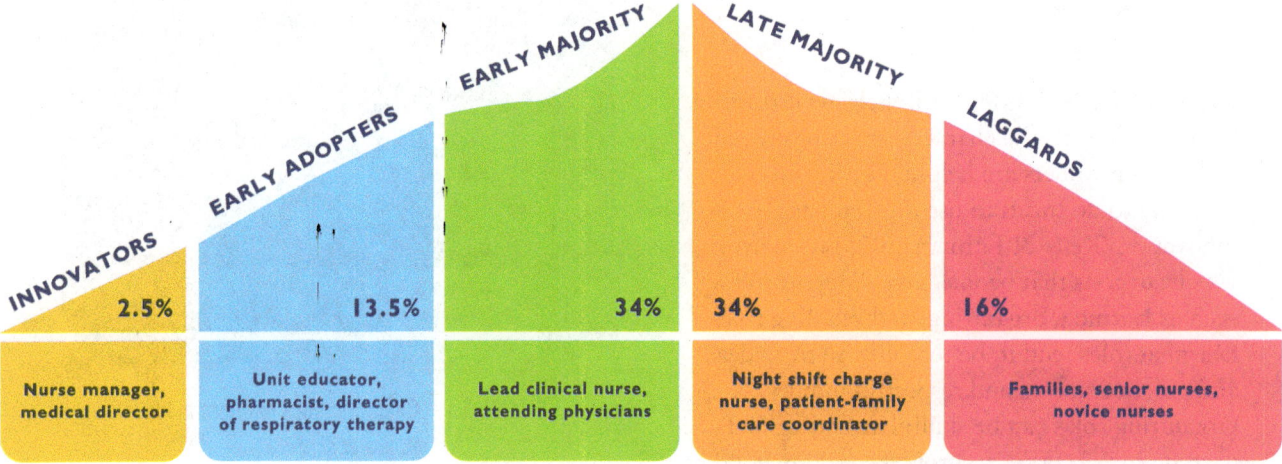

FIGURE 5.2 Example of PICU staff placement on the adopter curve.

subject matter expert may also be a learner and an informal leader in the unit. Investing time in building the right team is vital for an EBP project.

Action Item 2: Designate a Team Leader

The EBP team should also have a designated leader who can be assigned or chosen from the core team. The leader of the EBP team is essential for successful project implementation and long-term sustainability. The leader should know about the EBP process to ensure all steps are followed. They help establish a clear mission and vision for the team while ensuring alignment with evidence-based principles. Leaders maintain priorities, reinforce expectations, foster learning, and invest resources to support consistent EBP implementation. The leader will coordinate meetings, guide the project steps, and communicate the team's recommendations.

Action Item 3: Identify Impacted Groups

Once the core EBP team defines the problem and formulates the EBP question, they examine who the impacted groups are that can influence the EBP project's outcome by facilitating or hindering the implementation of the project recommendations. The choice of suitable impacted groups depends on who is affected by the problem or issue, where it happens, and when it occurs. Key impacted groups may belong to categories from the local or unit level to the institutional or health system level. Selecting impacted groups from all levels early on helps ensure the project's success by proactively assessing the impact and influence impacted groups may have. Table 5.1 helps differentiate between the role of an EBP team member versus an impacted group member. The project team should complete the Impacted Groups Analysis and Communication Resource (Hopkins.org/resources) to identify all possible impacted groups and ensure that appropriate communication strategies are started with each

TABLE 5.1 Team Members Versus Impacted Groups

	ROLE	RESPONSIBILITY	ENGAGEMENT	EXAMPLES
Team Member	Active involvement in the ongoing activities of the EBP project	Responsible for the tasks of the project Contributes to the completion of the project's goals	Attends team meetings Active in the planning and implementation of the project	Frontline interprofessional staff Clinical nurse specialists Nursing practice and professional staff Other interprofessional educators/specialists
Impacted Group Member	Has expertise or interest in the project's outcome May oversee the area where the project is being implemented	Acts as a consultant Provides feedback Grants approval at various stages of the project	Attends meetings when invited to participate in critical decision points	Interprofessional leaders Managers Directors Medical directors

one. As the EBP project advances, more needs may arise, and the EBP team should constantly evaluate the need for more impacted groups. Note: Consider involving a patient or family member as an impacted group or team member for patient-centered problems.

> **NOTE**
>
> **PATIENTS AND FAMILIES AS IMPACTED GROUPS** Bring diverse perspectives of lived experiences
> - Promote patient- and family-centered care
> - Help EPB team consider effect of proposed changes

EFFECTIVE TEAMWORK: COMPETENCIES OF AN INTERDISCIPLINARY TEAM

Group work can be notoriously difficult and tricky. While an interdisciplinary team is an essential component of a robust EBP project, it is still vulnerable to many of the threats that groups face when trying to produce meaningful work promptly.

Interdisciplinary teamwork is complex enough of a process to have an entire field devoted to its study. For example, healthcare workforce experts in England incorporated data from a study on interdisciplinary care teams with the results from a systematic review to create a set of competencies related to effective interdisciplinary team practices (Nancarrow et al., 2013). Themes were extracted from this paper and adapted to fit the process of EBP. The following list applies these critical concepts to the EBP team's strategy and will help the team function at the highest level:

1. Select a team leader who sets a clear direction and vision for the team while offering support and supervision to the EBP team members.
2. Include enough EBP core team members to ensure a suitable mix of skills, competencies, and personalities for smooth functioning.
3. Recruit core EBP team members who demonstrate interdisciplinary competencies such as collaborative leadership, communication, professional knowledge, and experience.
4. Support role interdependence while respecting individual roles and autonomy.
5. Adopt a set of values that guide the EBP team.
6. Use communication strategies that enhance intra-team communication, collaborative decision-making, and effective team processes.
7. Display an EBP team culture and interdisciplinary environment of trust where contributions are valued and consensus is fostered.
8. Ensure adequate time, resources, processes, and structures are in place to support the EBP team's vision.
9. Provide recommendations for high-quality EBP with measurable outcomes; utilize feedback for improvement.
10. Encourage personal development through appropriate training and opportunities for learning the EBP process.

Action Item 4: The First Meeting

Once the team has been assembled, the identified leader should orient the group to the EBP question and their role in the project. Different messaging may be necessary based on team members' or impacted groups' vested interests. The Impacted Groups Analysis and Communication Resource (Hopkins.org/resources) can help tailor messaging by identifying a person's role, authority, impact, influence, and engagement level at the project's beginning. These initial efforts will help achieve success and avoid potential obstacles that slow progress due to confusion, disagreement, or lack of buy-in.

Additionally, key team members producing action items throughout the project should be fully informed of their responsibilities as they agree to the work. It is highly recommended to build in time for questions to initial meeting agendas, as members will receive much information at once. To end the initial discussion, the team leader will work to coordinate the team's goals and agree on a tentative timeline with an awareness that it may change as priorities and assumptions change.

Action Item 5: Maintaining Team Engagement and Accountability

In the dynamic world of EBP project management, maintaining team engagement and accountability cannot be overstated. An engaged team drives successful project execution, fostering a positive work environment where creativity and productivity thrive. Accountability ensures that each member is responsible for their contributions, creating a sense of reliability and trust within the team. It helps set clear expectations and measurable goals, which are essential for tracking progress and achieving project milestones. Engagement and accountability form the backbone of a high-performing team, driving EBP projects toward successful completion and cultivating a culture of excellence.

Keeping the Team Engaged Forming the EBP team may seem complex, but it is easier than keeping the team members active and responsible for their work. Picking team members who are eager and have an interest or skill in the topic is only the beginning. Quality and safety work has shown that creating initial buy-in is crucial. Team leaders should ask themselves, "How can we engage hearts and minds equally?" Using powerful stories and relevant data to show the importance of the work has worked well in this effort (Pronovost et al., 2008).

Additionally, help team members create an individualized sense of ownership for their role in the initiative. Adapting the question "How do I make the world a better place?" for each impacted group will also encourage lasting commitment. For example, executive leaders want to know how they can make an organization safe for patients and rewarding for staff. They want to see how the changes and strategies align with the health system's mission and values. Unit leaders care most about the effects of the changes on their whole population and those caring for their patients. Frontline staff need to feel they can change the world, whether it be a safer unit or a more enjoyable workplace. With this feeling, they are more likely to be engaged as they can see the impact of their participation (Pronovost et al., 2008).

Another strategy to keep the team engaged is the 5 Cs: Care, Connect, Coach, Contribute, and Congratulate (see Table 5.2). This broad approach fosters employee engagement and can be adapted for EBP (Gratifi, 2023; Venier, 2023). Participating in the EBP work makes team members feel far more appreciated, involved, and aligned with the health system's mission.

Keeping the Team Accountable EBP team leaders will face challenges, and their members will be accountable for assigned tasks, deadlines, and meeting schedules. Many of the aforementioned tactics to engage the team will also help with accountability. Additional barriers and strategies to address them are included in Table 5.3. These can help ensure that the group stays on track with the project timeline and that tasks are done on time and well (Indeed Editorial Team, 2024; Maybray, 2023).

TABLE 5.2 The 5 Cs to Facilitate Team Engagement

	DESCRIPTION	TACTICS (EBP-RELATED EXAMPLES)
Care	Caring for your team members is the first and fundamental step in engaging them.	• Check in with team members to ensure they understand the assigned task, and offer additional support when needed. • Set clear expectations and deadlines. • Offer flexibility in workload and task assignment. • Ask team members how they prefer to receive communication (e.g., email, text, a communication platform, etc.). • Promote an equitable distribution of work. • Prevent power struggles among team members if working in groups.
Connect	Emphasizes the importance of building solid relationships within the workplace.	• Foster a culture of respect, trust, and belonging within the EBP team. • Build strong relationships among team members (consider having members work in pairs on assigned tasks). • Discuss diverse perspectives, values, and preferences. • Encourage collaboration and open communication when questions arise or deadlines are challenging.
Coach	Effective coaching and mentoring help employees reach their potential and boost engagement.	• Guide work. • Be available for regular touch-bases. • Support professional development, provide education on various EBP processes, etc. • Enlist mentors who have a strong EBP background.
Contribute	Empower employees to actively contribute and feel that their work is meaningful and benefits a larger purpose.	• Promote individual autonomy; help team members to take on new opportunities or develop new strengths in EBP competencies. • Create opportunities for staff to share ideas freely via team meetings or other communication channels. • Seek input from team members and involve them in critical decisions.
Congratulate	Recognizing and appreciating employees' efforts is vital to maintaining high levels of engagement.	• Recognize hard work. • Appreciate team members' contributions to the completed EBP project. • Celebrate achievements. • Make praise visible.

(Gratifi, 2023; Venier, 2023)

TABLE 5.3 Strategies to Ensure Efficiency and Accountability

BARRIER	STRATEGY
Ineffective leadership	Set a schedule of follow-ups and implement changes to the project plan as needed
Goal confusion	Establish a standardized protocol for setting goals, analyzing them, and outlining workflow to achieve them efficiently
Communication gaps	Unify the platform for communication and ensure all members of the team are included in communication (e.g., Reply All function in email)
Lack of trust	Effectively foster trustful relationships through team-building exercises and regular opportunities for collaboration
Team size issues: • Small: Too much work • Large: Challenges with sharing duties	Continuously reassess team size and the need for more or fewer impacted groups/team members
Underperformers	Address individual causes Enlist a mentor Reassign tasks as needed (not first choice)
Overperformers	Encourage equitable task assignments
Workflow mismanagement	Ensure the use of a project planning tool
Lack of commitment/ownership	Establish universal team norms/standards
Tolerating poor performance	Address poor performance with continuous feedback
Time management issues	Create processes for tracking workflow and keeping all team members accountable for their specific duties
Inadequate resource allocation	Determine ways to get additional support or change the project plan as needed
Poor planning	Utilize project planning tools from the beginning Revisit the project plan and make changes as needed

(Maybray, 2023)

SUMMARY

EBP requires interprofessional collaboration, enabling different health professionals to contribute their varied and specialized knowledge, skills, and approaches to the project. This chapter has discussed how to establish and manage an effective interprofessional EBP team that can implement evidence into practice and overcome the difficulties and obstacles that may occur along the way. The chapter has given practical advice on selecting the core EBP team members and the team leader, recognizing and involving other impacted groups, enhancing effective teamwork, and developing skills and strategies for successful interprofessional EBP teams. The chapter has also provided tips and tools for maintaining the team's engagement and accountability throughout the project. By following the recommendations and examples in this chapter, health professionals can form and lead interprofessional EBP teams that can improve health outcomes and patient care.

REFERENCES

CFAR Inc., Tomasik, J., & Fleming, C. (2015). *Promising interprofessional collaboration practices* [White paper]. Robert Wood Johnson Foundation. https://www.rwjf.org/content/dam/farm/reports/reports/2015/rwjf418568

Google re:Work. (2024). *Learn what an effective team is.* https://rework.withgoogle.com/jp/guides/understanding-team-effectiveness#help-teams-take-action

Gratifi. (2023, Nov. 8). *The 5Cs of employee engagement: A comprehensive guide.* https://www.gratifi.com/blog/the-5-cs-of-employee-engagement-a-comprehensive-guide/

Indeed Editorial Team. (2024, Aug. 15). *11 Common barriers to teamwork and how you can overcome them.* https://www.indeed.com/career-advice/career-development/barriers-to-teamwork

Institute of Medicine. (2003). *Health professions education: A bridge to quality.* National Academies Press. https://doi.org/10.17226/10681

Kelley, T., & Littman, J. (2005). *The ten faces of innovation: IDEO's strategies for beating the devil's advocate and driving creativity throughout your organization.* Currency.

Maybray, B. (2023). *Accountability in teams: 13 ways to build it.* HubSpot. https://blog.hubspot.com/marketing/how-to-inspire-accountability-in-your-virtual-startup-team

Morena, A. L., Gaias, L. M., & Larkin, C. (2022). Understanding the role of clinical champions and their impact on clinician behavior change: The need for causal pathway mechanisms. *Frontiers in Health Services, 2,* 896885.

Nancarrow, S. A., Booth, A., Ariss, S., Smith, T., Enderby, P., & Roots, A. (2013). Ten principles of good interdisciplinary team work. *Human Resources for Health, 11,* 19. https://doi.org/10.1186/1478-4491-11-19

Pronovost, P. J., Berenholtz, S. M., & Needham, D. M. (2008). Translating evidence into practice: A model for large scale knowledge translation. *BMJ, 337,* a1714. https://doi.org/10.1136/bmj.a1714

Rogers, E. M. (2003). *Diffusion of innovations* (5th ed.). Free Press.

Venier, G. (2023, Nov. 5). *The 5Cs of employee engagement – framework.* https://www.simpleworkapps.com/blog/5cs-of-employee-engagement/

OVERVIEW OF THE EVIDENCE PHASE

The preceding chapters highlighted the importance of exploring and defining the problem and developing a searchable evidence-based practice (EBP) question. With these two tasks completed, the teams must determine if EBP is the proper approach and what kind of search they need to conduct. In the last edition of this text, we presented an algorithm to determine the need for an EBP project. This decision tree assisted teams in determining if EBP was the correct approach or if another strategy or form of inquiry would be a better fit, such as quality improvement or research. For this fifth edition, we have revised the algorithm to indicate if EBP is the best option and the type of evidence search required. More detailed descriptions of the search techniques mentioned will follow in subsequent chapters. The following represents a brief overview of this decision-making process (see Figure 6.1). See the EBP Project Steps and Overview (Appendix A) for this decision tree.

Once the EBP team has sufficiently defined the problem and crafted a searchable EBP question, the next step is to ask if the problem meets the organization's strategic priorities. As discussed in Chapter 4, problems and projects that do not match the organization's priorities and focus may receive little support or traction. Teams should consider alternatives to conducting the EBP project. Perhaps there is another avenue to resolve the issue or a different aspect of the problem that would align with the strategic priorities.

Provided the problem aligns with the organization's priorities, the team should conduct a best-evidence search specifically for recent pre-appraised evidence:

- The EBP team should first search for clinical practice guidelines (CPGs), followed by literature reviews with a systematic approach (LRSAs), and finally, evidence summaries (see Chapters 6 and 7).

- Any pre-appraised evidence uncovered should be reviewed for suitability and quality (see Chapter 8).

- If there is suitable and adequate pre-appraised evidence, the team searches for any additional evidence published since the original review was conducted.

- If the team does not find additional evidence, or if additional evidence confirms the findings from the pre-appraised evidence, they do not need to conduct a full evidence review. They can proceed to identifying the best-evidence recommendations for the translation phase of the PET process.

- If newer evidence contradicts the original evidence, the team would need to convene impacted groups and determine recommendations to move into translation (see Chapters 8 and 9).

- Alternatively, if a best-evidence search fails to identify any suitable pre-appraised evidence of adequate quality, the team should conduct an exhaustive search of the literature with a systematic process to screen the results (see Chapter 7).

- If this thorough search reveals a lack of sufficient evidence related to the problem, an EBP project cannot be conducted. The team should consider whether a research study would be more appropriate to address the problem. Other options include maintaining the current organizational practice or investigating/confirming the community standard. Only when the literature's exhaustive search indicates that a body of evidence exists should the team proceed with the EBP project.

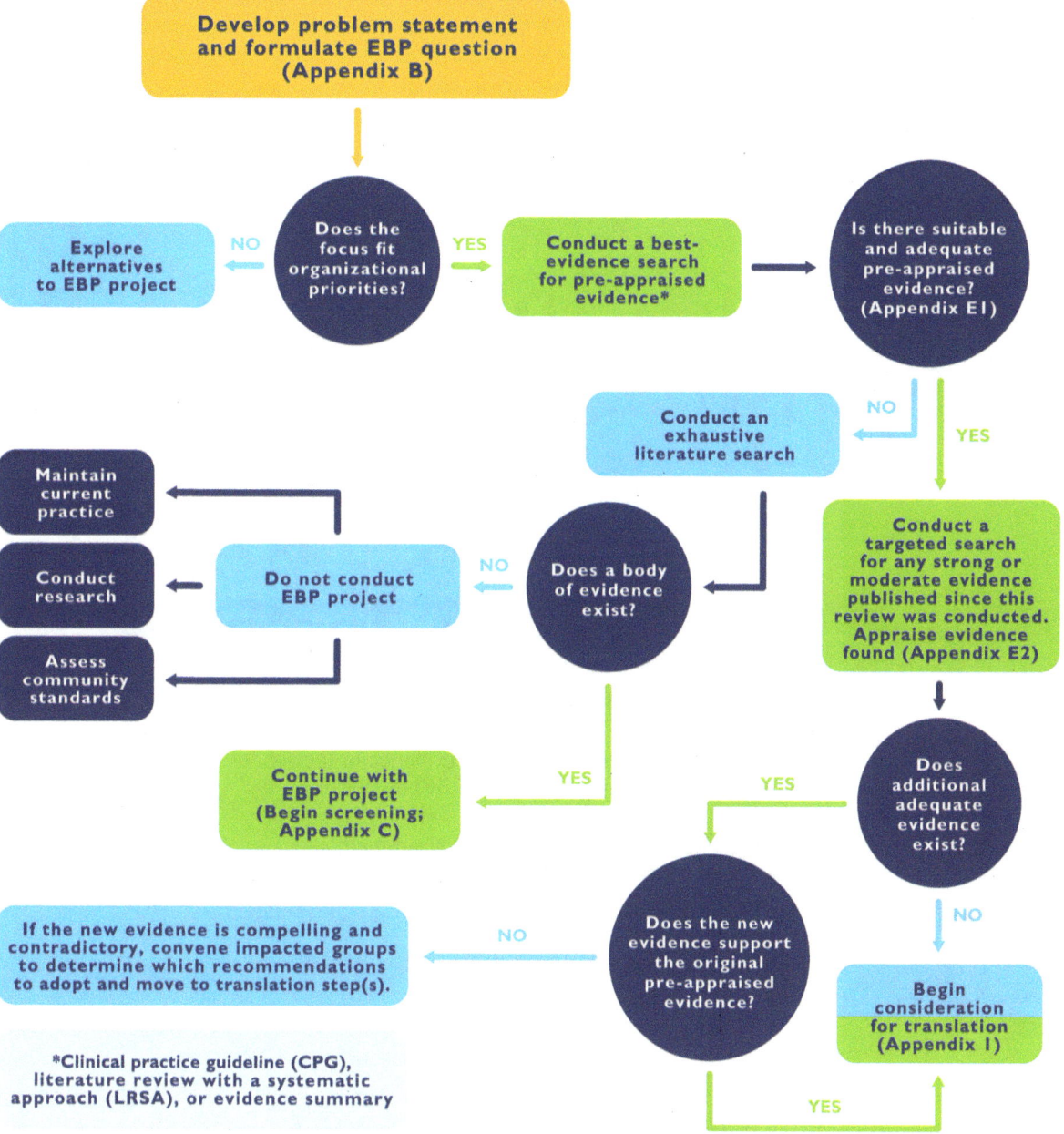

FIGURE 6.1 Determining the best course of action.

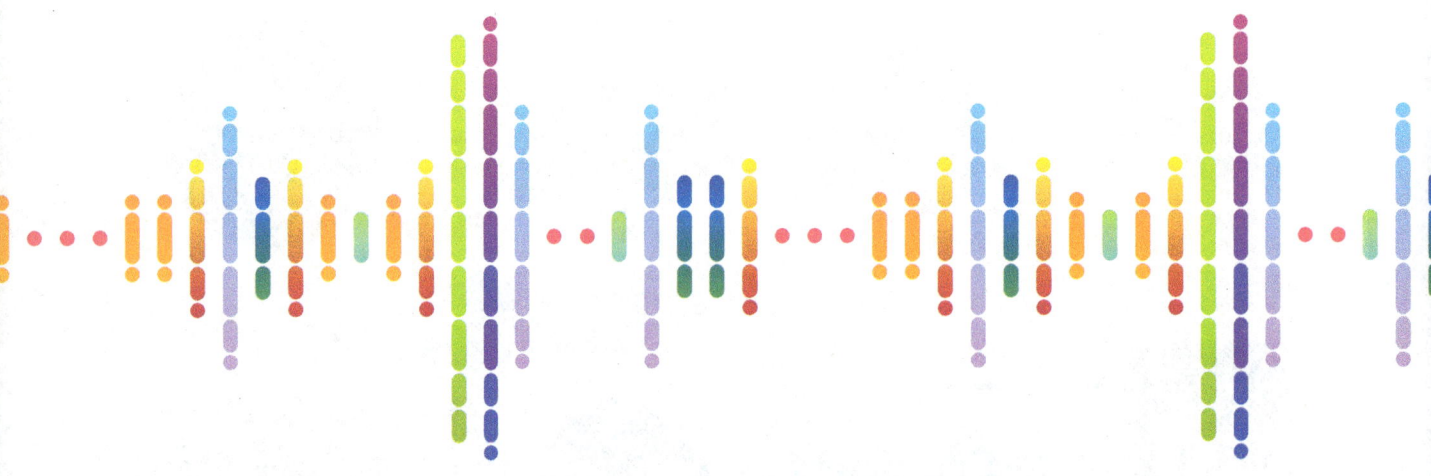

OBJECTIVES

- Define evidence and its role in EBP projects

- Define and describe the three types of evidence in the Johns Hopkins Evidence-Based Practice (JHEBP) model

- Describe quantitative, qualitative, and mixed-methods approaches to generate evidence

6

EVIDENCE PHASE: INTRODUCTION TO EVIDENCE

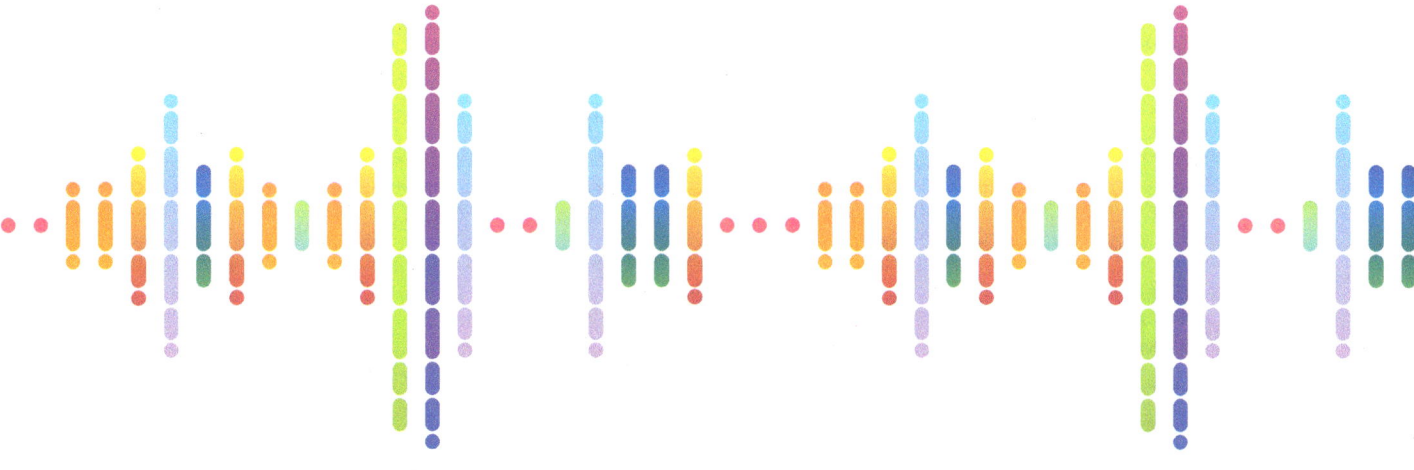

KEY POINTS

The evidence phase contains seven steps. This chapter gives an overview of the evidence that will be gathered and appraised in Steps 4, 5, and 6 (see Box 6.1).

Information in this chapter will assist the EBP evidence team in completing the JHEBP Searching and Screening Tool (Appendix C) and the Pre-appraised Evidence Appraisal Tool, Single Study Evidence Appraisal Tool, and Anecdotal Evidence Appraisal Tool (Appendices E1, E2, and E3, respectively).

- The JHEBP model has updated its approach to evidence appraisal.

- Pre-appraised evidence—such as clinical practice guidelines (CPGs), literature reviews with a systematic approach (LRSAs), and evidence summaries—can provide independent support for decision-making if they are suitable to the EBP question and of sufficient quality.

- There are various types of LRSAs, but all must meet specific criteria to be considered "systematic."

- Single studies with formal study designs can provide strong or moderate support for decision-making if they are of sufficient quality.

- Studies may follow qualitative, quantitative, or mixed-methods approaches.

- Anecdotal evidence—such as expert opinions, book chapters, position statements, case reports, programmatic experiences, and literature reviews without a systematic approach—provides limited support for decision-making.

> **BOX 6.1   STEPS IN THE EVIDENCE PHASE: THE E IN THE PET PROCESS**
>
> 4. Conduct best-evidence search and appraisal
> 5. Conduct targeted evidence search or conduct exhaustive search and screening
> 6. Appraise the evidence
> 7. Summarize the evidence
> 8. Organize the data
> 9. Synthesize the findings
> 10. Record best-evidence recommendations

> **NOTE**
>
> Terms that are bolded have associated definitions in the Evidence Terminology and Considerations Guide (Appendix F).

INTRODUCTION

Finding and evaluating evidence, the cornerstone of evidence-based healthcare, is the second phase of the JHEBP PET process. The team uses the EBP question generated in the previous phase to guide their collection and selection of evidence. This chapter describes what types of evidence the team may find during their exploration of the literature. This will lay the foundation for the next steps in the EBP process that include searching for evidence, screening the results, and appraising the applicable literature. Understanding these various types of evidence is crucial, as each contributes uniquely to the overall picture of best practices. For instance, qualitative studies offer insights into patient experiences and perspectives, while quantitative studies provide measurable data on treatment outcomes. Systematic reviews synthesize existing studies to present comprehensive conclusions, and clinical guidelines offer evidence-based recommendations for practice.

EVIDENCE DEFINED

The term *evidence* does not have a single definition, but in health sciences, it generally refers to information, findings, facts, knowledge, or data that are systematically obtained (Yu et al., 2024). *Evidence-based medicine* refers to clinically relevant research, but other approaches to evidence-based healthcare employ a wider definition and consider holistic sources beyond empirical research (Mackey & Bassendowski, 2017; Sackett et al., 1996; Yu et al., 2024).

> **NOTE**
>
> **ORIGINS OF EVIDENCE-BASED HEALTHCARE**
>
> Evidence-based healthcare began in the mid-1800s. What we now think of as evidence-based medicine got traction in the 1970s and was cemented in the 1990s, in large part due to the work of Dr. David Sackett. The term also became ubiquitous in the nursing profession and healthcare disciplines outside of medicine as they began developing their own approaches to identify clinical problems and evaluate evidence to find solutions (Mackey & Bassendowski, 2017).

Evidence is the information the team systematically gathers during their literature search and evaluates to determine how to address their EBP problem. Evidence comes in a variety of forms that dictate how the team can use it to inform their practice question. In the Johns Hopkins model, these are grouped into three types: pre-appraised, single studies, and anecdotal.

UPDATES IN EVIDENCE APPRAISAL IN THE 5TH EDITION OF THE JHEBP MODEL

In the past, the Johns Hopkins EBP model sorted evidence into a five-level hierarchy. While evidence hierarchies can be a helpful visual tool, there is no gold standard of how evidence should be ranked (Vere & Gibson, 2021). These rankings are ultimately subjective and may not be well-suited to the nuances of best-practice questions (Edmonds et al., 2024; Hammersley, 2013). For example, the implementation of a new nursing practice in the neonatal intensive care unit likely will not be well-informed by a **randomized control trial** but rather a pragmatic implementation study, which traditionally would be considered a "lower" level of evidence. The "value" of evidence or types of knowledge are not fixed but rather contextual.

In this edition of the JHEBP model, there are three types of evidence—pre-appraised, single studies, and anecdotal—that can provide independent, strong, moderate, or limited support for decision-making. The support for decision-making is based on the type of evidence and the details of the approach (design) the authors used to generate their findings and conclusions. This update acknowledges the subjective variations in evidence ranking of traditional hierarchies and increases efficiency for frontline clinicians by minimizing unnecessary decision-making during the appraisal process. These revisions are in line with a general movement in evidence-based healthcare and guidance from the Agency for Healthcare Research and Quality (2023) to question the use of a static hierarchy as the judge of "best" information (Booth et al., 2022; Clark et al., 2018; Edmonds et al., 2024; Hammersley, 2013, 2020; Murad et al., 2016; Parkhurst & Abeysinghe, 2016; Vere & Gibson, 2021).

TYPES OF EVIDENCE

Pre-appraised Evidence (Independent Support for Decision-Making)

Pre-appraised evidence, also referred to as *filtered* or *secondary* literature, describes a group of individual studies that have undergone a methodical process for collection and critical evaluation (filtering) by teams of investigators and content experts for quality and clinical utility (Polit & Beck, 2021). This type of evidence allows clinicians to rely on content and research methods experts to process literature and generate recommendations that serve as independent support for decision-making in healthcare. Identifying and applying pre-appraised evidence has been proposed as the 4S, 5S, and now 6S model. This is a hierarchical system that directs clinicians to seek the most integrated and rigorous available information and move sequentially down the list depending on the available information (DiCenso et al., 2009; Haynes, 2001, 2006). At the top of the pyramid is systems (e.g., computerized decision support systems), followed by summaries (e.g., evidence-based **CPGs**), synopses of syntheses (e.g., summaries of systematic reviews), syntheses (e.g., systematic reviews), synopses of studies (e.g., brief summaries of single studies), and individual single studies (DiCenso et al., 2009; Polit & Beck, 2021).

Examples of pre-appraised evidence include **CPGs** from professional organizations, **LRSAs,** and **evidence summaries** (DiCenso et al., 2009). In general, CPGs and LRSAs rely on more robust and exhaustive methodologies than evidence summaries. They may provide a more comprehensive synthesis of the literature and should be prioritized over evidence summaries. More information on the approach the team should use to identify the most compelling evidence is discussed in Chapter 7.

Clinical Practice Guidelines *CPGs* are reports that generate recommendations on a specific healthcare topic. They are based on a rigorous collection and appraisal of evidence by a group of experts. CPGs are systematic in their collection of evidence as well as their process for achieving consensus among contributors (DiCenso et al., 2009; Shekelle, 2022). Examples include the American Heart Association's 2023 Guidelines Update for Cardiopulmonary Resuscitation and Emergency Cardiovascular Care (Perman et al., 2024) or the 2021 Society of Critical Care Medicine and the European Society of Intensive Care Medicine's International Guidelines for Management of Sepsis and Septic Shock (Evans et al., 2021). See Chapter 7 for more information on accessing individual reports. Readers should note that **CPGs** are different from consensus statements. While both are frequently produced by a group of experts, consensus statements do not collect and critique the evidence with the same degree of rigor and do not provide independent support for decision-making. Common sources of **CPGs** include:

- Governmental organizations
  - National Institute for Health and Care Excellence (NICE)
  - US Preventive Services Task Force (USPSTF)
  - Agency for Healthcare Research and Quality (AHRQ)
  - World Health Organization (WHO)
- Regulatory bodies
  - The Joint Commission
  - US Government Centers for Medicare & Medicaid Services
- Professional organizations
  - American Heart Association
  - American Academy of Pediatrics
  - International Council of Cardiovascular Prevention and Rehabilitation
- Nonprofit healthcare organizations
  - Cochrane Library
  - Campbell Collaboration

Literature Reviews with a Systematic Approach *LRSAs* use explicit methods to search scientific evidence, assess and analyze the information, extract data, and summarize the included studies. To minimize bias, a group of experts, rather than individuals, apply these standards to the review process. A key requirement of systematically generated reviews is the transparency of methods to ensure that rationale, assumptions, and processes are open to scrutiny and can be replicated or updated. These reviews do not create new knowledge but rather provide a concise and relatively unbiased report of research evidence for a topic of interest (Aromataris et al., 2024). As of 2019, there were 48 types of reviews (Peters et al., 2020). See Table 6.1 for a more detailed description of literature reviews that meet the criteria for an **LRSA**.

TABLE 6.1 Reviews With a Systematic Approach

TYPE OF REVIEW	DESCRIPTION	TYPE OF SEARCH	GOALS	EXAMPLE
Systematic review	Systematically searches for, appraises, and synthesizes research evidence	Exhaustive	Identify what is known, gaps and recommendations for practice and future research	"Strategies to Mitigate Pain and Anxiety in Intrauterine Device Insertion: A Systematic Review" (Nguyen et al., 2020)
Systematic review with meta-analysis	Systematic reviews of quantitative research that statistically combine the results of multiple studies to create new summary statistics, often displayed in a forest plot	Exhaustive, limited to quantitative research	Identify the true relationship between variables through pooling of smaller data sets	"Is Family Caregiving Associated with Inflammation or Compromised Immunity? A Meta-Analysis" (Roth et al., 2019)
Systematic review with meta-synthesis	Systematic reviews of qualitative research that integrate findings from multiple studies to produce a high-level narrative and generate deeper understanding	Exhaustive, limited to qualitative research	Generate new theories, develop conceptual models, identify gaps, add depth of understanding to existing knowledge	"The Nurse's Role in Palliative Care: A Qualitative Meta-Synthesis" (Sekse et al., 2018)
Integrative review	Broadly gathers and evaluates information from a wide variety of sources, including empirical (based on facts or observations) and theoretical (based on concepts) sources	Exhaustive, includes both research and non-research materials	Provide the state of the evidence on a topic, contribute to theory development, and inform best practices	"Best Practices for Promoting Safe Patient Care Delivery by Hospital-Based Traveling Clinical Staff: An Integrative Review" (Krzyzewski et al., 2024)

continues

TABLE 6.1 Reviews With a Systematic Approach (cont.)

TYPE OF REVIEW	DESCRIPTION	TYPE OF SEARCH	GOALS	EXAMPLE
Rapid review	Accelerated traditional systematic review through simplifications or methodological shortcuts; assesses what is known about a policy or practice issue to provide timely recommendations	Systematic, may be exhaustive if time allows	Summarize evidence to allow for rapid clinical or policy-related decisions	"Coronavirus in Pregnancy and Delivery: Rapid Review" (Mullins et al., 2020)
Umbrella review	Compiles and summarizes results from multiple systematic reviews (a systematic review of systematic reviews)	Exhaustive, limited to systematic reviews	Present an overview of evidence on a broad topic (e.g., medical conditions or risk factors) to allow for comparison and recommendations for practice and research	"Risk Factors for Postpartum Depression: An Umbrella Review" (Hutchens & Kearney, 2020)

(Belbasis et al., 2022; Booth et al., 2022; Grant & Booth, 2009; Mohammed et al., 2016; Polit & Beck, 2021; Smela et al., 2023; Whittemore & Knafl, 2005)

What Is a Literature Review With a Systematic Approach (LRSA)?

Systematic review refers to a specific type of literature review, but there are many other types of literature reviews that use a systematic approach and are rigorous and replicable. To be considered an **LRSA,** a review should include (Booth et al., 2022):

- A preplanned method or protocol that is explicitly provided
- A clear question the authors are attempting to answer
- Clear and explicit inclusion and exclusion criteria (which studies will be included and which will be excluded)
- A documented **search strategy,** including sources and terms
- Use of tables to provide pertinent characteristics of the studies included
- An explicit approach to assess the quality (risk of bias) of included evidence
- Exploration of the data to identify consistencies as well as gaps
- Use of tables or figures to support interpretation of data
- Appendices or supplemental files to provide further details regarding methods, such as the specific search strategy or quality assessment tools

Keep in mind that it is not the title of a review that determines if it was done systematically but the methods used to execute the investigation and how well they were reported. The EBP team should evaluate the methods of each literature review to determine if it used a systematic approach.

Evidence Summaries *Evidence summaries* are a type of pre-appraised or synthesized evidence written by organizations for researchers, healthcare professionals, and policymakers to make decisions on time-sensitive topics. **Evidence summaries** are often intended to support point-of-care decision-making by presenting information in a succinct and actionable way for a broad audience (Jordan et al., 2019; Petkovic et al., 2016). Because, in many cases, the goal is to provide timely information, they tend not to be based on an exhaustive search of the literature but rather a targeted search looking for the highest levels of evidence (Jordan et al., 2019). While this is less rigorous than a systematic review, organizations known for producing this type of evidence follow predetermined methods to ensure the best information drives recommendations and the reports undergo peer review (Munn et al., 2015). **Evidence summaries** may also include contextual information related to a particular decision being informed by the summary. For instance, SUPPORT summaries were developed for policymakers in low- and middle-income countries to support decision-making for maternal and child health programs (http://supportsummaries.org/). Other well-known organizations that produce evidence summaries are JBI (the Joanna Briggs Institute), UpToDate, and BMJ Best Practice.

Many clinicians have access to online healthcare resources for clinical decision support and point-of-care resources. While some of these platforms follow a rigorous process for producing summaries, the approach is not always transparent, and the underlying evidence can vary widely by topic. The EBP team should investigate the underlying methods to determine if these entries meet the requirements of a pre-appraised **evidence summary**. If they do not, the EBP team may want to go to the source material for a specific recommendation to evaluate how it was generated and the level of support for decision-making it was based on.

Single Studies With a Formal Study Design (Strong and Moderate Support for Decision-Making)

Single studies with a formal study design use systematic inquiry to answer questions or solve problems (Polit & Beck, 2021). Reports are written by an author or team of authors and recount their scientific or clinical experience. This evidence comes in many forms that can be categorized by both the methodologic approach (quantitative, qualitative, or mixed-methods) and the design. The EBP team's ability to use evidence to make changes is determined by the design. See Chapter 8 for details on determining support for decision-making.

> **NOTE**
>
> **RESEARCH OR QUALITY IMPROVEMENT (QI)?**
>
> Evidence can also be grouped by intent (research vs. QI). Research's goal is to generate new, generalizable knowledge, while QI aims to improve local systems and processes. In previous editions, QI was treated differently than research. In this edition, evidence is categorized by the design, not the intent. This means that QI projects that have a formal design should be evaluated the same as traditional research. See Chapter 2 for further details on the differences between QI, research, and EBP.

Evidence that has a formal study design generates scientific data in two forms: *quantitative* data, or data from numbers, and *qualitative* data, or data from words.

Quantitative and **qualitative** methods are foundational approaches in the field of scientific investigation, each with distinct approaches, tools, and outcomes. Sometimes study teams combine qualitative and quantitative methods within a single study to benefit from the strengths of both. This approach, known as mixed-methods, allows for comprehensive analysis that addresses complex questions by exploring different dimensions of the problem. See Table 6.2 for an overview of the features and characteristics of quantitative, qualitative, and mixed-methods approaches.

Quantitative methods involve the collection and analysis of number-based data to quantify a problem by generating numerical information or data that can be transformed into usable statistics (Polit & Beck, 2021).

Qualitative designs collect and analyze narrative data to gain an in-depth understanding of a social phenomenon or experience, including opinions, meanings, and motivations. They provide insights into the problem or help to develop ideas or hypotheses for potential quantitative research (Polit & Beck, 2021).

Mixed methods combine the approach and strengths of both qualitative and quantitative approaches for a broader and more comprehensive understanding of complex topics. They may explain if an intervention works and why. **Data collection** and analysis can occur concurrently (at the same time) or sequentially (one followed by the other; Creswell & Plano, 2011; Guetterman et al., 2015). Of note, to be truly considered mixed methods, the team must employ the data collection and analysis methods of both types of studies. Simply asking a numerical question (such as demographic information) in a qualitative study or an open-ended question (such as allowing for a free text response) in a quantitative study does not necessarily constitute a mixed-methods approach.

TABLE 6.2 Overview of the Features and Characteristics of Quantitative, Qualitative, and Mixed-Methods Approaches

	QUANTITATIVE	QUALITATIVE	MIXED-METHODS
Unit of analysis	Numbers and statistics	Text, words, or narratives	Combination of numbers and narratives
Focus	Who, what, and when	Why and how	Who, what, when, why, or how
Scope	Concise and focused	Complex and broad	Complex and focused
Goal	Establish patterns and relationships among variables to describe, predict, test hypotheses, classify features, and construct models	Thoroughly describe a phenomenon or topic of interest	Explore various facets of complex topics for a more nuanced understanding of the phenomenon
Data collection	Structured methods such as surveys, questionnaires, or experiments where the data can be numerically assessed	Unstructured or semi-structured techniques such as interviews, observations, or focus groups	Integration of both qualitative and quantitative methods in a single study or series of studies
Examples of metrics	Biometric data, responses to multiple-choice questions, Likert scales, time markers, or morbidity and mortality rates	Thoughts, experiences, attitudes, interpretations, or opinions	Numerical rankings followed by open-ended interviews, experiences, or thoughts related to an intervention and related biometric data

Data analysis	Statistical, mathematical, or computational techniques	Thematic analysis, content analysis, or narrative analysis to interpret a phenomenon and bring meaning	Analytic techniques of both qualitative and quantitative methods with an integration of findings
Sample sizes	Larger sample sizes, driven by "power" or other measures related to determining statistical significance	Smaller sample sizes, driven by "saturation"	Varies by how data is gathered and how quantitative and qualitative data inform one another
Results	Reported in terms of statistical significance	Reported in the form of quotes or narratives	Ideally reported as a joint display of quantitative and qualitative information
Generalizability	Statistical generalization (representativeness)	Analytic generalization (conceptual power)	Based on sampling
Example	"A Scoring Tool That Identifies the Need for Positive-Pressure Ventilation and Determines the Effectiveness of Allocated Respiratory Therapy" (Vines et al., 2022)	"In-Hospital Education of Parents of Newborns May Benefit From Competency-Based Education: A Qualitative Focus Group and Interview Study Among Health Professionals" (Stelwagen et al., 2023)	"Confronting Systemic Racism in Occupational Therapy: A Mixed Methods Study" (Murphy et al., 2024)

(Creswell & Plano, 2011; Guetterman et al., 2015; Onwuegbuzie & Collins, 2007; Polit & Beck, 2021)

Anecdotal Evidence (Limited Support for Decision-Making)

Anecdotal evidence is published information that was not generated from a research study but rather from personal, professional, or clinical experience. It may or may not be peer-reviewed. Common sub-types of anecdotal evidence include:

- **Expert opinion:** This type of evidence consists of insights or conclusions based on the professional or personal experiences of an individual recognized as an authority in a topic or field. While expert opinions are valuable for their depth of experience and knowledge, they may be biased and lack empirical testing or peer validation. Example: "Artificial Intelligence in Nursing: From Speculation to Science" (Nilsen, 2024).

- **In-print and online book chapter:** Entries in a text or manual written by experts providing an overview of a topic, often reflecting the views and professional experience of the author. While they may reference other literature, these entries are primarily treated as expert opinions. For example, Chapter 1: "Introduction to Nursing Research in an Evidence-Based Practice Environment" in *Nursing Research: Generating and Assessing Evidence for Nursing Practice* (11th ed.; Polit & Beck, 2021).

- **Position statement:** Issued by organizations or expert groups, position statements reflect a consensus or official stance on issues. While they are based on evidence and expert consensus, they do not usually provide detailed methodologies for how the evidence was reviewed and are not peer-reviewed in the traditional sense. Example: "Emergency Nurses Association Firearm Safety and Injury Prevention: Position Statement" (Peta et al., 2023).

- **Case report:** This evidence reflects a presentation of a single patient's medical history, symptoms, diagnosis, treatment, and follow-up. These tend to provide in-depth details about the clinical management of an individual, including unique or rare conditions, using a narrative structure. This description may include the patient's response to treatment, which can highlight new insights or unexpected outcomes. This is distinct from case study or case report research. Example: "Supporting the HIV+ Mother with Breastfeeding in the United States: A Case Report" (Rosenblum & Sturdivant, 2023).

- **Programmatic experience:** This literature describes a project or program implemented by a healthcare individual or team. Although it lacks the formal study design of a robust quality improvement project, it offers a narrative account of the successes and opportunities for improvement of the initiative. These reports typically detail experiences after the project is underway without a prior plan for implementation and evaluation. They often lack data, and the authors are usually the program leaders rather than independent researchers. Example: "Answering the Call: Impact of Tele-ICU Nurses During the COVID-19 Pandemic" (Arneson et al., 2020).

- **Literature reviews without a systematic approach:** As discussed in the pre-appraised literature section, there are dozens of approaches to summarize existing evidence. These reviews lack both a formal search technique and/or a system to evaluate the quality of the information. The reader is unable to track how the author(s) selected the literature they included and excluded. The reviews may provide some background information, but because they provide an incomplete picture of the state of the evidence on a topic, they need to be used with caution. See Table 6.3 for further details on types of non-systematic reviews.

TABLE 6.3 Reviews With an Unsystematic Approach

TYPE OF REVIEW	DESCRIPTION	TYPE OF SEARCH	GOALS	EXAMPLE
Scoping review	Exploratory effort to identify key concepts, types of evidence, and gaps in research related to specific topics that may be new, complex, or heterogeneous (diverse in character or content)	Varies, can be targeted or exhaustive	Identify and map available evidence, including working definitions and concepts, to gain a greater understanding of available knowledge and gaps	"Effects of Virtual Learning Environments: A Scoping Review of the Literature" (Caprara & Caprara, 2022)
Critical review	Evaluate and critique the limitations of existing research; often discuss assumptions, practices, and implications of existing studies to provide a deep understanding of the topic	Targeted, focused on the most significant literature in the field	Generate a hypothesis or model	"Gamifying Education: What Is Known, What Is Believed, and What Remains Uncertain: A Critical Review" (Dichev & Dicheva, 2017)
Literature review	Summarize existing information on a topic without a clear methodology	Varies, may range from exhaustive to author-driven selection of preferred evidence	Provide an overview of published information on a topic; may advocate for a specific stance or practice	"Music in Waiting Rooms: A Literature Review" (Lai & Amaladoss, 2022)

(Grant & Booth, 2009; Munn et al., 2018; Peters et al., 2020; Polit & Beck, 2021; Sataloff et al., 2021)

SUMMARY

This chapter provides a comprehensive introduction to the concept of evidence and the various types the EBP team may uncover during their literature search. It begins by defining evidence in the context of EBP and explores the details of various types of evidence.

The chapter also explains recent changes to the JHEBP model's approach to assessing evidence and contextualizes these updates within broader trends and advancements in evidence-based healthcare, emphasizing the model's alignment with contemporary standards and practices. This information serves as the basis for the next steps in the evidence phase: literature search and screening, and appraisal.

REFERENCES

Agency for Healthcare Research and Quality. (2023, Oct. 18). *Fact sheet: Rating the strength of scientific research findings*. AHRQ Publication No. 02-P022. https://archive.ahrq.gov/clinic/epcsums/strenfact.pdf

Arneson, S. L., Tucker, S. J., Mercier, M., & Singh, J. (2020). Answering the call: Impact of tele-ICU nurses during the COVID-19 pandemic. *Critical Care Nurse, 40*(4), 25–31.

Aromataris, E., Lockwood, C., Porritt, K., Pilla, B., & Jordan, Z. (Eds.). (2024). *JBI manual for evidence synthesis*. JBI. https://doi.org/10.46658/JBIMES-24-01

Belbasis, L., Bellou, V., & Ioannidis, J. P. A. (2022, Nov. 22). Conducting umbrella reviews. *BMJ Medicine, 1*(1). https://doi.org/10.1136/bmjmed-2021-000071

Booth, A., Sutton, A., Clowes, M., & Martyn-St James, M. (2022). *Systematic approaches to a successful literature review* (3rd ed.). Sage.

Caprara, L., & Caprara, C. (2022). Effects of virtual learning environments: A scoping review of literature. *Education and Information Technologies, 27*(3), 3683–3722.

Clark, E., Draper, J., & Taylor, R. (2018). Healthcare education research: The case for rethinking hierarchies of evidence. *Journal of Advanced Nursing, 74*(11), 2480–2483.

Creswell, J. W., & Plano, V. L. (2011). *Designing and conducting mixed methods research* (2nd ed.). Sage.

DiCenso, A., Bayley, L., & Haynes, R. B. (2009). Accessing pre-appraised evidence: Fine-tuning the 5S model into a 6S model. *Evidence-Based Nursing, 12*(4), 99–101.

Dichev, C., & Dicheva, D. (2017). Gamifying education: What is known, what is believed and what remains uncertain: A critical review. *International Journal of Educational Technology in Higher Education, 14*, 1–36.

Edmonds, S., Cullen, L., & DeBerg, J. (2024). The problem with the pyramid for grading evidence: The evidence funnel solution. *Journal of PeriAnesthesia Nursing, 39*(3), 484–488.

Evans, L., Rhodes, A., Alhazzani, W., Antonelli, M., Coopersmith, C. M., French, C., & Levy, M. (2021). Surviving sepsis campaign: International guidelines for management of sepsis and septic shock. *Critical Care Medicine, 49*(11), e1063–e1143.

Grant, M. J., & Booth, A. (2009). A typology of reviews: An analysis of 14 review types and associated methodologies. *Health Information & Libraries Journal, 26*(2), 91–108.

Guetterman, T. C., Fetters, M. D., & Creswell, J. W. (2015). Integrating quantitative and qualitative results in health science mixed methods research through joint displays. *Annals of Family Medicine, 13*(6), 554–561. https://www.annfammed.org/content/13/6/554

Hammersley, M. (2013). *The myth of research-based policy and practice*. Sage. https://doi.org/10.4135/9781473957626

Haynes, R. B. (2001, May). Of studies, summaries, synopses, and systems: The "4S" evolution of services for finding current best evidence [Editorial]. *Evidence-Based Mental Health, 4*(2), 37–39. https://doi.org/10.1136/ebmh.4.2.37

Haynes, R. B. (2006, December). Of studies, syntheses, synopses, summaries, and systems: The "5S" evolution of information services for evidence-based healthcare decisions. *Evidence-Based Medicine, 11*(6), 162–164. https://doi.org/10.1136/ebm.11.6.162-a

Hutchens, B. F., & Kearney, J. (2020). Risk factors for postpartum depression: An umbrella review. *Journal of Midwifery & Women's Health, 65*(1), 96–108.

Jordan, Z., Lockwood, C., Munn, Z., & Aromataris, E. (2019). The updated Joanna Briggs Institute model of evidence-based healthcare. *JBI Evidence Implementation, 17*(1), 58–71.

Krzyzewski, J., Cook, M., Memken, A., Johnson, M., Francis, S. E., Romao, B., & Whalen, M. (2024). Best practices for promoting safe patient care delivery by hospital-based traveling clinical staff: An integrative review. *Journal of Nursing Care Quality, 39*(2), 144–150.

Lai, J. C. Y., & Amaladoss, N. (2022). Music in waiting rooms: A literature review. *HERD: Health Environments Research & Design Journal, 15*(2), 347–354.

Mackey, A., & Bassendowski, S. (2017). The history of evidence-based practice in nursing education and practice. *Journal of Professional Nursing, 33*(1), 51–55.

Mohammed, M. A., Moles, R. J., & Chen, T. F. (2016). Meta-synthesis of qualitative research: The challenges and opportunities. *International Journal of Clinical Pharmacy, 38*, 695–704.

Mullins, E., Evans, D., Viner, R. M., O'Brien, P., & Morris, E. (2020). Coronavirus in pregnancy and delivery: Rapid review. *Ultrasound in Obstetrics & Gynecology, 55*(5), 586–592.

Munn, Z., Lockwood, C., & Moola, S. (2015). The development and use of evidence summaries for point of care information systems: A streamlined rapid review approach. *Worldviews on Evidence-Based Nursing, 12*(3), 131–138.

Munn, Z., Peters, M. D., Stern, C., Tufanaru, C., McArthur, A., & Aromataris, E. (2018). Systematic review or scoping review? Guidance for authors when choosing between a systematic or scoping review approach. *BMC Medical Research Methodology, 18*, 1–7.

Murad, M. H., Asi, N., Alsawas, M., & Alahdab, F. (2016). New evidence pyramid. *BMJ Evidence-Based Medicine, 21*(4), 125–127.

Murphy, R., Park, K., Billock, C., Becerra-Culqui, T., Perkins, N. A., & Bains, R. (2024). Confronting systemic racism in occupational therapy: A mixed methods study. *Open Journal of Occupational Therapy, 12*(1), 1–16. https://doi.org/10.15453/2168-6408.2167

Nguyen, L., Lamarche, L., Lennox, R., Ramdyal, A., Patel, T., Black, M., & Mangin, D. (2020). Strategies to mitigate anxiety and pain in intrauterine device insertion: A systematic review. *Journal of Obstetrics and Gynaecology Canada, 42*(9), 1138–1146.

Nilsen, P. (2024, February). Artificial intelligence in nursing: From speculation to science. *Worldviews on Evidence-Based Nursing, 21*(1), 4–5. https://doi.org/10.1111/wvn.12706

Onwuegbuzie, A. J., & Collins, K. M. (2007). A typology of mixed methods sampling designs in social science research. *Qualitative Report, 12*(2), 281–316.

Parkhurst, J. O., & Abeysinghe, S. (2016). What constitutes "good" evidence for public health and social policymaking? From hierarchies to appropriateness. *Social Epistemology, 30*(5–6), 665–679.

Perman, S. M., Elmer, J., Maciel, C. B., Uzendu, A., May, T., Mumma, B. E., & American Heart Association. (2024). 2023 American Heart Association focused update on adult advanced cardiovascular life support: An update to the American Heart Association guidelines for cardiopulmonary resuscitation and emergency cardiovascular care. *Circulation, 149*(5), e254–e273.

Peta, D., Vanairsdale, S., & Stone, E. (2023). *Firearm safety and injury prevention* [Position statement]. Emergency Nurses Association. https://enau.ena.org/URL/FirearmSafetyandInjuryPreventionPositionStatement

Peters, M. D., Marnie, C., Tricco, A. C., Pollock, D., Munn, Z., Alexander, L., McInerney, P., Godfrey, C. M., & Khalil, H. (2020). Updated methodological guidance for the conduct of scoping reviews. *JBI Evidence Synthesis, 18*(10), 2119–2126.

Petkovic, J., Welch, V., Jacob, M. H., Yoganathan, M., Ayala, A. P., Cunningham, H., & Tugwell, P. (2016). The effectiveness of evidence summaries on health policymakers and health system managers use of evidence from systematic reviews: A systematic review. *Implementation Science, 11*, 1–14.

Polit, D., & Beck, C. (2021). *Nursing research: Generating and assessing evidence for nursing practice* (11th ed.). Wolters Kluwer.

Rosenblum, N., & Sturdivant, H. (2023). Supporting the HIV+ mother with breastfeeding in the United States: A case report. *Clinical Lactation, 3*, 141–147. https://doi.org/10.1891/cl-2023-0003

Roth, D. L., Sheehan, O. C., Haley, W. E., Jenny, N. S., Cushman, M., & Walston, J. D. (2019). Is family caregiving associated with inflammation or compromised immunity? A meta-analysis. *The Gerontologist, 59*(5), e521–e534.

Sackett, D. L., Rosenberg, W. M., Gray, J. M., Haynes, R. B., & Richardson, W. S. (1996). Evidence-based medicine: What it is and what it isn't. *BMJ, 312*(7023), 71–72.

Sataloff, R. T., Bush, M. L., Chandra, R., Chepeha, D., Rotenberg, B., Fisher, E. W., Goldenberg, D., Hanna, E. Y., Kerschner, J. E., Kraus, D. H., Krouse, J. H., Li, D., Link, M., Lustig, L. R., Selesnick, S. H., Sindwani, R., Smith, R. J., Tysome, J., Weber, P. C., & Welling, D. B. (2021, July 1). Systematic and other reviews: Criteria and complexities [Editorial]. *World Journal of Otorhinolaryngology—Head & Neck Surgery, 7*(3), 236–239. https://doi.org/10.1016/j.wjorl.2021.04.007

Sekse, R. J. T., Hunskår, I., & Ellingsen, S. (2018). The nurse's role in palliative care: A qualitative meta-synthesis. *Journal of Clinical Nursing, 27*(1–2), e21–e38.

Shekelle, P. (2022). *Overview of clinical practice guidelines.* UpToDate. Wolters Kluwer. https://dsp.facmed.unam.mx/wp-content/uploads/2022/07/Lectura-complementaria.-Shekelle-P.-Overview-of-clinical-practice-guidelines.-abril-2022.pdf

Smela, B., Toumi, M., Świerk, K., Francois, C., Biernikiewicz, M., Clay, E., & Boyer, L. (2023). Rapid literature review: Definition and methodology. *Journal of Market Access & Health Policy, 11*(1), 2241234.

Stelwagen, M., Westmaas, A., Van Kempen, A., & Scheele, F. (2023). In-hospital education of parents of newborns may benefit from competency-based education: A qualitative focus group and interview study among health professionals. *Journal of Clinical Nursing, 32*(7/8), 1076–1088. https://doi.org/10.1111/jocn.16334

Vere, J., & Gibson, B. (2021). Variation amongst hierarchies of evidence. *Journal of Evaluation in Clinical Practice, 27*(3), 624–630.

Vines, D. L., Tangney, C., Meksraityte, E., Scott, J. B., Fogg, L., Burd, J., Yoder, M. A., & Gurka, D. P. (2022). A scoring tool that identifies the need for positive-pressure ventilation and determines the effectiveness of allocated respiratory therapy. *Respiratory Care, 67*(2), 167–176. https://doi.org/10.4187/respcare.08555

Whittemore, R., & Knafl, K. (2005). The integrative review: Updated methodology. *Journal of Advanced Nursing, 52*(5), 546–553.

Yu, X., Wu, S., Sun, Y., Wang, P., Wang, L., Su, R., & Chen, Y. (2024). Exploring the diverse definitions of 'evidence': A scoping review. *BMJ Evidence-Based Medicine, 29*(1), 37–43.

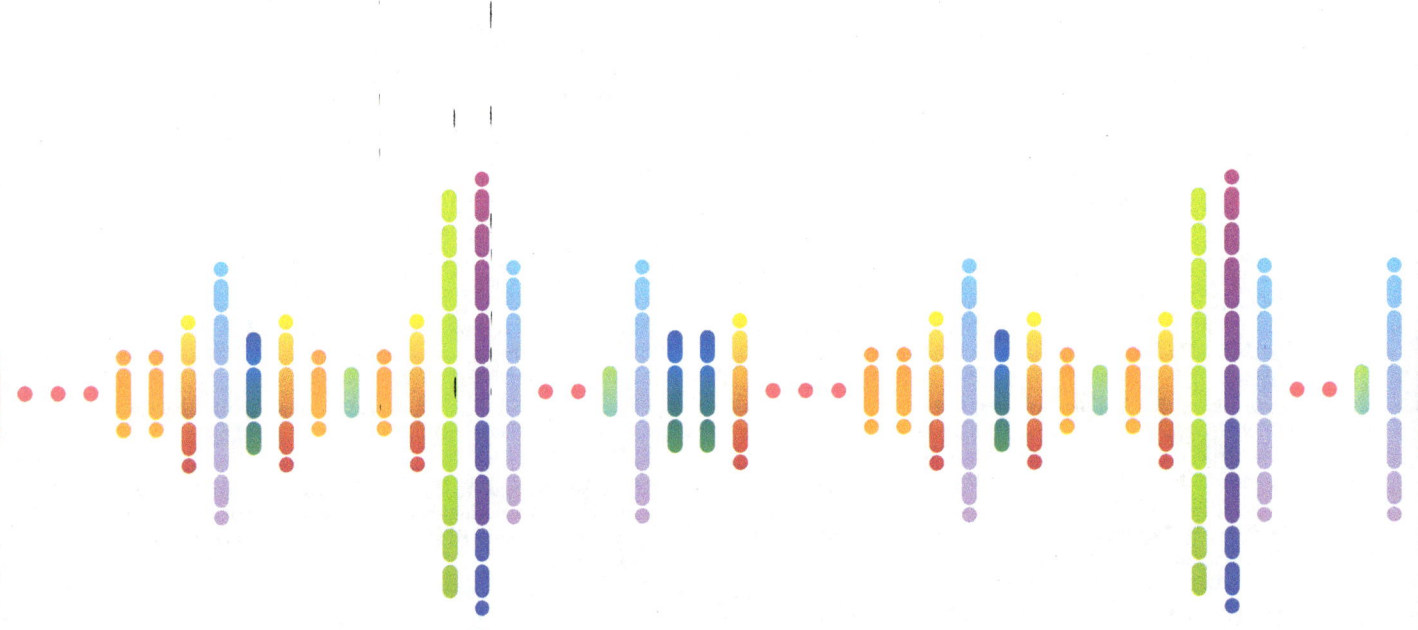

OBJECTIVES

- Define types of literature searches and their context in an EBP project
- Describe the action items in a best-evidence literature search
- Describe the action items in an exhaustive literature search, including building key concepts
- Identify common databases for best-evidence and exhaustive literature searches on healthcare topics
- Identify tools to conduct a literature search, such as controlled vocabulary, Boolean operators, truncation, exact phrasing, and title/abstract limiters
- Define literature screening and its context within an EBP project
- Describe the process and considerations for conducting a high-quality literature screening
- Review special considerations for minimizing bias in literature searching and screening

7

EVIDENCE PHASE: THE EVIDENCE SEARCH AND SCREENING

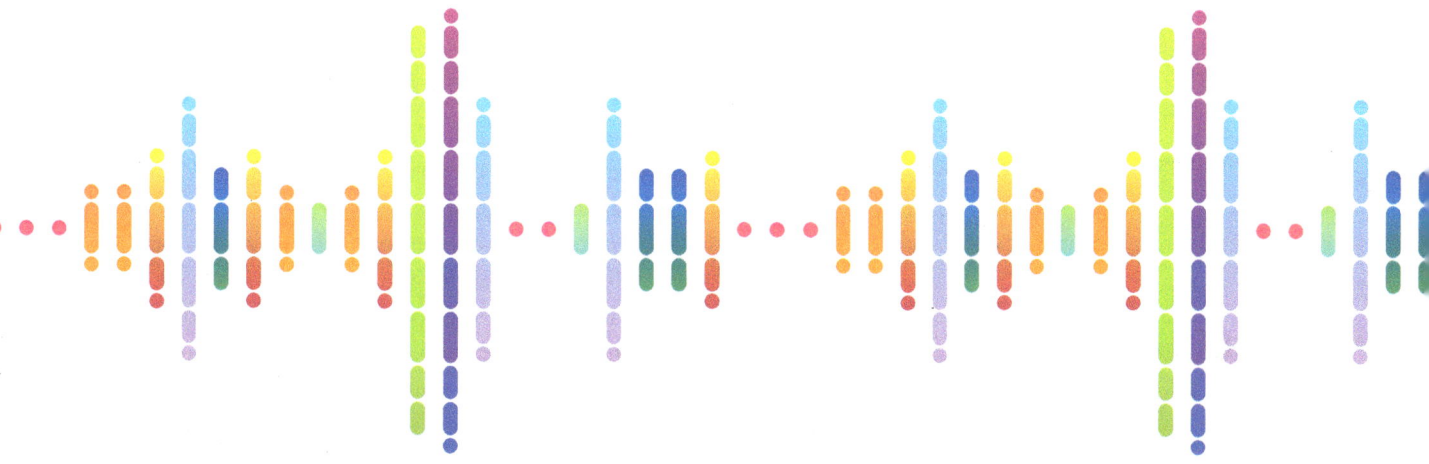

KEY POINTS

The evidence phase contains seven steps. This chapter covers the first two (see Box 7.1). The Johns Hopkins Evidence-Based Practice (JHEBP) Searching and Screening Tool (Appendix C) facilitates these steps.

- There are various types of literature searches an EBP team can conduct, yet all should follow a systematic process to promote efficiency and minimize bias.
- Best-evidence literature searches concentrate on gathering foundational information and pre-appraised evidence. Various databases specialize in providing this type of evidence.
- Exhaustive evidence literature searches attempt to gather all literature on a topic within predetermined parameters. EBP teams design search strategies to conduct these searches.
- The EBP question guides the literature search. EBP teams will need to isolate the elements of their EBP question to create search concepts and build search strings.
- Additional tools to create search strings include truncation, Boolean operators, controlled vocabulary, exact phrasing, and title/abstract limiters.
- Literature screening is a systematic process to winnow down the results of an exhaustive search in an unbiased manner to only those that answer the EBP question and meet inclusion/exclusion criteria.
- Documenting the search and screening process is an important element to establish rigor and replicability.
- Various forms of bias can influence the trustworthiness of the results of a team's literature search. Bias should be recognized and minimized.

> **BOX 7.1** STEPS IN THE EVIDENCE PHASE: THE E IN THE PET PROCESS
>
> 4. **Conduct best-evidence search and appraisal**
> 5. **Conduct targeted evidence search or conduct exhaustive search and screening**
> 6. Appraise the evidence
> 7. Summarize the evidence
> 8. Organize the data
> 9. Synthesize the findings
> 10. Record best-practice recommendations

INTRODUCTION

Conducting a search for evidence is the first step of the "E" phase of the PET process. While there are innumerable sources of healthcare information, the evidence-based practice (EBP) team's ability to efficiently and systematically identify relevant and representative evidence will dictate the success of all future steps of the project. Teams will need to have knowledge of both the subject matter as well as information literacy, which refers to an individual's ability to "recognize when information is needed and have the ability to locate, evaluate, and use effectively the needed information" (American Library Association, 1989, para. 3). Not only will this make the team more successful in their EBP efforts, but increased information literacy skills can also increase appreciation and application of research (McCulley & Jones, 2014).

Healthcare providers have unprecedented access to information. While this means there are more resources than ever to deliver high-quality care, it also means there is more data to collect, assess, and eventually apply. Fortunately, clinical resources and databases are also evolving, giving teams more tools to identify information more easily and efficiently.

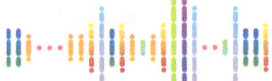

"Knowledge is of two kinds. We know a subject ourselves, or we know where we can find information on it."
–Samuel Johnson

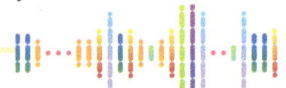

SEARCHING THE LITERATURE

A *literature search* is a systematic and structured approach to query databases to identify information of interest to the EBP team. Various types of literature searches can fulfill a variety of needs. Regardless of the approach, all searches should be iterative and follow a systematic process to promote efficiency, minimize bias, and ensure the evidence retrieved truly reflects the state of the literature on a subject (Booth et al., 2021). Types of evidence searches and their characteristics are displayed in Table 7.1. All literature searches are focused on the EBP question. The EBP team will use their EBP question (see Chapter 4) to identify key concepts that will drive the search (see Appendices B and C).

Before conducting an exhaustive literature review, the EBP team should first seek information that has already been assessed and synthesized by reputable sources (pre-appraised evidence). This may save the team many hours of work and take advantage of the expertise of professional organizations who are well-equipped to generate guidance based on high-quality and rigorous investigations of literature.

Best-evidence searches leverage the work of other experts in gathering and assessing the literature. This means that, while systematic reviews are the gold standard for generating recommendations for practice change, the EBP team does not necessarily need to conduct their own. By conducting a focused

TABLE 7.1 Types of Literature Searches and Their Characteristics

TYPE OF SEARCH	DEFINITION	EXAMPLES OF REVIEWS THAT USE THIS TYPE OF SEARCH	BEST USE
Best-evidence	Focused process to identify key foundational articles and existing syntheses (pre-appraised evidence), but not all articles on a topic	Evidence scan, evidence summary, rapid*	Time-sensitive decision-making, guiding internal decisions, informing larger research projects
Exhaustive	Gold standard: systematically identifies all relevant literature with structured, comprehensive, and reproducible methods	Systematic, integrative, rapid*	Informing clinical questions or practice

*There is no universal definition or protocol for completing a rapid review. The team may use a best-evidence or exhaustive search depending on the goals of the project, the timeline, and available resources (Booth et al., 2021; Henrikson & Blasi, 2023).

search and identifying pre-appraised evidence that addresses all components of the EBP question, the team may be able to simply look for any relevant updates and begin translation to their practice setting. If there is no high-quality, recent, and relevant pre-appraised evidence, the EBP team undertakes a full literature search.

Best-Evidence Search

Action Item 1: Identify the Elements of the EBP Question to Search While best-evidence searches are less structured than exhaustive searches, the EBP team must still determine the elements of the EBP question that need to be searched to ensure the results address the EBP problem as thoroughly as possible. The team does this by reviewing the EBP question they created in Step 3 (see Chapter 4) and isolating the population, setting, topic or intervention, and in some cases an outcome. See the Question Development Tool (Appendix B) for further guidance.

Action Item 2: Identify Resources for Pre-appraised Evidence As discussed in the previous chapter, some well-known groups generate high-quality literature syntheses. These sources of pre-appraised evidence (sometimes referred to as "filtered" or "secondary literature") include the Cochrane Library, JBI, National Institute for Health and Care Excellence (NICE), US Preventive Services Taskforce (USPSTF), Agency for Healthcare Research and Quality (AHRQ), and World Health Organization (WHO), as well as professional organizations such as the American Academy of Pediatrics, the American Heart Association, and the International Council of Cardiovascular Prevention and Rehabilitation. The EBP team can access each of these databases by visiting their individual websites. Additionally, websites such as the ECRI (Emergency Care Research Institute) Guidelines Trust, Guideline Central, and others serve as repositories for hundreds of vetted clinical practice guidelines from dozens of global organizations. Each database includes a search function similar to an internet search engine and options to explore publications by topic or type. While these are reputable sources, the EBP team should always evaluate their results using the Pre-appraised Evidence Appraisal Tool (Appendix E1, reviewed in the next chapter) to ensure it is independently actionable. See Table 7.2 for more information on resources to identify pre-appraised evidence during a best-evidence search.

TABLE 7.2 Resources for Pre-appraised Evidence

SOURCE	FOCUS	SUBSCRIPTION REQUIREMENTS (LINK)
ORIGINAL SOURCES OF PRE-APPRAISED EVIDENCE		
Cochrane Library	Systematic reviews and control trials	Reviews are freely available 12 months after publication (https://www.cochranelibrary.com)
JBI (Joanna Briggs Institute)	Evidence summaries and other actionable sources of best practices for clinical implementation	Requires subscription (https://jbi.global/jbi-ebp-database)
National Institute for Health and Care Excellence (NICE)	Practice guidelines, quality standards and indicators to measure quality in healthcare from the United Kingdom	Freely available (https://www.nice.org.uk)
US Preventive Services Taskforce (USPSTF)	Evidence-based recommendations on clinical preventive services	Freely available (https://www.uspreventiveservicestaskforce.org/uspstf/)
AHRQ Evidence-based Practice Center (EPC) Reports	Evidence reports released by the AHRQ's EBP Center on common or priority medical conditions, healthcare technology, and strategies	https://www.ahrq.gov/research/findings/evidence-based-reports/index.html
World Health Organization (WHO) Guidelines	Recommendations for clinical practice or public health policy	Freely available (https://www.who.int/publications/who-guidelines)
REPOSITORIES OF CLINICAL PRACTICE GUIDELINES FROM PROFESSIONAL ORGANIZATIONS		
ECRI Guidelines Trust	Clinical practice guidelines	Repository freely available, individual guideline(s) may require subscription (https://guidelines.ecri.org/)
Guideline Central	Evidence-based clinical support tools including guidelines, calculators, drug libraries, and clinical trial registries	Repository freely available, individual guideline(s) may require subscription (https://www.guidelinecentral.com)

Physiotherapy Evidence Database (PEDro)*	Randomized control trials, systematic reviews, and CPGs to inform physiotherapy interventions	Repository freely available, texts may require subscription (https://pedro.org.au/)
Trip Database*	Clinical guidance using high-quality research evidence with leveling and bias indicators, including guidelines, regulatory guidance, clinical calculators, primary research, and textbooks	Repository freely available, texts may require subscription (https://www.tripdatabase.com)

*Also provides citations for single studies

In some cases, systematic reviews produced outside of formal organizations may also provide sufficient support for practice change. They can be accessed using the same action items as those outlined below for locating primary sources.

Action Item 3: Execute the Search Using the elements of the EBP question identified during Action Item 1, query relevant databases. The EBP team should focus on first identifying clinical practice guidelines (CPGs), then literature reviews with a systematic approach (LRSAs), followed by evidence summaries (adapted from DiCenso et al., 2009 6S model for pre-appraised evidence). This is an iterative process, and there is not a predetermined number of databases that need to be explored, but the EBP team should ensure they have identified work from the professional organizations and other resources specific to their practice area. This will rely on the professional experience of the group. For example, if the EBP team is asking a question related to infection control, they would want to ensure they have reviewed any recent guidance from the Society for Healthcare Epidemiology of America (SHEA). More novice teams may want to consider speaking with experienced colleagues if they are unsure of the relevant organizations. Visiting repositories, such as Trip Database, ECRI Guidelines Trust, or Guideline Central, can be a good strategy for identifying relevant publications from multiple organizations within one search.

Action Item 4: Evaluate the Search Results The EBP team should review the information they were able to gather in their best-evidence search to ensure it addresses all aspects of their EBP question and is of sufficient quality. If the EBP team finds multiple reports, they can decide as a group which to include. They may want to consider the best fit for the clinical problem and practice setting. They should also consider the possibility of overlapping evidence between the sources and determine if they truly represent unique information by looking at the reference lists. See Chapter 8 for more information on evaluating and appraising literature found during the searching stage.

> **NOTE**
> **HEALTH INFORMATIONIST/HEALTH SCIENCES LIBRARIANS**
>
> *Health informationists,* also known as *health science librarians,* can be an essential part of an EBP team. They are trained professionals who have special education in, and focus on, sources of high-quality health information. They work in hospitals, clinics, universities, research centers, and more (Medical Library Association, 2024). Their participation in literature searching has been shown to produce better quality search strategies, less risk of bias, and better reporting of the search methods used (Lefebvre, 2023). When possible, the EBP team should engage their librarian early and often.

Action Item 5: If Applicable, Conduct a Targeted Search If the team can locate a source of high-quality, pre-appraised evidence that addresses all aspects of their EBP question, they should then conduct a targeted literature search. This action item is intended to identify additional evidence that offers new and compelling information that has been published since the search date provided in the pre-appraised evidence. Teams should focus on evidence that provides strong or moderate support for decision-making. Evidence that provides limited support for decision-making does not need to be reviewed because it cannot be used to change practice alone. More information on conducting searches for primary sources is included below.

Exhaustive Search

After assessing the availability of high-quality pre-appraised evidence that answers the EBP question, the team may need to move on to conducting an exhaustive, systematic literature search. During this step, the EBP team will develop and implement a literature search strategy to identify relevant literature on their topic. A search strategy is a formal process used to retrieve evidence by identifying databases and creating search strings that include key concepts and synonyms with database-specific syntax (Booth et al., 2021; Bramer et al., 2018). A good search strategy identifies all pertinent articles while minimizing superfluous results. See Figure 7.1 for a visual representation of the sensitivity and precision considerations of a high-quality literature search.

Each action item to create and execute the search is described below.

> **EXAMPLE**
>
> **BROAD EBP SEARCH QUESTION**
> To further explore the action items for searching and screening the literature, we will be using the broad EBP question example, "Among hospitalized pediatric patients on invasive mechanical ventilation, what are best practices regarding the administration of nebulized medications?"

Action Item 1: Determine Which Databases to Search The first action item in an exhaustive literature search is determining what types of information are needed to answer the EBP question and which databases will provide that information. Databases are standardized and searchable repositories of indexed citations (some with full-text access), usually focusing on a specific subject, such as biomedicine, nursing, physiotherapy, psychiatry, and others (Welsh, 2010). While always evolving, these databases all now include options for filters by date, article type, language and more. Of note, access to a database allows the team to search indexed citations, but access to full text will depend on their institution's subscriptions and the availability of Open Access (OA) articles.

	Reports Retrieved	Reports Not Retrieved
Relevant Reports	Relevant reports retrieved (a)	Relevant reports not retrieved (b)
Irrelevant Reports	Irrelevant reports retrieved (c)	Irrelevant reports not retrieved (d)

Sensitivity: fraction of relevant reports retrieved from all relevant reports (a/(a+b))
Precision: fraction of relevant reports retrieved from all reports retrieved (a/(a+c))

FIGURE 7.1 Literature search sensitivity and precision.
Lefebvre et al., 2023

There are various core databases and database interfaces in healthcare that each consist of hundreds of journals and millions of records. Of note, PubMed is a well-known name in healthcare; however, it is not a database itself, but rather an *interface* maintained by the National Library of Medicine to search the *databases* MEDLINE and PubMed Central. MEDLINE comprises 92% of the citations available through PubMed. MEDLINE can also be accessed by other fee-based platforms, including Ovid or EBSCO. See Table 7.3 for further details on common healthcare databases, including when to use each.

> **NOTE**
>
> **OPEN ACCESS ARTICLES**
>
> Open access (OA) is a growing publishing model in which a reader has "free access, without subscription, payment or registration to the full text of a scientific journal article" (Björk, 2017, p. 247). While there are various tiers of OA, in short, anyone with the internet can access an article at no cost. This is made possible by bypassing subscription fees to the journal itself (which were once necessary to print and distribute physical journals) and passing the responsibility to authors in the form of publication charges. While there are some inherent risks to this approach, overall, it is beneficial to consumers of evidence and a future direction in publishing (Björk, 2017).

TABLE 7.3 Common Healthcare Databases and Their Characteristics

	NAME	USE WHEN…	TYPES OF INDEXED RESOURCES	SUBSCRIPTION REQUIREMENTS (LINK)
	CINAHL database	Seeking literature focused on nursing and allied health; it also contains information on biomedicine, alternative or complimentary medicine	Textbooks, nursing dissertations, conference abstracts, peer-reviewed journals, legal cases, and clinical trials	Requires subscription (consult your institution's library website or resources)
PubMed Interface	MEDLINE database	Looking to answer EBP questions focused on healthcare science, with a focus on biomedical research	Peer-reviewed journals, ahead of print citations, conference abstracts, online books, and clinical trials	PubMed interface is freely searchable. Access to full text to articles in MEDLINE will depend on the institution's subscriptions and availability of OA publications (https://pubmed.ncbi.nlm.nih.gov/).
	PubMed Central	Looking to answer EBP questions focused on healthcare science, with a focus on biomedical research; offers free access to full-text articles	Peer-reviewed journals, pre-prints	Freely searchable with access to full text (https://www.ncbi.nlm.nih.gov/pmc/)

continues

TABLE 7.3 Common Healthcare Databases and Their Characteristics (cont.)

NAME	USE WHEN…	TYPES OF INDEXED RESOURCES	SUBSCRIPTION REQUIREMENTS (LINK)
Embase database	Looking to answer EBP questions focused on biomedical research; provides citations beyond what is covered in PubMed, including a focus on medical devices, drugs, diseases, and chemicals	Peer-reviewed journals, conference abstracts, and online books	Requires subscription (consult your institution's library website or resources)
American Psychological Association PsychINFO database	Focusing on evidence in psychology, behavior, and social sciences	Peer-reviewed journals, book chapters, and book reviews	Requires subscription (consult your institution's library website or resources)
Epistemonikos database	Looking for scientific evidence with an international lens, including publications in multiple languages and systematic reviews	Peer-reviewed journals, evidence-based policy briefs, guidelines, and structured summaries of evidence	Freely searchable. Access to full text articles will depend on the institution's subscriptions and availability of OA publications.
Google Scholar search engine*	Gathering preliminary background information on a broad range of topics	Peer-reviewed journals, grey literature, books, white papers, unpublished trial data, government publications and reports, court opinions, dissertations, and theses	Freely searchable. Access to full text articles will depend on the institution's subscriptions and availability of OA publications.

*See the "Using Google Scholar" sidebar on the next page.

> **EXAMPLE**
>
> **SEARCHING ACTION ITEM 1: DETERMINE WHICH DATABASES TO SEARCH**
>
> "Among hospitalized pediatric patients on invasive mechanical ventilation, what are best practices regarding the administration of nebulized medications?"
>
> This question crosses several disciplines, including nursing and respiratory therapy. All the above databases may be appropriate, but the team should include CINAHL with its emphasis on nursing and allied health.

USING GOOGLE SCHOLAR

Google Scholar is a common and simple-to-use tool because of most people's familiarity with the use of Google as a search engine. Google Scholar can be a helpful place to start a search to get a better idea of available information and terminology associated with the topic or cast a broad net without a structured search strategy. Unfortunately, search algorithms change daily, making it impossible to replicate a search. Despite this drawback, it has additional features that make it a useful tool for EBP teams, including:

My profile: A tool for authors to track their work, number of citations, and other details. There is also a feature to create alerts for pre-selected search terms that will trigger a notification via email when the terms are published online. This is helpful to keep up to date with literature as it is published on a topic or area of interest.

Cite: A feature that can generate citations and export citations to reference managers. By clicking on the closed quotation icon (") under a listing, a pop-up box will appear with a citation in a variety of styles. Teams can directly copy/paste the entry or export it into a citation manager.

Cited by: This option allows a reader to see other publications that have cited a given source. This can be helpful when trying to identify recent literature or other articles that may have used similar methods. There is an additional feature to search within this generated list.

Action Item 2: Build the Search—Identify Key Concepts After identifying appropriate resources, the team uses their EBP question to create database-specific search strings. It can be helpful to focus on the search for one database and once that has been piloted, adjust it for other databases. The first part of building these structured queries is to create search concepts using various tools, including keywords, controlled vocabulary, exact phrasing, truncation, and title or abstract limits.

Search concepts are clusters (or "buckets") of keywords or phrases that describe each core element of the EBP question which are then linked to produce a search string. Historically, this process has been guided by the PICO (Population, Intervention, Comparison, Outcome) format; however, PICO questions are essentially just a tool to build a search, and the same approach can be applied to any well-written EBP question. To complete this action item, the EBP team should isolate each element of their question and identify synonyms and alternative spellings for the word or phrase listed. For example, the term "geriatric" can also be described as "elderly," "senior," or "aged." Additionally, American English only represents a portion of English-language articles, and alternative spellings (e.g., "pediatric" and "paediatric" or "behaviour" and "behavior") or names (e.g., "emergency department" and "accident and emergency") are important to capture. Keep in mind, there may be several concepts within a component of the question (e.g., the population of pediatric oncology patients will need two search concepts, one for pediatrics and the other for oncology). Essentially, the team is trying to brainstorm all the alternative terms authors could have used to describe the same idea they are interested in.

While creating these buckets, the team should also identify any controlled vocabulary associated with their keywords. Controlled vocabulary is the use of specific, standardized words to index and catalog concepts within a database based on a common scheme (Booth et al., 2021). All citations tagged with a term from the pre-defined vocabulary list will be retrieved when that controlled vocabulary term is searched, like searching a hashtag in social media. This is helpful to ensure consistency and reduce ambiguity when the same concept may have different names, or one word has several meanings (e.g., "nursing" can refer to both the healthcare profession as well as the act of breastfeeding; Booth et al., 2021; Bramer et al., 2018). Controlled vocabulary systems all follow a similar process but have slightly different names and ways to denote the specific search, depending on the database. For advanced users, there are many different database-specific field codes that can be used to further refine a search (see Bramer et al., 2018 for more information). If the team is not sure which terms may be associated with their EBP question, it can be helpful to retrieve a highly relevant article and then see which controlled vocabulary has been assigned to it. See Table 7.4 for a list of common healthcare databases and their use of controlled vocabulary and how to operationalize them.

Additional tools to define key concepts are the use of truncation, exact phrasing, and field tags.

When an asterisk (*) is placed at the end of a word, the database will search just the provided root with all possible permutations (e.g., nurs* → nurses, nursing, nursed). Exact phrasing is indicated by placing single or double quotation marks (depending on the database) around a word or phrase. This directs the database to only retrieve that specific set of words (e.g., nursing ethics vs. "nursing ethics"). Finally, each database has characters, called *field tags*, that can be used to limit queries of words or phrases to the title, abstract, or keywords fields. Adding "[tiab]" after a term or phrase in PubMed (e.g., hospital*[tiab]) or the letters "TI" OR "AB" before a series of words enclosed by parentheses (e.g., TI(hospital* OR ward OR inpatient)) in CINAHL directs a database to only look for the given word or term in the title or abstract. Similarly, using the letters ":ti," ":ab," or ":kw" after a term (e.g., hospital*:ti,ab,kw) directs Embase to only look for that term in the title, abstract, or keywords, respectively.

TABLE 7.4 Common Databases and Their Use of Controlled Vocabulary

DATABASE	CONTROLLED VOCABULARY SYSTEM	EXAMPLE FOR THE TERM "SWALLOWING" (THE ACT OF SWALLOWING, MOVING SOMETHING FROM THE MOUTH TO THE STOMACH)
PubMed	Medical Subject Headings (MeSH)	Deglutition [MeSH]
CINAHL	Subject Headings (MH), including Major (MM) and Minor (DH)	Major subject: Deglutition Minor subjects: Human; Adult; Deglutition Disorders
Embase	Emtree Explode (exp), No Explode (/de), and As Major Focus (/mj)	'swallowing'/exp, 'dysphagia'/exp

EXAMPLE

SEARCHING ACTION ITEM 2: BUILD THE SEARCH—IDENTIFY KEY CONCEPTS

"Among <u>hospitalized</u> <u>pediatric patients</u> on invasive <u>mechanical ventilation,</u> what are best
                 1   2   3

nursing practices regarding the administration of <u>nebulized medications</u>?"
                                                                             4

The EBP team isolates four elements of their EBP question they will need to search to gather relevant literature. They have two concepts that fall into the "population" category because they are looking for pediatric patients that are on invasive mechanical ventilation. Pediatrics and patients on mechanical ventilation will each need to be an independent search concept.

CONCEPT	SYNONYMS (INCLUDING USE OF TRUNCATION OR EXACT PHRASING)	CONTROLLED VOCABULARY		
		PUBMED	CINAHL	EMBASE
Concept 1 (setting): Hospital	• hospital* • ward* • "acute care" • "critical care" • in-patient • inpatient • ICU	• "hospitals" [MeSH] • "hospital units" [MeSH] • "inpatients" [MeSH]	• MH "inpatients" • MH "hospital units" • MH "hospitals"	• 'hospital patient'/exp • 'hospital'/exp
Concept 2 (population): Pediatric patients	• pediatric* • adolescen* • child* • infant • kid • paediatric* • juvenile* • baby • teen*	• "adolescent" [MeSH] • "child" [MeSH] • "infant" [MeSH] • puberty" [MeSH]	• MH "adolescence" • MH "child" • MH "infant" • MH "puberty"	• 'adolescent'/exp • 'child'/exp • 'infant'/exp • 'puberty'/exp
Concept 3 (population): Patients on invasive mechanical ventilation	• "invasive mechanical ventilation" • IMV • ventilat* • intubat* • "artificial ventilation"	• "respiration, artificial"[MeSH] • "intubation"[MeSH] • "ventilators, mechanical"[MeSH]	• MH "respiration, artificial" • MH "intubation" • MH "ventilators, mechanical"	• 'artificial ventilation'/exp • 'mechanical ventilator'/exp • 'intubation'/exp
Concept 4 (topic): Administration of nebulized medications	• nebuliz* • nebulis* • aerosol* • vaporiz*	• "nebulizers and vaporizers" [MeSH] • "aerosols" [MeSH] • "administration, inhalation" [MeSH]	• MH "nebulizers and vaporizers" • MH "aerosols" • MH "administration, inhalation"	• 'nebulizer'/exp • 'inhalational drug administration'/exp • 'aerosol'/exp • 'bronchodilating agent'/de

Keep in mind, not all elements of an EBP question should be used to generate search concepts. When a search term concept is added, the database will only retrieve articles that contain the exact provided words or phrases. The EBP team will not want to use the "best strategies" or "best practices" portion of a question because it will only yield results that have that specific phrase, meaning an article may help establish what a best practice is, but unless the authors used that exact wording, an article would not be identified. Likewise, the team should not include terms that indicate directionality (e.g., increase, decrease, improve, reduce) because the results may exclude evidence that provides a complete picture of the impact of a change or intervention. For example, if the EBP team searches "decrease" with a concept related to non-slip socks and fall rates, they may retrieve five articles that state non-slip socks *decrease* fall rates but could miss another 10 articles that state non-slip socks *increase* fall rates. Similarly, in many cases, the same outcome can be described from multiple angles (e.g., increase safe ambulation vs. decrease fall rates), and the use of a directional term will bias the search (Bramer et al., 2018).

Action Item 3: Build the Search—Create Search Strings Once the EBP team has developed a concept for each element of the EBP question, they will use Boolean logic to create associations both *within* and *between* the concepts. Boolean operators, named after the English mathematician George Boole, are conjunctions (AND, OR, and NOT) to define relationships between terms in a literature search (Britannica, 2021). Within each concept, the team uses the term "OR" to link synonyms. The EBP team indicates the beginning and end of the list of synonyms using open and closed parentheses. They then connect this set of synonyms to other sets with the word "AND." The word "NOT" is used to exclude concepts but should be used with caution as it may omit relevant results. See Table 7.5 for a visual example of each Boolean operator with explanations.

Keep in mind that if the team is investigating an EBP question comparing one intervention to another, they will likely need to conduct two independent searches, one for each intervention to gather all relevant information. If the team only looks for articles containing all interventions of interest (linked with an AND), they will miss evidence that has information for each individually that could be used to generate a comparison.

TABLE 7.5 Boolean Operators

BOOLEAN OPERATOR	VENN DIAGRAM	EXPLANATION
AND	(Venn diagram with intersection highlighted in yellow)	Use AND to link concepts where you want to see both ideas in your search results. The area in yellow on the diagram highlights the results when AND is used to combine words or concepts. AND narrows the search.

OR

Use OR between similar keywords, like synonyms, acronyms, and variations in spelling within the same idea or concept.

The area in yellow on the diagram highlights the results when OR is used to combine words or concepts.

OR broadens the search.

NOT

NOT is used to exclude specific keywords from the search; however, use NOT with caution because you may end up missing something important.

The yellow area on the diagram shows the results you will get when you combine two concepts using NOT.

NOT is used to make broad exclusions.

> **EXAMPLE**
>
> ### SEARCHING ACTION ITEM 3: BUILD THE SEARCH—CREATE SEARCH STRINGS
> "Among hospitalized pediatric patients on invasive mechanical ventilation, what are best practices regarding the administration of nebulized medications?"
>
> By combing the terms identified in Action Item 2 with the Boolean operators "AND" and "OR," the EBP generates the following database-specific queries.
>
> **PubMed Search String:**
>
> (Hospital* OR ward OR "acute care" OR "critical care" OR in-patient OR inpatient OR ICU OR "hospitals"[MeSH] OR "hospital units"[MeSH] OR "inpatients"[MeSH])
>
> AND
>
> (Pediatric* OR adolescen* OR child*OR infant OR kid OR paediatric* OR juvenile* OR baby OR teen* OR "Adolescent"[MeSH] OR "Child"[MeSH] OR "Infant"[MeSH] OR "Puberty"[MeSH])
>
> AND
>
> ("invasive mechanical ventilation" OR IMV OR ventilat* OR intubat* OR "artificial ventilation" OR "respiration, artificial"[MeSH] OR "intubation"[MeSH] OR "ventilators, mechanical"[MeSH])
>
> AND
>
> (Nebuliz* OR nebulis* OR aerosol* OR vaporiz* OR "nebulizers and vaporizers"[MeSH] OR "aerosols"[MeSH] OR "Administration, Inhalation"[MeSH])
>
> **CINAHL Search String:**
>
> (Hospital* OR ward OR "acute care" OR "critical care" OR in-patient OR inpatient OR ICU OR MH "Inpatients" OR MH "hospital units" OR MH "hospitals")
>
> AND
>
> (Pediatric*OR adolescen*OR child*OR infant OR kid OR paediatric* OR juvenile* OR baby OR teen* OR MH "Adolescence" OR MH "Child" OR MH "Infant" OR MH "Puberty")
>
> AND
>
> ("invasive mechanical ventilation" OR IMV OR ventilat* OR intubat* OR "artificial ventilation" OR MH "respiration, artificial" OR MH "intubation" OR MH "ventilators, mechanical")

AND

(Nebuliz* OR nebulis* OR aerosol* OR vaporiz* OR MH "nebulizers and vaporizers" OR MH "aerosols" OR MH "Administration, Inhalation")

Embase Search String:

(Hospital* OR ward OR "acute care" OR "critical care" OR in-patient OR inpatient OR ICU OR 'hospital patient'/exp OR 'hospital'/exp)

AND

(Pediatric* OR adolescen* OR child* OR infant OR kid OR paediatric* OR juvenile* OR baby OR teen* OR 'adolescent'/exp OR 'child'/exp OR 'infant'/exp OR 'puberty'/exp)

AND

('invasive mechanical ventilation' OR IMV OR ventilat* OR intubat* OR 'artificial ventilation' OR 'artificial ventilation'/exp OR 'mechanical ventilator'/exp OR 'intubation'/exp)

AND

(Nebuliz* OR nebulis* OR aerosol* OR vaporiz* OR 'nebulizer'/exp OR 'inhalational drug administration'/exp OR 'aerosol'/exp OR 'bronchodilating agent'/de)

Action Item 4: Execute the Search Using the search strings created in the previous action item, navigate to each of the databases identified in Action Item 1 and perform the search. This can be done by copying/pasting the search strings from a Word document or typing them into the search bar provided by the database. Some people search all concepts (connected with the word "AND") at once, while others prefer to search each independently and then use the "advanced search" function available in most databases to combine each independent concept.

EXAMPLE

SEARCHING ACTION ITEM 4: EXECUTE THE SEARCH

"Among hospitalized pediatric patients on invasive mechanical ventilation, what are best practices regarding the administration of nebulized medications?"

The EBP team copy/pasted their terms into the PubMed search bar. See screenshot below. Because the search bar is short, they are only able to see the first few words, although all are present.

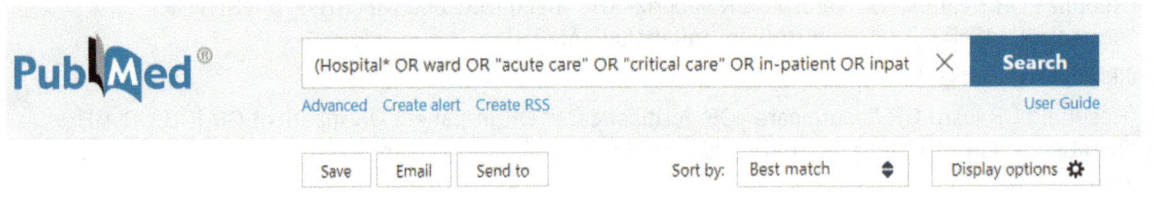

Action Item 5: Apply Initial Limits or Filters, When Appropriate After executing the search, the EBP team can immediately apply limits or filters to the results to narrow the amount of literature that will need to undergo screening. Beyond the confines of the population, topic, and setting, common initial filters include year and language. In addition to exclusion criteria based on the content of the article, teams can also exclude based on the type of article itself—for example, conference abstracts. These limits are a subset of the inclusion/exclusion criteria the team will formally establish in the screening phase; however, establishing a cut-off date, or other initial criteria that can be objectively filtered within a database, will limit the number of superfluous results. For example, searching "telemedicine" in PubMed yields 54,719 results between 1962 and 2024. When this is shortened to the last five years (2019–2024), the number of results drops to 29,731. All limits should include a justification (Bramer et al., 2018). See the later section "Minimizing Bias in Literature Search and Screening" for more considerations.

> **EXAMPLE**
>
> **SEARCHING ACTION ITEM 5: APPLY INITIAL LIMITS OR FILTERS, WHEN APPROPRIATE**
>
> "Among hospitalized pediatric patients on invasive mechanical ventilation, what are best practices regarding the administration of nebulized medications?"
>
> The EBP team is updating a policy that included an exhaustive literature search conducted in 2019. They are trying to determine if any new information has come out in the interim that indicates they should update their policy. Because of this they decide to limit the search from 2019 to the present. In CINAHL, this reduces their initial search from 251 results to 55. They also do not have two people on the team who are able to read medical literature in a language other than English and don't have the resources for translation. They decide to also limit their search to English-language only. This further reduces the CINAHL search from 55 to 54 articles.
>
> Finally, the team notices a large number of results in their Embase search are conference abstracts only. They decide to exclude these articles because they do not provide sufficient information to complete an adequate quality appraisal. Applying the language and year filters to exclude conference abstracts reduces their Embase search results from 975 to 734.

Action Item 6: Evaluate, Revise, and Refine the Search As the team moves through the search process, they will likely identify gaps in their initial approach as well as opportunities to optimize the results. This may include adding new keywords within a concept, or additional concepts. The process is iterative and flexible, but it is important to document all changes as they happen.

> **EXAMPLE**
>
> **SEARCHING ACTION ITEM 6: EVALUATE, REVISE, AND REFINE THE SEARCH**
>
> "Among hospitalized pediatric patients on invasive mechanical ventilation, what are best practices regarding the administration of nebulized medications?"
>
> During review of the results of their initial search, the team notices they may be inadvertently missing some important literature because they are missing a term. In reviewing a highly relevant article, they notice an additional controlled vocabulary term they think will improve their search. They rerun the search with the addition of the controlled vocabulary term "Bronchodilator Agents/administration and dosage" in PubMed and "Bronchodilator Agents/AD" in CINAHL. This brings their search results from 54 to 61 in CINAHL.

Action Item 7: Document the Search Once the team has decided on a final search strategy, they need to document the strategy. Most databases have a feature that allows saving a search within the database; however, it is always a good idea to keep multiple copies of searches. Microsoft Word documents or emails are a great way to keep a record of work. Be sure to include the databases included in the search, search string for each database, number of citations retrieved from each database, and the search date (Booth et al., 2016).

> **TIP**
>
> **CITATION MANAGEMENT TOOLS**
>
> In addition to the tools within some databases to save searches and set alerts, *citation management tools*, also called *reference management software*, are programs used to store and organize literature citations as well as generate bibliographies. Options include EndNote, RefWorks, Zotero, Mendeley, Papers, and others. The functions and capabilities of the various programs are similar. Some citation management programs are free, whereas others need to be purchased; some may be provided at no cost by an organization.

> **EXAMPLE**
>
> **SEARCHING ACTION ITEM 7: DOCUMENT THE SEARCH**
>
> "Among hospitalized pediatric patients on invasive mechanical ventilation, what are best practices regarding the administration of nebulized medications?"
>
> Search run June 27, 2024
>
> Limits: English only, 2019–2024
>
> **CINAHL Search:**
>
> 61 results
>
> (Hospital* OR ward OR "acute care" OR "critical care" OR in-patient OR inpatient OR ICU OR MH "Inpatients" OR MH "hospital units" OR MH "hospitals") AND (Pediatric* OR adolescen* OR child*OR infant OR kid OR paediatric* OR juvenile* OR baby OR teen* OR MH "Adolescence" OR MH "Child" OR MH "Infant" OR MH "Puberty") AND ("invasive mechanical ventilation" OR IMV OR ventilat* OR intubat* OR "artificial ventilation" OR MH "respiration, artificial" OR MH "intubation" OR MH "ventilators, mechanical") AND (Nebuliz* OR nebulis* OR aerosol* OR vaporiz* OR MH "nebulizers and vaporizers" OR MH "aerosols" OR MH "Administration, Inhalation" OR MH "Bronchodilator Agents/AD")

PubMed Search:

215 results

(Hospital* OR ward OR "acute care" OR "critical care" OR in-patient OR inpatient OR ICU OR "hospitals"[MeSH] OR "hospital units"[MeSH] OR "inpatients"[MeSH]) AND (Pediatric*OR adolescen*OR child*OR infant OR kid OR paediatric* OR juvenile* OR baby OR teen* OR "Adolescent"[MeSH] OR "Child"[MeSH] OR "Infant"[MeSH] OR "Puberty"[MeSH]) AND

("invasive mechanical ventilation" OR IMV OR ventilat* OR intubat* OR "artificial ventilation" OR "respiration, artificial"[MeSH] OR "intubation"[MeSH] OR "ventilators, mechanical"[MeSH]) AND (Nebuliz* OR nebulis* OR aerosol* OR vaporiz* OR "nebulizers and vaporizers"[MeSH] OR "aerosols"[MeSH] OR "Administration, Inhalation"[MeSH] OR "Bronchodilator Agents/administration and dosage"[MeSH])

Embase Search:

734 results

(Hospital* OR ward OR "acute care" OR "critical care" OR in-patient OR inpatient OR ICU OR 'hospital patient'/exp OR 'hospital'/exp) AND (Pediatric*OR adolescen*OR child*OR infant OR kid OR paediatric* OR juvenile* OR baby OR teen* OR 'adolescent'/exp OR 'child'/exp OR 'infant'/exp OR 'puberty'/exp) AND ("invasive mechanical ventilation" OR IMV OR ventilat* OR intubat* OR "artificial ventilation" OR 'artificial ventilation'/exp OR 'mechanical ventilator'/exp OR 'intubation'/exp) AND (Nebuliz* OR nebulis* OR aerosol* OR vaporiz* OR 'nebulizer'/exp OR 'inhalational drug administration'/exp OR 'aerosol'/exp OR 'bronchodilating agent'/de)

Additional Search Techniques

It is important to note that not all literature is found through database searching, either due to indexing or to outliers not captured by the original search strategy. Because of this, the team can gain valuable information by:

- Table of contents scanning: Hand searching the table of contents of peer-reviewed journals that cover the subject area the EBP team is focusing on
- "Snowballing": Evaluating the reference list of books and articles retrieved during the formal search
- "Cited by" searching: Moving forward in the publication timeline to find articles that cited a highly relevant article identified during the search process

SYSTEMATIC LITERATURE SCREENING

Literature screening is the systematic process of winnowing down search results to include only articles that answer the EBP question and meet inclusion and exclusion criteria.

Once the team downloads and stores exhaustive search results, the next step is screening those results. Much like the systematic approach to conduct the literature search, using a methodical and rigorous approach to screen the result ensures a comprehensive and unbiased picture of the state of the evidence on a given topic. This lends credence to the eventual recommendations from the project (Lefebvre et al., 2023; Whittemore & Knafl, 2005).

In addition to minimizing *selection bias*—when a reviewer selects studies that support their previously held beliefs—a systematic screening process also saves the team time and effort (Booth et al., 2016). Completing an exhaustive literature review that truly reflects the state of the evidence can be a large undertaking with hundreds, if not thousands, of results. Screening is a necessary step to narrow the results of a search to only those that are pertinent. Note that very large search results may be a sign that the search strategy or the EBP question needs to be revised. Employing a team-based literature screening protocol and tracking mechanism helps to establish clear documentation of the process and makes screening more efficient and reliable. Following a methodical approach of reviewing titles and abstracts, then full-text reading, conservatively allows a team to screen 500–1,000 articles over an eight-hour period (Lefebvre et al., 2023). Quickly culling superfluous results helps the team to home in on information truly relevant to the identified problem. With many competing priorities, EBP teams should avoid spending time considering articles that do not answer the EBP question through thoughtful approaches to the process.

The following action items outline how teams can create a reliable and well-documented literature screening process. The evidence phase of the EBP process mirrors that of conducting an integrative review, and the steps for searching and screening can be applied accordingly (Lawless & Foster, 2020).

> **NOTE**
>
> Reviewers should be attentive in identifying duplicate publications that may be included in other research studies, such as a primary research study that is then referenced in a literature review or a professional organization's position statement. The team should discuss how to handle such duplications on a case-by-case basis, acknowledging the risk of skewing the overall evidence by overrepresenting one source (Lefebvre et al., 2023).

Action Item 1: Establish Inclusion and Exclusion Criteria for the Literature Screening

Establish and write down inclusion and exclusion criteria. Copy the EBP question and place it in a visible location to view during screening. Commonly used exclusion criteria include population, language, date, intervention, outcomes, or setting. See the later "Minimizing Bias in Literature Search and Screening" section to explore these potential parameters. Keep in mind, as the team delves deeper into the literature, they will gain a greater understanding of the available knowledge on a topic, and the need to establish new limitations may surface. They should communicate throughout the process to adjust inclusion and exclusion criteria as needed.

> **EXAMPLE**
>
> **SCREENING ACTION ITEM 1: ESTABLISH INCLUSION AND EXCLUSION CRITERIA FOR THE LITERATURE SCREENING**
>
> "Among hospitalized pediatric patients on invasive mechanical ventilation, what are best practices regarding the administration of nebulized medications?"
>
> As the team begins to screen their results, they notice there is specific information for neonates as well as a concentration on safe administration of medications as it relates to spreading of infectious materials to healthcare workers. The EBP team meets to discuss which population they want to concentrate on. In addition to the parameters identified in the EBP question, the team decides that because they do not treat intubated neonates, and this is a very specific sub-population with unique needs, they want to only include patients outside of the neonatal intensive care unit. Additionally, they decide that ensuring safe and effective administration from the healthcare provider point-of-view is a different focus and choose to only include articles that speak to the well-being of the patients.

Inclusion criteria:

Pediatric patients on invasive mechanical ventilation ages

Hospitalized patients

Administration outcomes as it relates to the patient

Nebulized medication administration

Exclusion criteria:

Adult patients

Neonates in the NICU

Outside the hospital setting

Patients with other types of respiratory support (e.g., non-invasive)

Non-nebulized medication

Conference abstracts

Action Item 2: Determine a Plan for Performing the Literature Screening

To screen the search results in a systematic manner, the team should determine a process prior to starting, including the number of reviewers and tracking mechanism. Best practice is to have at least two people independently review records during title/abstract and full-text screen to decrease the odds of erroneously including or excluding an entry (Lefebvre et al., 2023; Polanin et al., 2019). A recent study found single reviewers erroneously excluded on average 13% of relevant citations, while dual reviewers missed only 3% (Gartlehner et al., 2020). Tools such as Excel, Google Forms, or Covidence (Veritas Health Innovation, Melbourne, Australia) can assist in tracking the screening process. Many databases and reference management software can produce a file to facilitate importing citations into the selected program. Other free tools available online include Rayyan or Abstrackr.

> **EXAMPLE**
>
> **SCREENING ACTION ITEM 2: DETERMINE A PLAN FOR PERFORMING THE LITERATURE SCREENING**
>
> "Among hospitalized pediatric patients on invasive mechanical ventilation, what are best practices regarding the administration of nebulized medications?"
>
> The team does not have access to a free software program to screen evidence through their organization. They decide to use an Excel spreadsheet to screen the articles. They export the citations from Embase, CINAHL, and PubMed and convert them into a spreadsheet with table headers. They assign codes to "duplicates," "include" and "exclude," and move through the titles, abstract, and full text sequentially, filtering out the excluded articles at each stage to create a final list. Each reviewer has their own assigned column to enter decisions so the team leader can review to identify and resolve any discrepancies.

Action Item 3: Begin by Screening Only the Title and Abstracts Produced From the Search

Performing a title screening and then returning to the remaining articles for an abstract screening can save time and distraction; however, the ability to screen titles only may be limited based on the type of screening software the team is using (Mateen et al., 2013). Exclude only those articles that concretely meet one of the exclusion criteria or do not answer the EBP question. Note that "a single failed eligibility criterion is sufficient for a study to be excluded from a review" (Lefebvre et al., 2023, 6.4). A key idea to remember here is that the article is included until proven otherwise. There is no right or wrong answer, only a consistent answer. The team should apply criteria uniformly regardless of who is screening each record.

> **EXAMPLE**
>
> **SCREENING ACTION ITEM 3: BEGIN BY SCREENING ONLY THE TITLE AND ABSTRACTS PRODUCED FROM THE SEARCH**
>
> "Among hospitalized pediatric patients on invasive mechanical ventilation, what are best practices regarding the administration of nebulized medications?"
>
> After completing a title and abstract screening, the team is left with 41 unique articles that may answer their EBP question. These articles advance to the full-text screening phase.

Action Item 4: Complete Full-Text Screening for All Articles That Remain After Screening the Titles and Abstracts

EBP team members should continue to independently screen the full text of the remaining articles to determine whether they answer the EBP question and meet all inclusion criteria. This is an objective assessment and does not yet consider the evidence's quality. It is normal to continue to exclude articles throughout this stage. If full text is not available, you may be able to submit an interlibrary loan request or access the article through one of the free databases mentioned earlier in the chapter. As the team is unable to determine inclusion or quality from an abstract alone, if you have exhausted all resources and are unable to locate the article, it can be designated as "unable to retrieve."

> **EXAMPLE**
>
> **SCREENING ACTION ITEM 4: COMPLETE FULL-TEXT SCREENING FOR ALL ARTICLES THAT REMAIN AFTER SCREENING THE TITLES AND ABSTRACTS**
>
> "Among hospitalized pediatric patients on invasive mechanical ventilation, what are best practices regarding the administration of nebulized medications?"
>
> After completing the full-text screening, the team is left with nine unique articles that answer their EBP question. These articles can now be appraised to ensure they are of adequate quality to continue through the EBP process.

Action Item 5: Document the Screening Process

Record the number of articles removed throughout each level of screening. Tools such as the PRISMA flow diagram provide structure and prompts for the required information. Fields include the number of records identified from each database, the number of duplicates, the number of titles and abstracts screened, and the number of records that underwent full-text review with reasons for exclusion, if applicable (Lawless & Foster, 2020, p. 21). The diagram also provides space to note the number of records obtained through alternative means (e.g., hand searching, "snowballing" searching).

EXAMPLE

SCREENING ACTION ITEM 5: DOCUMENT THE SCREENING PROCESS

"Among hospitalized pediatric patients on invasive mechanical ventilation, what are best practices regarding the administration of nebulized medications?"

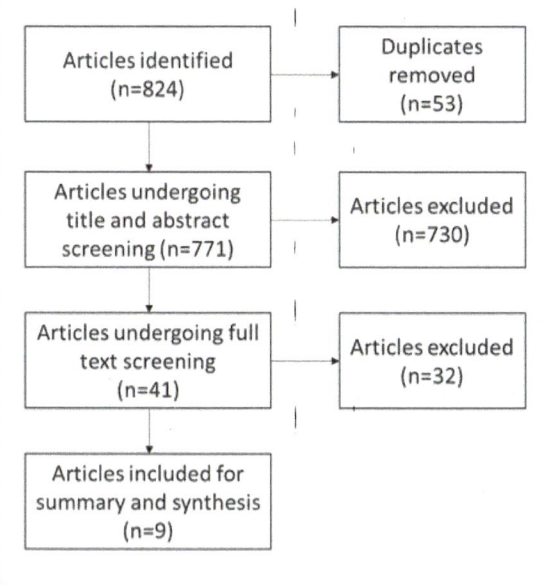

TIP

The EBP team should keep an eye out for warning signs that their evidence search or screening may have some fundamental flaws (adapted from Booth et al., 2021). They include:

The team has not shown why some studies were included or excluded. The decisions seem arbitrary.

The team has identified primary web sources (e.g., blogs, webpages) and not sufficient peer-reviewed evidence.

Key items are missing; the search was too narrow.

MINIMIZING BIAS IN LITERATURE SEARCH AND SCREENING

Bias is an influence that produces a distortion or error and results in a systematic alteration from the truth (McDonagh et al., 2013; Polit & Beck, 2021). Bias can occur at any stage of the EBP process, and the team should be aware of how the design of search strategy (including databases selection and key terms identification) and screening of subsequent results can lead to perpetuation of existing biases.

Some common biases to be aware of when developing the search strategy include spectrum bias, random error, search satisficing, premature closure, confirmation bias, attribute substitution, and "not invented here" (Gluck, 2020; McDonagh et al., 2013):

- *Spectrum bias* concerns the inclusion or exclusion of a specific population. For example, when looking for studies regarding treatment for women, focusing the results on studies of only women eliminates those studies that looked at both men and women and could potentially be relevant.

- *Random error* occurs from simple mistakes from individuals when reading or reviewing information and is more likely to occur with more subjective decision-making—for example, misclicking or miscoding an article. Independent double-check can reduce random errors.

- *Search satisficing* describes the tendency to consider a search finished once anything is found, regardless of whether the references are the best answer. It happens most commonly when a team only looks for a few good articles. For example, the EBP team conducts a search, and the top five articles on the page seem highly relevant, so they do no further gathering of information.

- *Premature closure* occurs most commonly in searches where little or no relevant information is found. Rather than reframing the question or trying a different source, the search is ended. For example, an EBP team searches "nursing report cards" and gets few results. They stop their search and assume there is little information on the topic. However, they did not realize the common term to refer to the same idea in the literature is "audit and feedback," which retrieves dozens of articles.

- *Confirmation bias* is the tendency to weigh more heavily on sources that confirm one's beliefs or reject sources that contradict beliefs. Many search teams tend to look for information that confirms and reinforces existing beliefs, structuring the search so that non-confirming sources may be missing. For example, excluding an article during the screening process because it indicates the intervention the team hopes to implement is not effective.

- *Attribute substitution* occurs commonly with complex questions and can occur when the question is overly simplified and leads to the loss of small but necessary nuances within the search parameters. This relies on using an easily accessible attribute as a proxy for a more complex one—for example, assuming that an article with many citations is better than one with fewer. Quantity is a proxy for quality.

- *"Not invented here"* refers to the tendency to focus searches on only literature written in the EBP team's country or geographic area. While this may be relevant for quality and policy questions, it is less suitable for clinical questions and could exclude relevant evidence. The team should always have a strong and well-documented rationale for including or excluding evidence based solely on geographic area. When possible, it should be based on objective criteria—for example, the World Health Organization's categories of economies, reference to laws or regulations, or scope of practice of healthcare providers in question. Another example is limiting a search to only articles reporting studies conducted in the same country as the EBP team's home country.

Additional sources of potential bias are the application of common strict exclusion criteria such as "ageism of knowledge" or the five-year rule (Truex et al., 2022), publication preference, and language restrictions, such as English only. The five-year rule is commonly used, though there is no literature to support or debunk it. It is important to remember that the older literature can be equally crucial for established topics or research areas. As a rule, year criteria can be valuable but should have an accompanying rationale for how it was determined by the EBP team. Publication preference can create bias when a reviewer gives greater weight to some articles over others, based solely on the journals in which they appear. This can happen due to personal relationships with authors or editors or perceptions of the quality of the journals. Although prevailing advice has been to include all languages to reduce the risk of bias, this advice can present problems for the team that does not have the resources to translate foreign language articles of relevance. There has been some research that suggests that systematically omitting non-English language articles does not have a meaningful effect on literature review findings (Morrison et al., 2012).

> **NOTE**
>
> **AI SEARCHING**
>
> Artificial intelligence (AI) is an emerging technology in almost all fields, including literature search and screening. While this is a rapidly changing tool, EBP teams should be aware of the use of AI to not only create search concepts but also screen retrieved literature (Wagner et al., 2021). Research is being done to determine the effectiveness of AI in completing either of these tasks. Current literature (as of 2024) suggests that AI can be a helpful tool but should be used in complement of, not in lieu of, human efforts (Feng et al., 2022; Gwon et al., 2024). However, it should be acknowledged that this technology is becoming more advanced very quickly, and the role and effectiveness of AI will continue to evolve.

SUMMARY

This chapter reviews types of literature searches; when, where, and how to conduct them; and the process of screening results to generate an accurate and manageable representation of the literature. The goal of these steps is to identify actionable information in the most efficient way possible. This may be in the form of accessible pre-appraised evidence or through an EBP team's own exhaustive literature search to find answers to their EBP question. Finally, as with all healthcare decisions, the team should be cautious of introducing biases while collecting evidence and the potential this has to perpetuate skewed perspectives.

REFERENCES

American Library Association. (1989). *Presidential committee on information literacy: Final report*. http://www.ala.org/acrl/publications/whitepapers/presidential

Björk, B. C. (2017). Open access to scientific articles: A review of benefits and challenges. *Internal & Emergency Medicine, 12*, 247–253. https://doi.org/10.1007/s11739-017-1603-2

Booth, A., Sutton, A., Clowes, M., & Martyn-St. James, M. (2021). *Systematic approaches to a successful literature review* (3rd ed.). Sage.

Booth, A., Sutton, A., & Papaioannou, D. (2016). *Systematic approaches to a successful literature review* (2nd ed.). Sage.

Bramer, W. M., De Jonge, G. B., Rethlefsen, M. L., Mast, F., & Kleijnen, J. (2018). A systematic approach to searching: An efficient and complete method to develop literature searches. *Journal of the Medical Library Association, 106*(4), 531.

Britannica. (2021, Dec. 4). George Boole. *Encyclopedia Britannica*. https://www.britannica.com/biography/George-Boole

DiCenso, A., Bayley, L., & Haynes, R. B. (2009). Accessing pre-appraised evidence: Fine-tuning the 5S model into a 6S model. *Evidence-Based Nursing, 12*(4), 99–101.

Feng, Y., Liang, S., Zhang, Y., Chen, S., Wang, Q., Huang, T., Sun, F., Liu, X., Zhu, H., & Pan, H. (2022). Automated medical literature screening using artificial intelligence: A systematic review and meta-analysis. *Journal of the American Medical Informatics Association, 29*(8), 1425–1432.

Gartlehner, G., Affengruber, L., Titscher, V., Noel-Storr, A., Dooley, G., Ballarini, N., & König, F. (2020). Single-reviewer abstract screening missed 13 percent of relevant studies: A crowd-based, randomized controlled trial. *Journal of Clinical Epidemiology, 121*, 20–28.

Gluck, J. C. (2020). How searches fail: Cognitive bias in literature searching. *Journal of Hospital Librarianship, 20*(1), 27–37. https://doi.org/10.1080/15323269.2020.1702839

Gwon, Y. N., Kim, J. H., Chung, H. S., Jung, E. J., Chun, J., Lee, S., & Shim, S. R. (2024). The use of generative AI for scientific literature searches for systematic reviews: ChatGPT and Microsoft Bing AI performance evaluation. *JMIR Medical Informatics, 12*, e51187.

Henrikson, N. B., & Blasi, P. R. (2023). Rapid evidence synthesis: A toolkit for finding and summarizing evidence on short timelines. *Implementation Science Methods*. https://impscimethods.org/application/files/3316/9705/5659/ImpSci_Methods-Toolkit_Rapid-Evidence-Synthesis.pdf

Lawless, J., & Foster, M. J. (2020). Searching systematically and comprehensively. In C. E. Toronto & R. Remington (Eds.), *A step-by-step guide to conducting an integrative review* (pp. 21–44). Springer.

Lefebvre, C., Glanville, J., Briscoe, S., Featherstone, R., Littlewood, A., Metzendorf, M-I., Noel-Storr, A., Paynter, R., Rader, T., Thomas, J., & Wieland, L. S. (2023, October). Searching for and selecting studies. In J. P. T. Higgin & J. Thomas (Senior Eds.), *Cochrane handbook for systematic reviews of interventions*, (Ed. 6.4., Sec. 2 Ch. 4). www.training.cochrane.org/handbook

Mateen, F., Oh, J., Tergas, A., Bhayani, N., & Kamdar, B. (2013). Titles versus titles and abstracts for initial screening of articles for systematic reviews. *Clinical Epidemiology, 5*(1), 89–95. https://doi.org/10.2147/CLEP.S43118

McCulley, C., & Jones, M. (2014). Fostering RN-to-BSN students' confidence in searching online for scholarly information on evidence-based practice. *The Journal of Continuing Education in Nursing, 45*(1), 22–27. http://dx.doi.org/10.3928/00220124-20131223-01

McDonagh, M., Peterson, K., Raina, P., Chang, S., & Shekelle, P. (2013). Avoiding bias in selecting studies. In *Methods guide for effectiveness and comparative effectiveness reviews.* Agency for Healthcare Research and Quality. https://www.ncbi.nlm.nih.gov/books/NBK126701/

Medical Library Association. (2024). *Explore a career in health sciences information.* https://www.mlanet.org/page/explore-this-career

Morrison, A., Polisena, J., Husereau, D., Moulton, K., Clark, M., Fiander, M., Mierzwinski-Urban, M., Clifford, T., Hutton, B., & Rabb, D. (2012). The effect of English-language restriction on systematic review-based meta-analyses: A systematic review of empirical studies. *International Journal of Technology Assessment in Health Care, 28*(2), 138–144.

Polanin, J. R., Pigott, T. D., Espelage, D. L., & Grotpeter, J. K. (2019). Best practice guidelines for abstract screening large-evidence systematic reviews and meta-analyses. *Research Synthesis Methods, 10*(3), 330–342. https://doi.org/10.1002/jrsm.1354

Polit, D., & Beck, C. (2021). *Nursing research: Generating and assessing evidence for nursing practice* (11th ed.). Wolters Kluwer.

Truex, E. S., Spinner, E., Hillyer, J., Ettien, A., Wade, S., Calhoun, C., Wolf, G., Hedreen, R., Heimlich, L., Nickum, A., & Vonderheid, S. (2022). Exploring the use of common strict search criteria in nursing literature searches. *Nurse Educator, 48*(4), 182–186. https://doi.org/10.1097/NNE.0000000000001353

Wagner, G., Lukyanenko, R., & Paré, G. (2022). Artificial intelligence and the conduct of literature reviews. *Journal of Information Technology, 37*(2), 209–226.

Welsh, T., & Wright, M. (2010). *Information literacy in the digital age: An evidence-based approach.* Elsevier.

Whittemore, R., & Knafl, K. (2005). The integrative review: Updated methodology. *Journal of Advanced Nursing, 52*(5), 546–553.

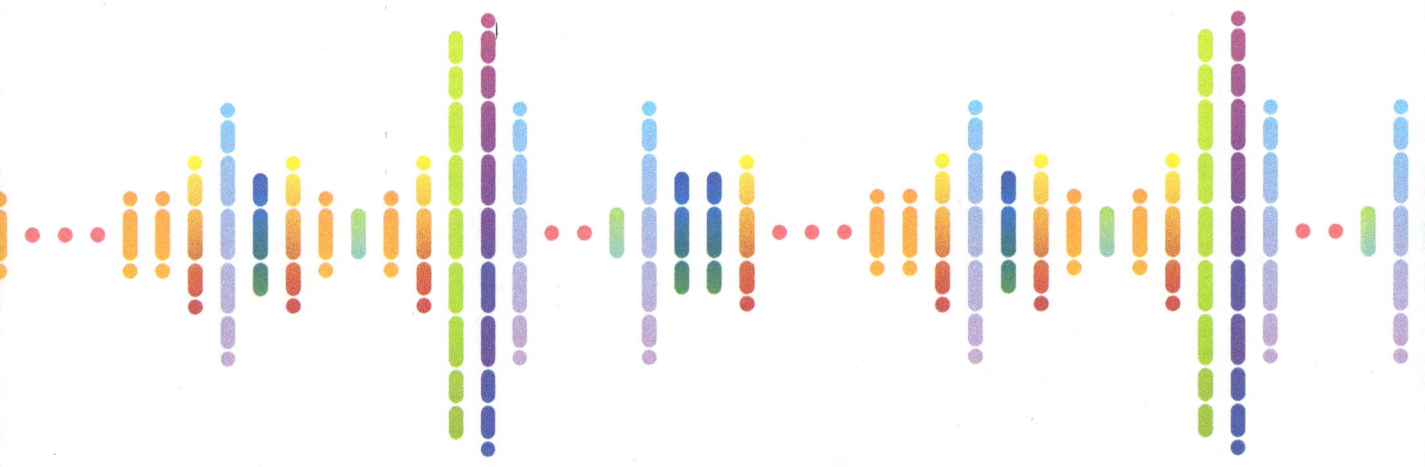

OBJECTIVES

- Discuss the purpose and fundamental components of evidence appraisal in the Johns Hopkins Evidence-Based Practice (JHEBP) model, including determining the level of support for decision-making and quality

- Review specific evidence appraisal action items for each type of evidence

- Discuss suitability considerations for pre-appraised evidence

- Describe single study designs and how they contribute to support for decision-making

8

EVIDENCE PHASE: APPRAISING THE EVIDENCE

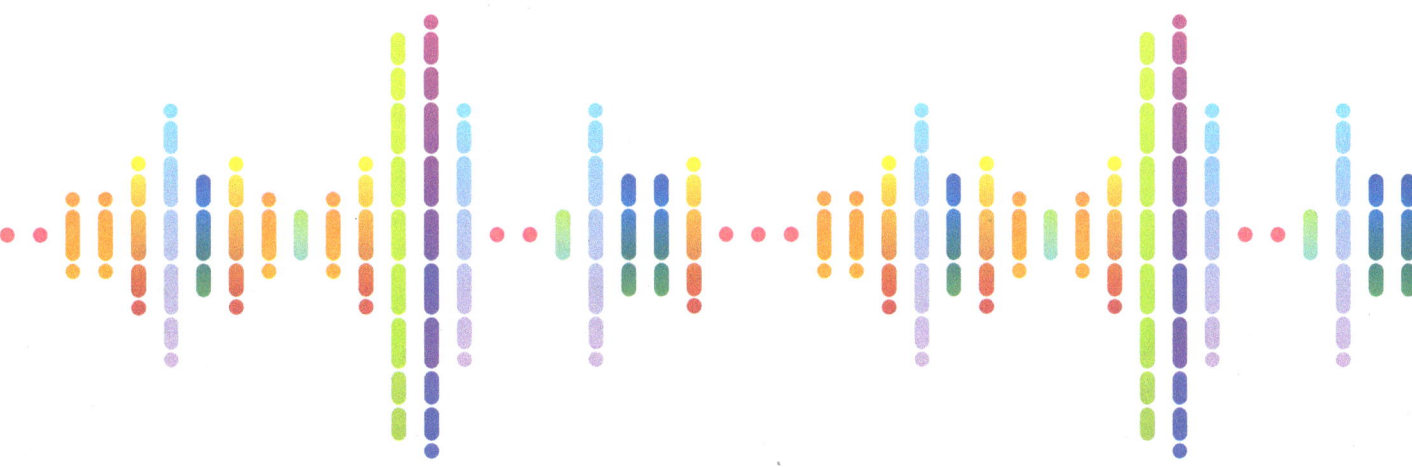

KEY POINTS

The evidence phase contains seven steps. This chapter discusses Step 6 (see Box 8.1). The JHEBP Appraisal Tool Selection Algorithm (Appendix D), Pre-appraised Evidence Appraisal Tool (Appendix E1), Single Study Evidence Appraisal Tool (Appendix E2), Anecdotal Evidence Appraisal Tool (Appendix E3), and Evidence Terminology and Considerations Guide (Appendix F) facilitate these steps.

- The appraisal process consists of determining the level of support for decision-making provided by evidence and assessing the quality of that evidence to ensure it is adequate.

- The specific action items of the process will vary depending on the type of evidence the team is appraising.

- Pre-appraised evidence requires a suitability assessment and a quality assessment.

- Single studies with a formal study design require an assessment of the design to determine the level of support for decision-making, followed by a quality assessment.

- Anecdotal evidence requires a quality assessment.

> **BOX 8.1** **STEPS IN THE EVIDENCE PHASE: THE E IN THE PET PROCESS**
>
> 4. Conduct best-evidence search and appraisal
> 5. Conduct targeted evidence search or conduct exhaustive search and screening
> 6. **Appraise the evidence**
> 7. Summarize the evidence
> 8. Organize the data
> 9. Synthesize the findings
> 10. Record best-practice recommendations

INTRODUCTION

Once the evidence-based practice (EBP) team has gathered all pertinent evidence through a structured search process, they need to assess that information to determine how it can contribute to answering their EBP question through a formal appraisal process. In the JHEBP model, this appraisal process is facilitated by a series of decision trees, tables, and checklists that provide systematic guidance to help the EBP team to determine if and how they should use each piece of gathered evidence.

> **NOTE**
>
> The bolded terms throughout the chapter are defined and discussed in the Evidence Terminology and Considerations Guide (Appendix F).

OVERVIEW OF THE APPRAISAL PROCESS

In the JHEBP model, the appraisal process has two fundamental components: 1) determine the level of support for decision-making, and 2) assess the quality of evidence to ensure it is adequate. These two assessments will tell the team if and how the evidence can influence decisions to change practice. Specific action items will vary for each type of evidence and are discussed below. See Figure 8.1 for an overview of the process.

Like the screening process, it is best practice to have at least two people independently review each article and then meet to establish a consensus on the level of support for decision-making and quality. Note that during any part of these steps, the EBP team may realize the evidence does not answer their EBP question or meets the exclusion criteria established in Step 5 and should be set aside. To be responsible consumers and critics of evidence, the EBP team needs a basic understanding of research methods and study design.

> **TIP**
>
> Many professionals devote years to understanding study design, research, and research methodologies. The information covered in this chapter should be considered a basic introduction to concepts related to research and other types of evidence. For more in-depth information, refer to a research text, organizational training, or mentorship resources.

> **NOTE**
>
> **QUALITY ASSESSMENT & RISK OF BIAS ASSESSMENT**
>
> The terms *quality assessment* and *risk of bias assessment* are often used interchangeably in the literature. While both address the efforts (or "safeguards") teams take in the design, conduct, and analysis of a study to ensure the findings are valid and reliable, quality assessment evaluates the inclusion of these efforts, and risk of bias evaluates their implications for the study results. In other words, quality assessment refers to efforts to avoid systematic errors, and risk of bias refers to how study flaws impact results. Quality assessments can be used to produce a judgment on the risk of bias (Banzi et al., 2018; Furuya-Kanamori et al., 2021).

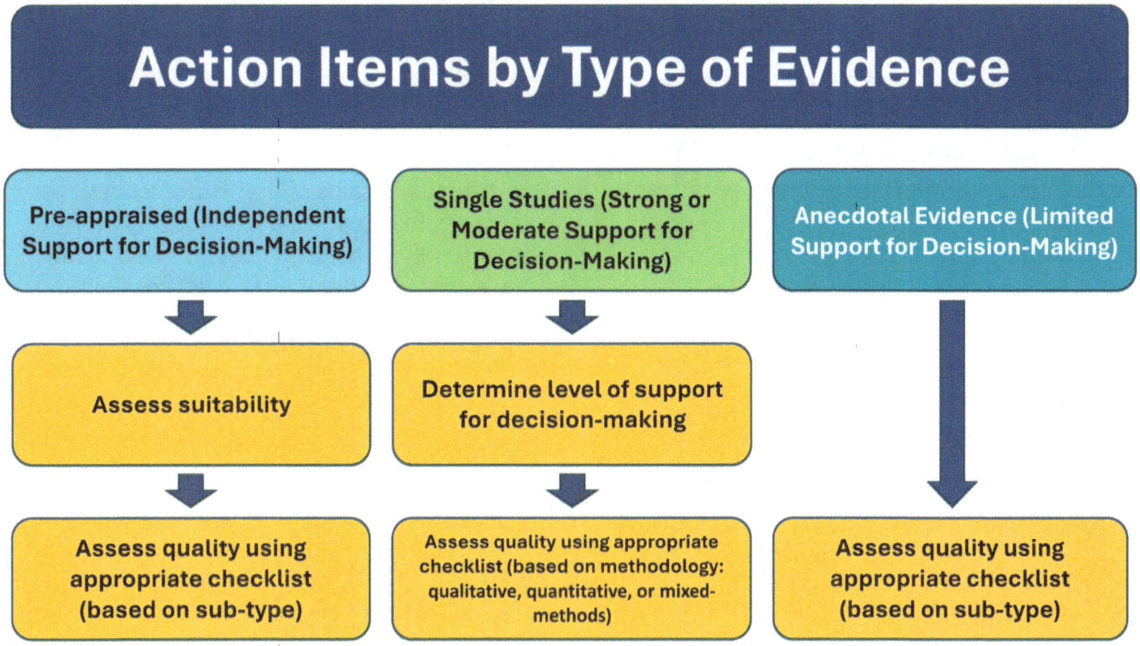

Action Items by Type of Evidence

Pre-appraised (Independent Support for Decision-Making) → Assess suitability → Assess quality using appropriate checklist (based on sub-type)

Single Studies (Strong or Moderate Support for Decision-Making) → Determine level of support for decision-making → Assess quality using appropriate checklist (based on methodology: qualitative, quantitative, or mixed-methods)

Anecdotal Evidence (Limited Support for Decision-Making) → Assess quality using appropriate checklist (based on sub-type)

FIGURE 8.1 Overview of the evidence appraisal process.

Level of Support for Decision-Making

The level of support for decision-making is determined by the type of evidence and for strong and moderate support, the details of the study design. See Table 8.1 for a summary of levels of support for decision-making and associated designs.

Quality Appraisal

The level of support that evidence can provide for decision-making only holds true if the quality of the information is sufficient. To determine this, the EBP team conducts a quality appraisal of all evidence to critique not only how well a study or project was executed but also how well it was

TABLE 8.1 Levels of Support for Decision-Making and Associated Designs

TYPE OF EVIDENCE	LEVEL OF SUPPORT FOR DECISION-MAKING	DESIGN
Pre-appraised	Independent	N/A
Single studies with a formal study design	Strong	**Controlled** trials with or without **randomization**
	Moderate	Interventional studies without **control** or **randomization** and observational designs
Anecdotal	Limited	N/A

reported. Like many other EBP models, in the JHEBP model, this is facilitated by a checklist for each type of evidence (the Pre-appraised Evidence, Single Study Evidence, and Anecdotal Evidence Appraisal Tools; Appendices E1, E2, and E3). The Appraisal Tool Selection Algorithm (Appendix D) aids the team in selecting the correct appendix. These tools have a series of "yes" or "no" questions to aid in critically evaluating the article. It is important to note that there is not a predetermined number of "yes" or "no" responses to establish quality. These are rather a list of items to consider for specific evidence the team is reviewing. The process is subjective and should be based on individual review followed by team discussion. The ultimate goal is to determine if the evidence is of sound quality and should be included or is too flawed and should be excluded. If included, the team should complete the data collection tool on the first page of the tool to gather pertinent information for the subsequent steps of the EBP process (evidence summary). If excluded, the EBP team should note that the article has been omitted and do not need to perform further evaluation.

> **NOTE**
>
> **WHAT IS EQUATOR?**
>
> The Enhancing the QUAlity and Transparency Of health Research (EQUATOR) network (https://www.equator-network.org) is a repository of reporting guidelines organized by study type. These guidelines provide a road map for the required steps to conduct and report a robust study. While ideally authors are using standard reporting guidelines, the degree to which journals demand adherence to these standards varies. Regardless of the specifics of the report, classic elements of published research include *title, abstract, introduction, method, results, discussion,* and *conclusion* (Hall, 2012).

All tools, definitions, and related quality considerations are indexed in the Evidence Terminology and Considerations Guide (Appendix F).

> **NOTE**
>
> In previous versions of the JHEBP model, the team would determine a letter quality rating (A, B, or C). Now, the team does not need to rank the evidence in these three categories but rather only decide if it is of sufficient quality to inform their EBP project. If the quality is adequate, it is included, and if it is inadequate, the article is excluded.

APPRAISAL PROCESS BY TYPE OF EVIDENCE

Pre-appraised Evidence (Independent Support for Decision-Making)

As discussed in Chapter 6, pre-appraised evidence, also known as *filtered* or *secondary* literature, is a group of individual studies that has undergone critical evaluation (filtering) by a team of investigators to ensure both quality and representation of the most rigorous research methods (DiCenso, 2009; Polit & Beck, 2021). The team should always confirm that their article, report, or guidelines meet the requirements of pre-appraised evidence. See Chapter 6 for more information about the sub-types of pre-appraised evidence (**clinical practice guidelines, (CPGs) literature reviews with a systematic approach (LRSAs),** and **evidence summaries**).

Although the evidence is pre-appraised, the EBP team still conducts their own assessment of how the literature was generated and reported. To complete the appraisal process, the EBP team uses the JHEBP Pre-appraised Evidence Appraisal Tool (Appendix E1) to evaluate two key aspects: 1) the suitability to their EBP question, and 2) its quality. This serves as a final "filter" before translation to the team's setting. If the evidence is deemed suitable and to be of adequate quality, the evidence can be used as independent support for decision-making. The EBP team then should conduct a search for any new evidence that has come out since the original publication (see the decision tree in the "Overview of the Evidence Phase" section in Chapter 6). If the evidence is unsuitable or of inadequate quality, the EBP team will continue with an exhaustive literature search (see Chapter 7).

> **NOTE**
>
> The EBP team does not need to do a deep dive regarding the designs of the individual studies included in the pre-appraised evidence because the associated findings should be based on the authors' own critical evaluation schema. This should result in recommendations or guidance provided with a level of certainty, confidence, or strength. The EBP team should consider these when translating the information to address their EBP problem.

Action Item 1: Determine the Suitability of the Evidence for the Team's EBP Question

Section I of the Pre-appraised Evidence Appraisal Tool (Appendix E1) contains a series of questions to help the EBP team determine if their evidence is recent enough (the age of the evidence) and is the same, or similar enough, to their topic of interest or intervention, population, setting, and, if applicable, outcomes to be a reasonable solution to their EBP problem. All these considerations are subjective, and there is not a single "correct" answer; however, the EBP team should provide a rationale for any decisions.

Age of Evidence

During the EBP process, teams often question how recent a literature review needs to be for it to be considered "recent enough." While five years is a common threshold, this is an arbitrary cutoff, and the team should evaluate their topic to determine whether the practice change should be informed by older (especially seminal) work. Some information suggests that 10–15 years provides an optimal balance between the quantity of information and time considerations (Furuya-Kanamore, 2023; Xu, 2022). Topics that are quickly changing (e.g., technology) or have a large amount of new information emerging (e.g., COVID-19) will need to be much more recent than more static topics (e.g., location of peripheral IV placement) or those that do not have significant new research or publication (e.g., Benner's Novice to Expert model). For example, five years may be too broad a range for a question related to artificial intelligence but too narrow for a question related to electronic health records. A couple of other things to keep in mind include:

- Do not identify the year the pre-appraised evidence was published but rather the year the search was conducted. This will likely push back how recent the evidence is by several years, and the team will need to make a judgment on whether important new information may have become available in the interim.

- Older citations in the reference list are not necessarily a red flag for an outdated review. References that are highly impactful or foundational to the topic can and should be included to establish the background for a topic. See **current literature** in the Evidence Terminology and Considerations Guide (Appendix F).

Topic, Population, Setting, and Outcomes

When writing their EBP question, the team identified the specifics of their topic, including who the group of interest is (population), where any solution would need to be implemented (setting), and, if applicable, why the group is undertaking the project (outcomes). These elements should be compared to the details provided in the pre-appraised evidence to ensure that they cover the same concepts or could be reasonably translated from one to the other. Often, the EBP team will need to do a deep dive into the methods of included evidence, often described in the form of a table and supplemental documents. See Tables 8.2 and 8.3 for examples of evaluating the suitability to the practice question.

TABLE 8.2 Example #1 of Suitability Evaluation

EBP QUESTION: *According to the literature, does the use of individualized audit and feedback report tools for nurses improve compliance, adherence, and/or performance of nursing tasks?*

SUITABILITY CONSIDERATION	EBP TEAM'S ELEMENTS OF INTEREST	PRE-APPRAISED EVIDENCE (COCHRANE SYSTEMATIC REVIEW) ELEMENTS OF INTEREST	SUITABILITY DECISION AND RATIONALE
Age of evidence	Project initiated in 2019	Search conducted in 2010	Not suitable—not recent enough. With the rapid expansion and integration of the electronic health record, the 2010 search did not reflect current practice. Most included studies used audit and feedback done by hand.
Topic or intervention	Individualized audit and feedback	Individualized audit and feedback	Suitable—only evidence that included healthcare provider-level, formal feedback was included in the systematic review. This matched the EBP team's exact topic of interest.
Population	Nurses	Various healthcare professionals, including doctors, nurses, and pharmacists	Not suitable—population not similar enough. Of the 140 included studies, only 16 included nurses (11.4%). As financial compensation is often tied to audit and feedback provided to physicians, their successes may not be applicable to nurses.
Setting	Not specified	Not specified	Suitable—all settings were included in the EBP team's question.
Outcomes	Compliance, adherence, performance of nursing tasks	Large variation, included compliance with guidelines, professional practice	Suitable—many types of outcomes included. Of note, the EBP question was updated throughout the process to reflect outcomes available in the literature.

FINAL DECISION: ***Not suitable.*** *Not recent enough; populations not similar enough for a meaningful comparison. Complete exhaustive literature search.*

(Ivers et al., 2012; Whalen et al., 2021)

TABLE 8.3 Example #2 of Suitability Evaluation

EBP QUESTION: *According to the evidence, what are best nursing practices to prevent pressure injuries (PIs) in patients in the medical intensive care unit (MICU)?*

SUITABILITY CONSIDERATION	EBP TEAM'S ELEMENTS OF INTEREST	PRE-APPRAISED EVIDENCE (CLINICAL PRACTICE GUIDELINE) ELEMENTS OF INTEREST	SUITABILITY DECISION AND RATIONALE
Age of evidence	Project initiated in 2016	Search conducted in 2013	Suitable—conducted in the three years prior to project start; no major changes in the topic of pressure injuries in the interim.
Topic or intervention	Prevention of PIs	Prevention and treatment of PIs included	Suitable—50 recommendations related to prevention, and 130 related to prevention and treatment.
Population	Critically ill patients	Intended for all patients; special guidance for critically ill individuals	Suitable—general guidance given as well as special considerations for critically ill patients (20 of the 575 recommendations).
Setting	MICU	Intended for all clinical settings; no search limitations on setting	Suitable—recommendations are intended for all clinical settings, including the MICU.
Outcomes	N/A	N/A	N/A

FINAL DECISION: *Suitable. Recent and highly relevant to the topic, population, and setting. Translate to the team's setting, including use of organizational approaches to education.*

(Aquino et al., 2019; Haesler et al., 2016; National Pressure Ulcer Advisory Panel et al., 2014)

TIP

It is possible that a singular pre-appraised resource will not provide sufficient information for the comprehensive and informed implementation of a practice change. In this case, the team should formulate additional EBP questions to gather evidence related to putting a practice change into action. For example, pre-appraised evidence may indicate that the best practice for screening for depression in adults in the outpatient setting is the use of the Patient Health Questionnaire (PHQ)-2. The EBP team decides to adopt the change but needs further information on educating staff on its use as well as how to follow up with patients who screen positive. This generates a second and third question that require additional investigation.

If the evidence is suitable and answers all aspects of the EBP question, after ensuring quality (Action Item 2), the EBP team may be able to move forward with this as independent support for decision-making. If the evidence is relevant but only addresses some elements of the EBP question, this evidence is not independently actionable. However, it may still be value-added to addressing the practice problem and provide strong support for decision-making. The EBP team should conduct a quality assessment and continue on the exhaustive evidence search path (see the decision tree in the "Overview of the Evidence Phase" section in Chapter 6).

Action Item 2: Appraise the Quality of the Evidence

The general approach to quality appraisal is described in the "Quality Appraisal" section earlier in the chapter. Specifically, to conduct the assessment for pre-appraised evidence, the team will need to determine the sub-type of evidence they have (CPG, LRSA, or evidence summary) and use the corresponding checklist in Section II of the Pre-appraised Evidence Appraisal Tool (Appendix E1) to examine evidence-specific quality considerations.

> **TIP**
>
> **RESEARCHING METHODOLOGY**
>
> Frequently, evidence summaries, and occasionally clinical practice guidelines, follow a rigorous approach but do not publish the methods within the main document. This is usually to provide succinct, actionable information that is accessible to frontline clinicians. The EBP team should look closely at the evidence and may need to visit the organization's website to learn more about its process of generating appraisals of evidence.

Single Studies With a Formal Study Design (Strong or Moderate Support for Decision-Making)

As described in Chapter 6, single studies with a formal study design use systematic inquiry to answer questions or solve problems (Polit & Beck, 2021). Reports are written by an author or team of authors and recount their scientific or clinical experience. See Chapter 6 for more information on approaches to generating single studies.

Single studies require a different appraisal process than pre-appraised evidence. The applicability to the EBP question was assessed during the screening phase (Step 5). In Step 6, the team uses the Single Study Evidence Appraisal Tool (Appendix E2) to 1) determine the design and associated level of support for decision-making and 2) appraise the quality.

Action Item 1: Determine the Design and Associated Level of Support for Decision-Making

Levels of support for decision-making for single studies are determined by the design. The design is the overall plan or blueprint for the planning and conducting of a study. It outlines the strategy logically and effectively answers the research or clinical question (Creswell, 2014). The Single Study Evidence Appraisal Tool (Appendix E2) includes a decision tree to help the team make this determination.

> **NOTE**
>
> There are many terms to describe study designs and different ways to group or categorize the approaches (Hulme, 2021). Likewise, some terms are not mutually exclusive (meaning they can overlap, interrelate, or co-exist). The information that follows is not meant to comprehensively define all study designs but rather help the EBP team assess the evidence and provide justification for each level of support.

Controlled Trials With or Without Randomization (Strong Support for Decision-Making) Controlled trials with or without **randomization** provide strong support for decision-making because researchers produce sound information about cause-and-effect relationships between two or more variables by introducing an **intervention** under controlled conditions. These studies are defined by the manipulation of an **independent variable** within one group and comparing an outcome of interest (**dependent variable**) with a control group. Findings are likely due only to the intervention introduced by the study team and not by other **confounding** factors.

In the case of **randomized control trials (RCTs)**, participants are **randomly** assigned to the control or intervention group. RCTs are considered true experimental studies and the gold standard for establishing **causation**. However, they are not always feasible or ethical (Polit & Beck, 2021). Control trials without randomization are considered **quasi-experimental** studies and can be used to establish causal relationships but are not as compelling as true experiments.

Data is usually gathered and analyzed using **quantitative** methods; however, **mixed-methods** approaches can also be used (Polit & Beck, 2021; Ranganathan & Aggarwal, 2018).

See Table 8.4 for terms frequently associated with this study design.

For the EBP team to determine if they have evidence that falls in this category, they should ask:

- Was there a formal study design?
- Did the study team introduce an intervention (i.e., did they do something)?
- Was there a **control** group (a group that did not get the intervention but is otherwise similar to the group that did)?

If the answer is "yes" to all of the above questions, this is a controlled trial with or without randomization and strong support for decision-making.

Interventional Studies Without Control or Randomization and Observational Designs (Moderate Support for Decision-Making) Interventional studies without **control** groups or **randomization** and observational designs provide only moderate support for practice change because they cannot establish cause and effect. Rather, these studies describe characteristics of a group or suggest relationships (**correlations**) between variables without determining a causal relationship (Gray & Grove, 2021a; Ranganathan & Aggarwal, 2018).

See Table 8.4 for terms frequently associated with this type of evidence.

Interventional Studies Without Control or Randomization Interventional studies without **control** or **randomization** include **manipulation** of a **variable** but do not have an equivalent comparison group (control group) that does not receive the intervention, and participants self-select for the intervention (instead of random assignment by the study team). In other words, the study team intervenes ("does something") but does not have a group to benchmark against and doesn't decide who receives the treatment, care, or other service. These designs are also considered quasi-experimental and can use **qualitative**, **quantitative**, or **mixed-methods** approaches (Gray & Grove, 2021a; Polit & Beck, 2021).

Observational Studies In observational studies, also called *non-interventional* and *non-experimental*, the study team does not actively intervene because it is not possible, practical, or ethical to manipulate a variable of interest (e.g., birth weight, height, congenital conditions, introduction of a toxin or known carcinogen, long-term exposure to known risk; Gray & Grove, 2021b; Polit & Beck, 2021; Ranganathan & Aggarwal, 2018). In these studies, an **independent variable** of interest may already be decided naturally or by other factors (e.g., lung cancer in people exposed to secondhand smoke; Polit & Beck, 2021; Ranganathan & Aggarwal, 2018). Data can be collected in a **longitudinal** (over a longer period of time) or **cross-sectional** (one time, provides a "snapshot") way (Gray & Grove, 2021b). There are two types of observational studies: 1) **observational analytic** (sometimes called *inferential*) and 2) **descriptive**.

TABLE 8.4. Study Designs and Frequently Associated Terms

STUDY DESIGN	TERMS FREQUENTLY ASSOCIATED WITH THIS TYPE OF DESIGN
Control trials with and without randomization	**Randomized control trial** Cluster randomized control trial Comparative effectiveness research Clinical trial Cross-over
Interventional studies without control or randomization	Time series design Pretest/posttest
Observational (analytic and descriptive)	**Case-control** Cohort Predictive modeling Tool validation **Descriptive** **Correlational** Case series **Prevalence** Natural experiment **Retrospective** Phenomenology Ethnography Grounded theory Focus group Thematic

Observational analytic designs Observational analytic designs analyze or suggest relationships between **variables** that occur naturally and generally use **quantitative** methods (Centre for Evidence-Based Medicine, 2016; Ranganathan & Aggarwal, 2018). These are common in the field of epidemiology and seek to examine the changes that occur over time related to an exposure and **incidence** or **prevalence** of disease (Gray & Grove, 2021b).

Descriptive designs **Descriptive** studies describe the characteristics of a single group or **phenomenon** or compare one group to another (Centre for Evidence-Based Medicine, 2016). The purpose is to "observe, describe and document a situation as it naturally occurs" (Polit & Beck, 2021, p. 196). This can be done using **quantitative, qualitative,** or **mixed-methods** approaches.

For the EBP team to determine if they have evidence that falls in this category, they should ask:

- Was there a formal study design?

- Did the study team describe something that was happening naturally (without their intervention or interference) or did the study team intervene (do something) but without a **control** group?

If the answer is "yes" to both of the above questions, this is an interventional study without randomization or control or it's observational and provides moderate support for decision-making.

Action Item 2: Appraise the Quality of Evidence

The general approach to quality appraisal is described in the "Quality Appraisal" section earlier in the chapter. After determining the design and associated level of support for decision-making, the team will need to determine if the study used a **qualitative, quantitative,** or **mixed-methods** approach in order to fill out the correct quality checklist on the Single Study Evidence Appraisal Tool (Appendix E2). See Chapter 6 for more information on qualitative, quantitative, and mixed-methods approaches.

Anecdotal Evidence (Limited Support for Decision-Making)

As discussed in Chapter 6, anecdotal evidence is not based on research or a formal study design but rather a less structured account of an experience or opinion. This type of evidence provides limited support for decision-making because it includes a high level of **bias** introduced by the authors and lacks the rigor of scientific methods. Anecdotal evidence cannot establish causal or **correlational** relationships but may be helpful for providing background information or when there is limited investigation into a topic. This evidence can be **peer-reviewed** or come from **gray literature** sources.

For the EBP team to determine if they have evidence that falls in this category, they should ask: Was there a formal study design? If the answer is "no" to this question, this is anecdotal evidence and provides limited support for decision-making.

Action Item 1: Quality Assessment

The general approach to quality appraisal is described above. Specifically, to conduct the assessment for anecdotal evidence, the team needs to determine the sub-type of evidence they have (expert opinion, book chapter, position statement, case report, programmatic experience, literature reviews without a systematic approach, etc.) and use the corresponding checklist on the Anecdotal Evidence Appraisal Tool (Appendix E3). This will provide them with the relevant considerations for each iteration of this type of evidence.

SUMMARY

This chapter describes the process for determining if and how evidence can inform an EBP team's decision-making. It outlines the overall purpose and methodology of the appraisal process, emphasizing special considerations for each type of evidence. These steps ensure that the team advances with sound evidence in an efficient manner, preparing them for the subsequent steps of summarizing, synthesizing, and generating best-evidence recommendations.

REFERENCES

Aquino, C., Owen, A., Predicce, A., Poe, S., & Kozachik, S. (2019). Increasing competence in pressure injury prevention using competency-based education in adult intensive care unit. *Journal of Nursing Care Quality, 34*(4), 312–317. https://doi.org/10.1097/NCQ.0000000000000388

Banzi, R., Cinquini, M., Gonzalez-Lorenzo, M., Pecoraro, V., Capobussi, M., & Minozzi, S. (2018, July). Quality assessment versus risk of bias in systematic reviews: AMSTAR and ROBIS had similar reliability but differed in their construct and applicability. *Journal of Clinical Epidemiology, 99*, 24–32. https://doi.org/10.1016/j.jclinepi.2018.02.024

Centre for Evidence-Based Medicine. (2016). *Study designs*. https://www.cebm.net/2014/04/study-designs/

Creswell, J. W. (2014). *Research design: Qualitative, quantitative, and mixed methods approaches* (4th ed.). Sage.

DiCenso, A., Bayley, L., & Haynes, R. B. (2009). Accessing pre-appraised evidence: Fine-tuning the 5S model into a 6S model. *Evidence-Based Nursing, 12*(4), 99–101.

Furuya-Kanamori, L., Lin, L., Kostoulas, P., Clark, J., & Xu, C. (2023). Limits in the search date for rapid reviews of diagnostic test accuracy studies. *Research Synthesis Methods, 14*(2), 173–179. https://doi.org/10.1002/jrsm.1598

Furuya-Kanamori, L., Xu, C., Hasan, S. S., & Doi, S. A. (2021). Quality versus risk-of-bias assessment in clinical research. *Journal of Clinical Epidemiology, 129*, 172–175.

Gray, J., & Grove, S. K. (2021a). Quantitative methodology: Interventional designs and methods. In J. Gray & S. K. Grove (Eds.), *Burns and Grove's the practice of nursing research* (9th ed., pp. 261–313). Elsevier.

Gray, J., & Grove, S. K. (2021b). Quantitative methodology: Noninterventional designs and methods. In J. Gray & S. K. Grove (Eds.), *Burns and Grove's the practice of nursing research* (9th ed., pp. 234–260). Elsevier.

Haesler, E., Kottner, J., Cuddigan, J., & 2014 International Guideline Development Group. (2016). The 2014 international pressure ulcer guideline: Methods and development. *Journal of Advanced Nursing, 73*(6), 1515–1530. https://doi.org/10.1111/jan.13241

Hall, G. M. (Ed.). (2012). *How to write a paper*. Wiley.

Hulme, P. (2021). Introduction to quantitative research. In J. Gray & S. K. Grove (Eds.), *Burns and Grove's the practice of nursing research* (9th ed., pp. 46–74). Elsevier.

Ivers, N., Jamtvedt, G., Flottorp, S., Young, J. M., Odgaard-Jensen, J., French, S. D., O'Brien, M. A., Johansen, M., Grimshaw, J., & Oxman, A. D. (2012). Audit and feedback: Effects on professional practice and healthcare outcomes. *Cochrane Database of Systematic Reviews, 6*(CD000259). https://doi.org/10.1002/14651858.CD000259.pub3

National Pressure Ulcer Advisory Panel, European Pressure Ulcer Advisory Panel, & Pan Pacific Pressure Injury Alliance. (2014). *Prevention and treatment of pressure ulcers: Quick reference guide* (2nd ed.). Cambridge Media. https://web.archive.org/web/20180424024843id_/http://www.npuap.org/wp-content/uploads/2014/08/Quick-Reference-Guide-DIGITAL-NPUAP-EPUAP-PPPIA-Jan2016.pdf

Polit, D., & Beck, C. (2021). *Nursing research: Generating and assessing evidence for nursing practice* (11th ed.). Wolters Kluwer.

Ranganathan, P., & Aggarwal, R. (2018). Study designs: Part 1 – An overview and classification. *Perspectives in Clinical Research, 9*(4), 184–186. https://doi.org/10.4103/picr.PICR_124_18

Whalen, M., Maliszewski, B., Gardner, H., & Smyth, S. (2021). Audit and feedback: An evidence-based practice literature review of nursing report cards. *Worldviews on Evidence-Based Nursing, 18*(3), 170–179.

Xu, C., Ju, K., Lin, L., Jia, P., Kwong, J. S. W., Syed, A., & Furuya-Kanamori, L. (2022). Rapid evidence synthesis approach for limits on the search date: How rapid could it be? *Research Synthesis Methods, 13*(1), 68–76. https://doi.org/10.1002/jrsm.1525

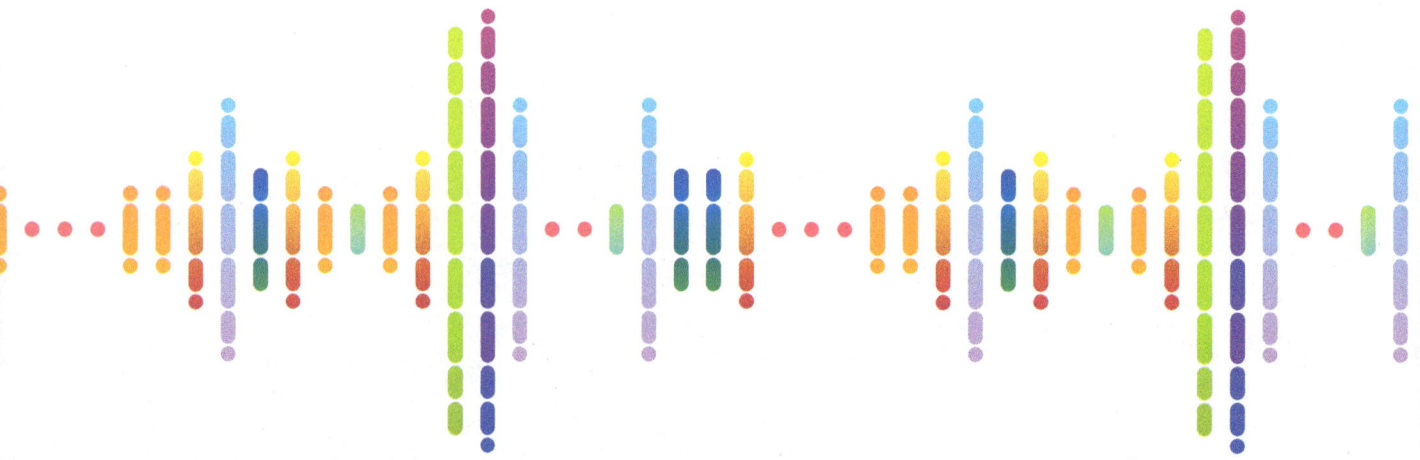

OBJECTIVES

- Define "summary" and "synthesis"

- Demonstrate understanding of the differences between summarizing and synthesizing literature

- Describe strategies to organize important information from the evidence to create greater meaning

- Explain the significance of the summary and synthesis steps in the overall context of a value-added EBP project

- State the process and purpose of establishing best-evidence recommendations based on the type of evidence the team has collected

9

EVIDENCE PHASE: SUMMARY, SYNTHESIS, AND BEST-EVIDENCE RECOMMENDATIONS

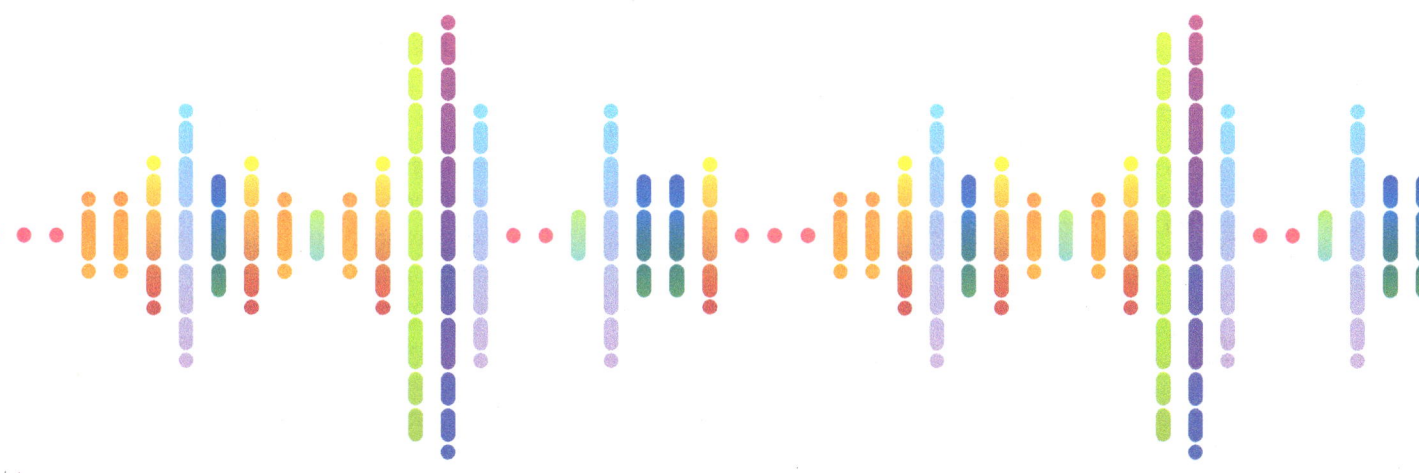

KEY POINTS

The evidence phase contains seven steps. This chapter provides an overview of Steps 7–10 (see Box 9.1). The Johns Hopkins Evidence-Based Practice (JHEBP) Best-Evidence Summary Tool (Appendix G1), Individual Evidence Summary Tool (Appendix G2), and Summary, Synthesis, & Best-Evidence Recommendations Tool (Appendix H) facilitate these steps.

- *Evidence summary* is the process of collating essential information from articles or reports into a central location. The EBP team uses a table with headers to provide pertinent data.

- Organizing or preparing the data from the evidence summary assists the team in conducting the next step of the process, evidence synthesis. This can be done with various visual and sorting tools.

- *Synthesis* is the process of creating greater meaning from the data provided by individual articles or reports.

- Synthesized evidence is used to generate best-evidence recommendations that answer the EBP question. Recommendations can be high, reasonable, reasonable-to-low, or low certainty.

> **BOX 9.1** STEPS IN THE EVIDENCE PHASE: THE E IN THE PET PROCESS
>
> 4. Conduct best-evidence search and appraisal
> 5. Conduct targeted evidence search or conduct exhaustive search and screening
> 6. Appraise the evidence
> 7. Summarize the evidence
> 8. Organize the data
> 9. Synthesize the findings
> 10. Record best-practice recommendations

INTRODUCTION

During the evidence phase of an EBP project, the EBP team not only needs to read and appraise all relevant evidence but also must begin to gather the information into a digestible form that lends itself to easy analysis and interpretation. The final steps of this phase include summarizing evidence, organizing the data, synthesizing findings, and developing best-practice recommendations. While all are interrelated, these are discrete steps that should build on one another and reflect an increasingly in-depth understanding of what literature means both independently and in a clinical context. One author refers to these steps as the "rule of rows and columns." The EBP team uses the "rule of rows" to compile information from each article in a table and the "rule of columns" to synthesize across the table of included evidence (Garrard, 2014).

Of note, these steps are meant to reflect the state of the evidence, and the EBP team does not yet consider their clinical context. These must be explicit and distinct processes because they form the foundation of eventual practice change recommendations for the team and possibly others with a similar clinical problem. Recording the objective findings from the evidence and the eventual best-evidence recommendations irrespective of the team's clinical environment allows other groups to confidently translate the recommendations to their own context and serves as a touchstone when the team's practice setting evolves.

EVIDENCE SUMMARY

Evidence summary, also known as *data tabulation*, is the process of collating essential information from articles or reports into a central location. Evidence summary does not involve drawing personal conclusions or opinions based on the literature. Rather, it is the process of extracting information, just as it is described in the source material, and collating it in a central document to lay the foundation for the next steps of an EBP project—organization, synthesis, best-evidence recommendations, and translation.

> **TIP**
>
> **HAVE CONTENT EXPERTS ON THE TEAM**
>
> It is important to have not only experts in the EBP process on a project team but also people who are highly knowledgeable regarding the content area. To promote accuracy and specificity, whenever possible, team members who have expertise in the topic at hand should complete the Evidence Summary Tools (Appendix G1 or G2). This ensures that information is relevant and meaningful to the end-users.

At this step, the EBP team has identified and evaluated literature either through a best-evidence and targeted search or an exhaustive search. The type of search and subsequent evidence collection from Steps 4, 5, and 6 will determine which tool the EBP team uses to complete the summary process. Best-evidence searches with pre-appraised evidence and supplementary literature use the Best-Evidence Summary Tool (Appendix G1). Exhaustive searches that have gathered pre-appraised evidence that doesn't fully answer the EBP question, single studies, and anecdotal evidence will use the Individual Evidence Summary Tool (Appendix G2). Regardless of the tool, the purpose and process are essentially the same.

The team completes this step by filling in the table on the tool using the prompts provided in the headers. This can be done during the literature appraisal process (while reading) or after all the articles have been reviewed. A single-row table with identical headers is provided on the appraisal tools to assist with collecting and compiling the information in real time. Each tool has a detailed set of instructions that provide further guidance on what data to include in each box. Of note, the EBP team can amend the evidence summary table to include headers that allow for a more thorough summary based on the scope of the EBP question. Consider brainstorming specific components of an intervention that would be helpful for designing implementation in the team setting; see Table 9.1 for an example.

As a continuation from the appraisal process, independent team members should also review and come to a consensus on the articles to be listed in the evidence summary (based on relevance and quality) and the pertinent information to include for each. Any discrepancies between reviewers must be resolved before the summary tool can be complete. The two reviewers should discuss the discrepancy and, if unable to resolve it, involve the EBP project leader for mediation (Li et al., 2023). Remember, any article that is considered inadequate quality should not be recorded in the Evidence Summary Tools.

Information included in the evidence summary should be accurate, complete, and accessible to all team members (Li et al., 2023). A robust evidence summary will include all necessary information to inform the EBP question without a simple restatement of the original source. For example, if only a small amount of a report applies to your EBP question, copying and pasting all the findings is not value-added. Inputting this information into a file-sharing software such as Google Forms, Microsoft Teams, or Covidence Systematic Review Software (Veritas Health Innovation, Melbourne, Australia) can help facilitate group review. Once all articles have been appraised and entered into the Evidence Summary Tools, the leader of the EBP project should plan to review, edit, and seek clarification on entries before moving on to the next step, organization.

SPECIAL CONSIDERATIONS FOR BEST-EVIDENCE SEARCHES WITH PRE-APPRAISED EVIDENCE

While the process and purpose of both versions of the Evidence Summary Tool are similar, there are several special considerations for the Best-Evidence Summary Tool (Appendix G1):

Depending on the comprehensiveness of the pre-appraised evidence and results of the targeted search, there may be as few as one entry in the tool.

The targeted search should focus only on evidence that provides strong and moderate support for decision-making. Only record evidence in Section II that is of sufficient quality and provides this level of support.

On the next tool, Summary, Synthesis, & Best-Evidence Recommendations Tool (Appendix H), skip to Section II.

TABLE 9.1 Examples of Additional Information in an Abbreviated Evidence Summary Table

EBP QUESTION: *According to the evidence, among pediatric patients in the critical care setting, what is the effect of music therapy on pain?*

AUTHOR, DATE, AND TITLE	TYPE OF EVIDENCE	POPULATION, SIZE, AND SETTING	INTERVENTION	FINDINGS THAT HELP ANSWER THE EBP QUESTION	MEASURES USED	SELECTION AND DELIVERY OF MUSIC	FREQUENCY AND DURATION OF MUSIC	MODE OF DELIVERY
Lombardi, 2021, "Music Therapy for Pediatric Pain"	Interventional study without control or randomization	Pediatric ICU, 20 beds, urban academic medical center in the Unites States	Recorded music therapy	Decreased pain reported in infants and school-age patients	Wong-Baker FACES Pain Rating Scale, r-FLACC, 0–10 pain scale	Patient selected for those able to participate over age 5; music therapist selected for those unable to participate and/or under age 5	Two times daily 20-minute sessions	Bluetooth speaker

ORGANIZATION/PREPARATION

Organization or preparation of the collated data involves sorting the information into various groups, clusters, or visual representations to aid the team in interpretation.

This step can occur during or after the data summary process to help the team understand the evidence for the next step, synthesis. Teams should always group and analyze evidence by level of support for decision-making (independent, strong, moderate, or limited). This is an essential step when preparing to synthesize the results of an exhaustive search on the Individual Evidence Summary Tool (Appendix G2) or a large amount of results from a targeted search in Section II of the Best-Evidence Summary Tool (Appendix G1).

Additionally, after reviewing and tabulating all the evidence, the team may have greater insights into the type of information available and can use other tactics to explore subtleties, such as sorting or assigning themes and labels. The team may want to compare specific aspects of each article side by side for more significant insights (e.g., perhaps the intervention worked well with students but not with post-licensure professionals, or audit and feedback improved performance with documentation but not performing a skill). The team may decide to analyze the evidence as a whole ("lumping") or break it into sub-groups ("splitting"; Booth et al., 2021). Splitting is a strategy to take a closer look at a population or intervention that was part of an EBP question that cast a wide net. This can be done within each level of support for decision-making or as a complete body of evidence. Finally, using data visualization tools such as color-coding themes, an evidence matrix, or a 2 x 2 table may also be helpful (see Tables 9.2 and 9.3 for examples; Booth et al., 2021; Efron & Ravid, 2018; Whittemore & Knafl, 2005).

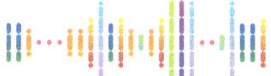

"Creativity and critical analysis of data and data displays are key elements in data comparison and the identification of important and accurate patterns and themes." (Whittemore & Knafl, 2005, p. 551)

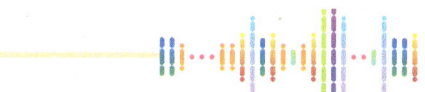

TABLE 9.2 Evidence Matrix Example of Included Populations

POPULATION INCLUDED	PATIENTS	VISITORS	STAFF
Liu et al., 2019	X	X	
Martinez & Young, 2020	X		X
Patel et al., 2021	X	X	
Johnson, 2020		X	
Baptiste et al., 2021		X	X

TABLE 9.3 Two by Two Table Example of the Effects of Gamification of Education

	HEALTHCARE STUDENTS	POST-LICENSURE HEALTHCARE WORKERS
Positive Effect	Henry & Williams, 2023 Rosenblum et al., 2020 Hawkins et al., 2021	Watson & AlJameel, 2019
No Effect or Negative Effect	Wills, 2020	Horton et al., 2019 Tschudin & Orem, 2018 Taylor et al., 2017 Baker & Chappell, 2022 Abron, 2020 Steinbrook et al., 2023

SYNTHESIS

Synthesis is the process of combining two or more elements to create a new idea or understanding, with the whole being greater than the sum of its parts. The basis of synthesis is pattern recognition, and specific strategies may include noting repetition and themes, clustering, counting, comparing and contrasting, exploring inconsistencies, and discerning common and unusual patterns. This means the literature synthesis is not a repetition of the data points in the Individual Evidence Summary Tool but rather the creation of an overall picture of the body of evidence. Synthesis generates new insights, perspectives, and understandings through group discussion and consensus building. Synthesis contains all the elements of summary, with greater context and connection, and is the opportunity to turn information into knowledge. See Table 9.4 for examples of information synthesis.

TABLE 9.4 Information Synthesis Examples

SUMMARY INFORMATION	SYNTHESIS
China, South Korea, Laos, Vietnam	A map of Asia
Nose, mouth, ears, eyes	A face
Birthday, you, to, happy, dear	The "Happy Birthday" song
Jersey, cleats, helmet, socks	An athletic uniform

> **NOTE**
>
> Traditionally, EBP projects use a narrative approach to this stage, which strives to "provide deep and 'rich' information . . . and seeks to remain faithful to the wholeness or integrity of the studies as a body while also preserving the idiosyncratic nature of individual studies" (Booth et al., 2016, p. 182). It is an iterative process and may require multiple passes to help the team truly glean everything the data has to offer. Just as determining a patient's diagnosis by synthesizing individual data points is an advanced skill for healthcare providers, so is interpreting individual evidence findings to determine how they contribute to answering the EBP question. Both require direct practice, experience, and critical thinking and benefit from mentorship.

Only EBP projects that used an exhaustive search and have gathered literature on the Individual Evidence Summary Tool (Appendix G2) will need to formally complete this step by filling out Section I of the Summary, Synthesis, & Best-Evidence Recommendations Tool (Appendix H). Of note, like the organization step, depending on the amount of information gathered from a targeted search to supplement pre-appraised evidence, the EBP team may benefit from synthesizing the information from collected individual studies to facilitate the next step, best-evidence recommendations. They can do so by annotating their entries in the Best-Evidence Summary Tool (Appendix G1).

> **TIP**
>
> **BE FLEXIBLE**
>
> Flexibility is key during this stage, as the team may need to undertake one approach and then re-analyze the evidence from a different perspective to have a true and complex understanding. Keep in mind that the team should approach the data from a standpoint of openness and curiosity. Remember that a lack of evidence or evidence that contradicts the proposed interventions is essential and should be explored and included in the final synthesis.

Action items for an exhaustive search with pre-appraised evidence that doesn't fully answer the EBP question, single studies, and anecdotal evidence are described here:

1. Review the Individual Evidence Summary Tool (Appendix G2) as a team to ensure all entries are complete and value-added. If needed, ask reviewers to clarify or update their article information.

2. Review the evidence that provides strong support for decision-making. Read the findings that help answer the EBP question and other important information. Annotate the table to help note patterns and themes.

3. Record the number of sources in the table.

4. As a group, discuss the pertinent findings.

5. In the "Strong Support for Decision-Making" row in Section I of the Summary, Synthesis, & Best-Evidence Recommendations Tool (Appendix H), record succinct statements that synthesize the information and help answer the EBP question. Note the author or assigned number of each article that supports the statement. In general, it is a good sign if you have multiple sources to support each statement.

6. Repeat Steps 2–5 for "Moderate" and "Limited Support" for decision-making.

7. As needed, analyze any additional evidence summary schema as described in the "Organization/Preparation" section earlier in the chapter and record the information in the provided extra table.

BEST-EVIDENCE RECOMMENDATIONS

Best-evidence recommendations are succinct statements, drawn from the synthesized evidence, that answer the practice question.

Generating the best-evidence recommendations is the final step of the evidence phase of the PET process and serves as the foundation for the next and final phase, translation. The team completes this step by filling out Section II of the Summary, Synthesis, & Best-Evidence Recommendations Tool (Appendix H). Many EBP questions will include multiple best-evidence recommendations with varying levels of support. Characterizing the individual recommendations, not the overall evidence, aids in determining specific best practices as well as interventions that do not have the requisite evidence to support moving forward with practice change. Recommendations can be put in one of four groups based on their characteristics:

- **High certainty recommendations:** Robust, well-documented, consistent, and persuasive evidence, based mostly on evidence that provides strong support for decision-making

- **Reasonable certainty recommendations:** Good, mostly compelling, consistent evidence, based mostly on evidence that provides moderate-to-strong support for decision-making

- **Reasonable-to-low certainty recommendations:** Good but conflicting evidence and inconsistent results, based mostly on evidence that provides moderate support for decision-making

- **Low certainty recommendations:** Little to no evidence; information is minimal, inconsistent, and/or based mostly on evidence that provides limited support for decision-making

Practice change can be based on recommendations with high and reasonable certainty. Recommendations with reasonable-to-low and low certainty do not provide adequate support for practice change. Keep in mind that an EBP team may recommend stopping or de-implementing a practice if there is high or reasonable certainty that it is *not* effective or if there is low certainty that it *is* effective.

The process for identifying best-evidence recommendations varies by the type of evidence the team is using and is discussed below.

Action Items for a Best-Evidence Search With Pre-appraised Evidence

1. In Section II of Appendix H, select the type of evidence used to generate the recommendations. The EBP team will select the first option, "pre-appraised evidence." They may also select the following option, "evidence from a targeted search," if they identified strong or moderate evidence in the supplementary search.

2. Record the best-evidence recommendations in the table as they (or the evidence they are based on) are characterized by the authors or organization of the report. This may be based on certainty, confidence, grade, or another categorization. Read the descriptions of each grouping on the tool to determine which is a best match for the way the recommendations are framed in the clinical practice guideline, literature review with a systematic approach, or evidence summary. See the example box on the next page.

3. If the team also identified strong or moderate evidence from their targeted search, they will record any necessary changes to the pre-appraised evidence in the corresponding row. When determining if a recommendation should be updated, consider the following: Does the new evidence provide results that are based on robust methods that the team considers compelling? How does the certainty of any new or altered recommendations compare to the certainty of the recommendation from the pre-appraised evidence? The recommendations may be unaltered or may undergo significant updates depending on the team's findings.

> **EXAMPLE**
>
> **BEST-EVIDENCE SEARCH WITH PRE-APPRAISED EVIDENCE**
>
> **Example:** JBI Evidence Summary: Pre-eclampsia Screening (Whitehorn, 2024)
>
> **Pre-appraised evidence review question:** What is the best available evidence regarding screening for pre-eclampsia in women?
>
> **Recommendations:**
>
> 1. Pregnant women should have their blood pressure measured and recorded at each antenatal visit (Grade A).
> 2. Urinalysis for protein should be offered to pregnant women at each antenatal visit (Grade B).
> 3. If available, algorithms that consider multiple factors such as maternal characteristics and history, mean arterial pressure, biochemical markers, and uterine artery pulsatility index may be considered for all pregnant women (Grade B).
>
> JBI considers Grade A recommendations "strong" (the desirable effects clearly outweigh undesirable effects; there is evidence of adequate quality supporting their use; there is a benefit or no impact on resource use and values; and preferences and the patient experience have been taken into account).
>
> Grade B recommendations are "weak" (the desirable effects appear to outweigh undesirable effects of the strategy, although this is not as clear; there is evidence supporting their use, although this may not be of high quality; there is a benefit, no impact, or minimal impact on resource use and values; and preferences and the patient experience may or may not have been taken into account).
>
> | JHEBP Model Characteristics of the Recommendations | Best-Evidence Recommendations |
> |---|---|
> | High certainty | 1) Pregnant women should have their blood pressure measured and recorded at each antenatal visit. |
> | Reasonable certainty | 2) Urinalysis for protein should be offered to pregnant women at each antenatal visit. |
> | | 3) If available, algorithms that consider multiple factors such as maternal characteristics and history, mean arterial pressure, biochemical markers, and uterine artery pulsatility index may be considered for all pregnant women. |
> | Reasonable-to-low certainty | |
> | Low certainty | |

Action Items for an Exhaustive Search With Single Studies and Anecdotal Evidence

1. In Section II of Appendix H, select the type of evidence used to generate the recommendations. The EBP team will select the last option, "evidence appraised by the EBP team from an exhaustive search."

2. Review the totality of the evidence presented in Section I of the tool. Consider the distribution across the levels of support for decision-making, consistency, quantity, and persuasiveness. There is not a predetermined number of articles needed to generate recommendations for practice change. The team must assess the available evidence and use clinical reasoning to make a determination on a case-by-case basis.

3. Record each individual recommendation in the box with a description that matches its characteristics.

See the sidebar on the next page for an example of generating best-evidence recommendations from the synthesis of individual evidence.

> **TIP**
>
> **A BUILDING ANALOGY**
>
> Here's another way to think about the summary, organization, and synthesis steps: When constructing a building, summary is considered dropping the building materials off at the site. Organization is the process of sorting the materials by room, size, type of material, etc. Synthesis is assembling the pieces into the final structure.

SUMMARY

The evidence portion of the EBP project is the crux of the EBP process. Without an in-depth understanding of the evidence related to the practice problem, organizational change can at best falter and at worst cause harm. Best-evidence recommendations based on a robust synthesis with careful consideration and highly developed critical thinking can make a good EBP project into a great EBP project. This builds a strong and reliable foundation for organizational translation, which builds on the process with the addition of organizational context, including patient and provider preference.

> **EXAMPLE**

GENERATING BEST-EVIDENCE RECOMMENDATIONS FROM SYNTHESIS OF INDIVIDUAL EVIDENCE

Example: Among hospitalized adult patients, what are best practices regarding maintaining peripheral IV catheters?

SUPPORT FOR DECISION-MAKING	SYNTHESIZED FINDINGS
Strong Number of sources = six	There is no difference in rates of infection or infiltration among adult patients who have their IV catheter changed based on a predetermined schedule as compared to those who only have the catheter changed when indicated when the site is inspected regularly (1, 4, 7). Hand hygiene before and after contact with an IV catheter has been shown to positively impact infection rates (1, 2, 3).
Moderate Number of sources = six	Assessing for patency prior to use of the IV catheter via aspiration is a reliable measure of functionality (5, 8). IV catheters should be assessed every two to four hours (6, 9). Hand hygiene before and after contact with an IV catheter positively impacts infection rates (11, 12). Regular inspection may or may not improve infection rates (11, 9).
Limited Number of sources = one	IV catheters should be assessed every shift (10). Regular inspection improves infection rates (10).

CHARACTERISTICS OF THE RECOMMENDATIONS	BEST-EVIDENCE RECOMMENDATION
High certainty	Rotate IV sites when indicated, not by a predetermined schedule. Inspect IV site at each shift change. Perform hand hygiene before and after contact with the IV catheter.
Reasonable certainty	The catheter should be assessed for patency via aspiration before each infusion.
Reasonable-to-low certainty	The IV catheter site should undergo regular inspection. Assessment should occur every two hours, every four hours, or every shift.
Low certainty	

REFERENCES

Booth, A., Sutton, A., Clowes, M., & Martyn-St James, M. (2021). *Systematic approaches to a successful literature review* (3rd ed.). Sage.

Booth, A., Sutton, A., & Papaioannou, D. (2016). *Systematic approaches to a successful literature review* (2nd ed.). Sage.

Efron, S. E., & Ravid, R. (2018). *Writing the literature review: A practical guide*. Guilford.

Garrard, J. (2017). *Health sciences literature review made easy: The matrix method* (5th ed.). Jones and Bartlett Learning.

Li, T., Higgins, J. P. T., & Deeks, J. J. (Eds.). (2023, August). Chapter 5: Collecting data. In J. P. T. Higgins, J. Thomas, J. Chandler, M. Cumpston, T. Li, M. J. Page, & V. A. Welch (Eds.), *Cochrane handbook for systematic reviews of interventions*, version 6.4. www.training.cochrane.org/handbook

Whitehorn, A. (2024). *Evidence summary. Pre-eclampsia: Screening*. The JBI EBP Database. JBI-ES-2594-5.

Whittemore, R., & Knafl, K. (2005). The integrative review: Updated methodology. *Journal of Advanced Nursing, 52*(5), 546–553.

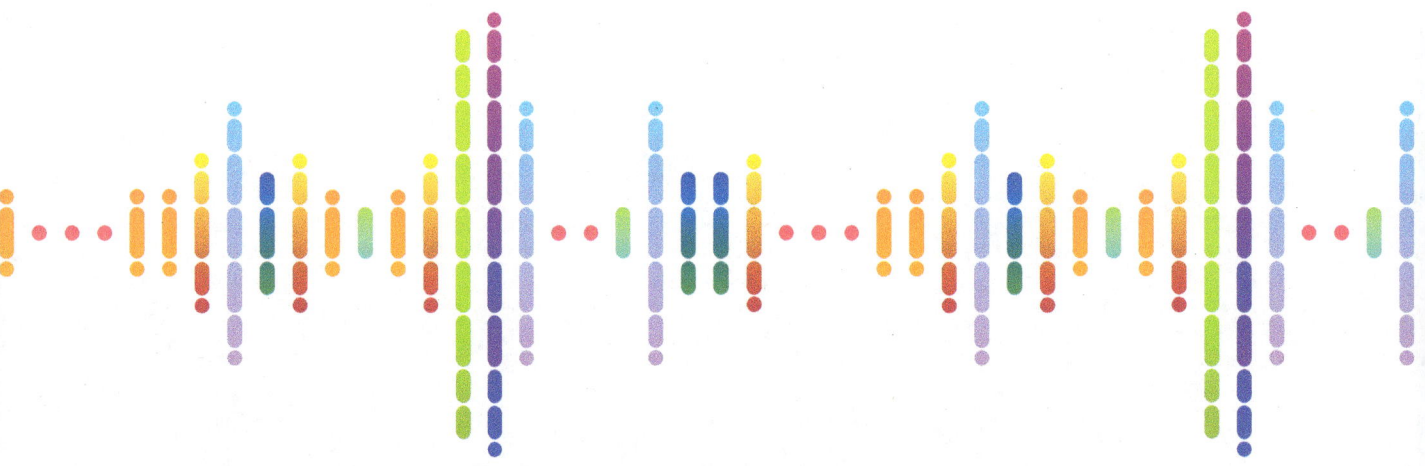

OBJECTIVES

- Review the steps to translate evidence
- Describe evidence-level characteristics that may influence practice-setting recommendations
- Describe organization-level characteristics that may influence practice-setting recommendations
- Discuss potential outcomes of the translation process

10
TRANSLATION PHASE: TRANSLATION

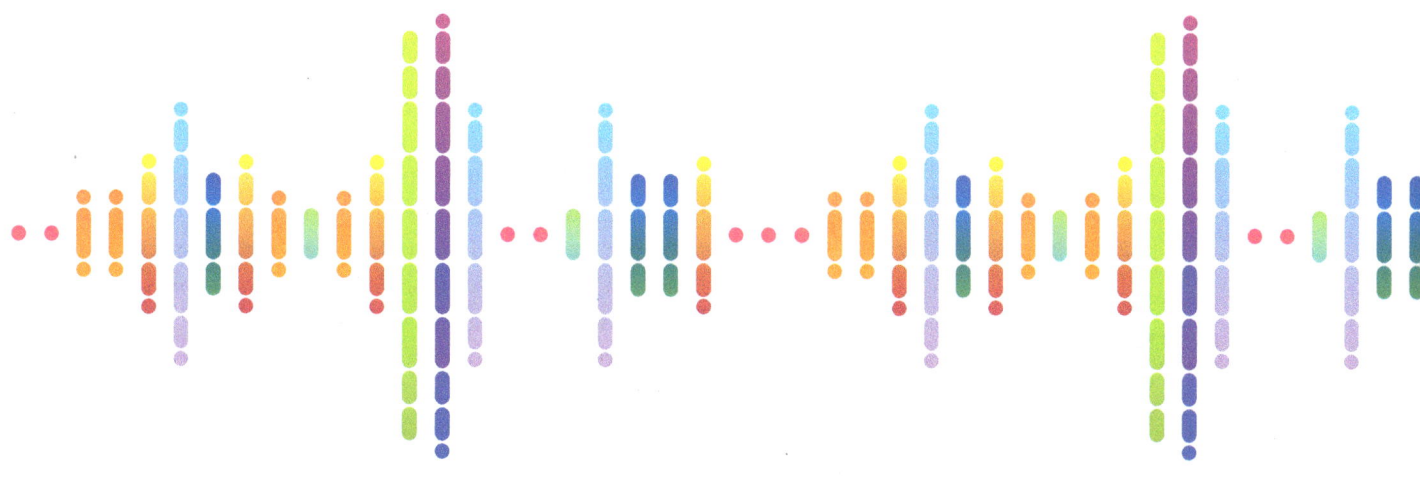

KEY POINTS

The translation phase contains six steps (see Box 10.1). This chapter gives an overview of Steps 11–12 to develop practice setting-specific recommendations from the evidence synthesis. Information in this chapter will assist the EBP team in completing the Translation Tool (Appendix I).

- *Translation* is the process of adapting or customizing evidence findings into the specific content in which they will be implemented.

- The EBP team needs to follow these steps to ensure that effective translation of each piece of evidence occurs:

  - Consider the certainty of each best-evidence recommendation.
  - Identify the potential negative impact on patient or staff safety.
  - *Fit* is accomplished by evaluating both the end-user and organizational characteristics.
  - Assessing the practice environment's readiness to change is critical to determining the *feasibility* of evidence translation.
  - Impacted groups are essential when establishing *acceptability* of the evidence.

- Tools exist that the EBP team can use to help inform organizational decision-making related to translation. The EBP team should make organization-specific recommendations and record them to ensure that all are clear so that implementation may proceed.

> **BOX 10.1 STEPS IN THE TRANSLATION PHASE: THE T IN THE PET PROCESS**
>
> 11. **Assess the risk, fit, feasibility, and acceptability of the best-evidence recommendations**
> 12. **Identify practice setting-specific recommendations**
> 13. Identify an implementation framework
> 14. Create an implementation/action plan
> 15. Implement
> 16. Monitor sustainability and identify next steps

INTRODUCTION

The final phase of the PET process is translation. This is the value-added step in an EBP project that could significantly impact clinical outcomes, patient safety and quality, leadership, and health policy (White et al., 2019). EBP teams may find evidence to support their current practice and continue without a change, or updates can occur in practice, process, or systems to influence targeted outcomes positively. Through the translation process, the EBP team evaluates the best-evidence recommendations (identified in the evidence phase) for transferability to a desired practice setting (Translation Tool, Appendix I). This step is followed by implementation, described in Chapter 11, with the potential for significant positive outcomes that can inspire and motivate the EBP team, revolutionizing healthcare practices and policies. The potential impact of the translation phase on healthcare practices and policies is significant, making the audience feel the importance and influence of their work in the EBP process.

The EBP process requires both critical thinking and clinical reasoning. While critical thinking is essential to the evidence phase of the PET process, clinical reasoning takes center stage in the translation phase. The EBP team engages in clinical reasoning to evaluate the relevance of the best-evidence recommendations to their practice setting. This process requires significant intellectual engagement and presents a substantial challenge, underscoring the complexity of the EBP process and keeping the team intellectually stimulated and engaged (Victor-Chmil, 2013).

In the EBP context, *translation* is the process of adapting or customizing evidence findings into the specific context in which they will be implemented. This involves assessing various components, including evidence-level factors such as strength, consistency, risk, and organizational readiness. *Organizational readiness,* or how prepared an organization is for translating evidence to practice, can be informed by assessing the intervention's fit, feasibility, and acceptability to produce setting-specific recommendations (Watson et al., 2022).

> **NOTE**
>
> **TERMS FOR THE TRANSLATION PHASE**
>
> The EBP team should remember that many related terms describe putting evidence or scientific findings into practice. These include *translation, knowledge translation, translation science, implementation science,* and *adoption.* All have distinct definitions and scopes but are meant to bridge the gap between evidence production and integration into healthcare (Titler, 2018). Titler (2018) describes translation as the use of evidence in a particular setting, adoption as the rate or "uptake" of evidence-based practices, and translational research as the application of research findings across a continuum (e.g., preclinical and animal studies, clinical trials, outcomes research).

CONTEXT IN THE EBP PROJECT

During the evidence phase, the team gathered information to answer their EBP question by identifying the best evidence (i.e., pre-appraised evidence) or an exhaustive literature review. Beyond the specific elements of the EBP question, this process was completed without interpreting the findings of the evidence for the team's context. This produces an objective literature picture that can be applied to various settings and re-translated based on changing circumstances. The EBP team introduces setting-specific considerations in the translation phase and generates concrete, actionable steps to otherwise theoretical recommendations. This is also how the team incorporates patient and healthcare provider preferences.

> **EXAMPLE**
>
> **TRANSLATING A BEST-EVIDENCE RECOMMENDATION**
>
> To further explore the translation process, we will use the example of translating the best-evidence recommendation to use a nurse-driven indwelling urinary catheter discontinuation algorithm to encourage prompt removal of urinary catheters to help prevent catheter-associated urinary tract infections (CAUTI) in the intensive care unit.

ASSESS THE RISK, FIT, FEASIBILITY, AND ACCEPTABILITY OF THE BEST-EVIDENCE RECOMMENDATIONS

Action Item 1: Establish Certainty

Even if based on compelling evidence, practice recommendations made in the evidence phase might not be suitable to implement in all settings. In the previous step, the EBP team characterized the evidence and its ability to inform their EBP question using the Summary, Synthesis, & Best-Evidence Recommendations Tool (Appendix H). They must use this categorization (high certainty recommendations, reasonable certainty recommendations, reasonable-to-low certainty recommendations, and low certainty recommendations) to determine the next steps:

- If the evidence is robust, strong, well-documented, consistent, and persuasive, based mostly on evidence that provides strong support for decision-making, change is indicated.

- If the evidence is good, mostly compelling, consistent, and based mostly on evidence that provides moderate to strong support for decision-making, change is indicated. However, the team must assess risk, fit, feasibility, and acceptability.

- If the evidence is good but conflicting with inconsistent results based mostly on evidence that provides moderate support for decision-making, the team should discuss discontinuing the project, waiting for more evidence, or conducting a research project to generate new information.

- If there is little to no evidence and the information is minimal, inconsistent, and/or based mostly on evidence that provides limited support for decision-making, the team should discuss discontinuing the project, waiting for more evidence, or conducting a research project to generate new information.

> **EXAMPLE**
>
> **TRANSLATION ACTION ITEM 1: ESTABLISH CERTAINTY**
>
> In our example of the indwelling urinary catheter nurse-managed discontinuation algorithm, there was strong and consistent evidence for using this practice, so the project team went forward with Action Item 3, determining fit, feasibility, and acceptability. If the evidence were moderate, the team would have needed to conduct a risk assessment to determine the next steps (Patel et al., 2023).

Action 2: Assessing Risk

Translation of evidence may introduce safety risks to patients, staff, or the environment. The EBP team completes a formal risk assessment during the translation phase. Risk tolerance may vary by organization and is an organization-level factor. For example, one organization may focus more on a problem area and, therefore, be more open to trying new solutions or may have resources to mitigate identified risks, while others may not. A risk assessment focuses on identifying, analyzing, and discussing safety vulnerabilities that a potential change may create for the organization.

In contrast, various risks are inherent to healthcare, such as clinical, financial, reputational, or technological. This step of the translation process focuses on safety risk identification. A *heat chart* is a helpful tool that shows a visual or graphical picture of complex dimensions of problems, or in this case, the risk consideration when determining if a change is indicated for translation. Figure 10.1 provides a color-coded representation of the interrelated role of risk and certainty of recommendations when the team determines whether the best-evidence recommendations should be implemented. Interventions with higher risk require more robust, higher certainty evidence than those with lower risk. With medium risk and reasonable certainty of the recommendations, a pilot or small test of change may be indicated. It is important to note that although an intervention with reasonable-to-low or low certainty of recommendations may be low risk, it should still be translated judiciously to ensure that the team is not wasting time and resources on a change not supported by the literature. On the opposite end of the spectrum, the team has an ethical obligation to put evidence that has high certainty into action to ensure that they are consistent with standards of care. The level of risk can also have a negative relationship with the uptake or adoption of an intervention (higher risk, lower adoption; Wisdom et al., 2013).

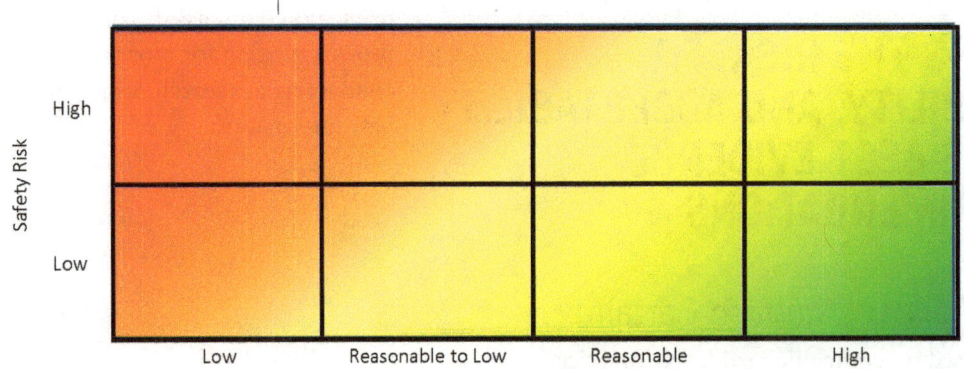

FIGURE 10.1 Heat chart for the interconnected role of safety risk and certainty of the recommendations.

Action Item 3: Assessing Fit, Feasibility, and Acceptability

To determine the likelihood of successful implementation of best evidence and generate guidance specific to their setting, the EBP team needs to formally assess each recommendation's fit, feasibility, and acceptability, which together take into consideration the practice setting's characteristics, such as culture, norms, beliefs, structures, priorities, workflow, and resources. Translation of best evidence may perfectly mirror the recommendations or vary drastically depending on various factors. Part of the core definition of EBP is integrating best evidence with clinical expertise and patient preferences. By assessing fit, feasibility, and acceptability in the translation phase, the EBP team incorporates organizational considerations (such as resources or priorities), patient preferences, and provider experiences. These can be overt or inferred attitudes, opinions, intentions, or behaviors (Proctor et al., 2011). This step also recognizes the multifaceted nature of health and healthcare by acknowledging that evidence does not accurately represent what is best for a person or a system. Beliefs, attitudes, values, perspectives, and experiences are all essential parts of the decision-making process and should be carefully integrated when operationalizing the best evidence (Siminoff, 2013). Note that there are a variety of terms in the literature that describe the components of a translation assessment. The following definitions are to help the EBP team operationalize the process and represent a comprehensive summary of considerations.

Fit *Fit,* sometimes called "goodness of fit," is how a change aligns with existing practices, norms, values, goals, and skills. The EBP team assesses this by evaluating both the end-user and organizational characteristics. The extent to which a change aligns with culture, abilities, values, knowledge, and current practice positively affects adoption (Wisdom et al., 2013).

> **EXAMPLE**
>
> **TRANSLATION ACTION ITEM 3: ASSESSING FIT**
>
> In our example of the nurse-managed discontinuation algorithm of indwelling urinary catheters, the fit assessment indicated that the change aligned with the organization's value of nurse autonomy, supported by the Professional Practice Model. In addition, preventing hospital-acquired infections, such as CAUTI, aligns with the organization's goals and strategic priorities. At the end-user level, the nurses have skills and experience following decision trees to guide clinical practice and value the ability to act independently to reduce patient harm. The change is a good fit.

Feasibility Determining the *feasibility* of implementing best-evidence recommendations within an organizational setting involves assessing the extent to which the team believes the change is doable and that barriers are realistic to overcome. The team should assess the practice environment's readiness for change, which includes the availability of human and material resources, support from decision-makers (individuals and groups), and budget implications. The project team may also request input from the frontline staff, impacted groups, and other individuals affected by the change to determine the change's feasibility.

> **EXAMPLE**
>
> **TRANSLATION ACTION ITEM 3: ASSESSING FEASIBILITY**
>
> The feasibility of implementing a nurse-managed indwelling urinary catheter discontinuation algorithm would likely require resources from nursing education and standards of practice to implement and sustain the practice. In addition, this nurse-managed practice would require buy-in from physicians and advanced practice providers to support the change. No additional supplies or equipment are needed, so there are no financial implications. The change is feasible.

Acceptability *Acceptability* refers to how impacted groups and organizational leadership perceive the EBP change as agreeable and palatable and trust that the change is reasonable. Leadership is critical in effectively implementing organizational innovations and change (Aarons et al., 2015; Warren et al., 2016). One strategy to promote the acceptability of an eventual change is to keep key impacted groups informed throughout the EBP project and to obtain their input and feedback. The EBP team should have identified impacted groups early in the process and should revisit the list as an ongoing consideration (see Chapter 5).

> **EXAMPLE**
>
> **TRANSLATION ACTION ITEM 3: ASSESSING ACCEPTABILITY**
>
> The EBP team determined that implementing a nurse-managed indwelling urinary catheter discontinuation algorithm was acceptable to leadership and frontline nurses. Leadership is invested in improving CAUTI rates and supporting opportunities for nurse autonomy. They believe this change is reasonable and will be impactful, with few unintended consequences. The change is acceptable.

ADDITIONAL TOOLS TO GUIDE ORGANIZATIONAL CONSIDERATIONS FOR THE TRANSLATION PHASE

Many tools can guide organizational considerations when translating evidence into practice. While the Translation Tool (Appendix I) guides the team through essential elements for evaluation, depending on the type of change being proposed, the EBP team may want to explore additional considerations. Each of the following tools is available in the reference list:

- For projects that change end-user workflows or propose end-user solutions (e.g., a new product for pressure injury prevention or a new procedure protocol), Quality Function Deployment (QFD) is a tool for analyzing organizational goals, identifying specific end-users, providing a voice for the customer, and addressing end-user/customer needs and priorities (Chan & Wu, 2002; Mazure, 2023).

- Projects that require behavior changes in the organization, customer, or patient (e.g., tobacco cessation, social distancing, shortening all meetings from one hour to 45 minutes) can be evaluated using the Capability, Opportunity, Motivation, and Behavior/Behavior Change Wheel as a tool (COM-B/BCW). COM-B/BCW posits that behavior change involves three conditions—capability, opportunity, and motivation—and the behavior change wheel offers interventions addressing the barriers (Michie et al., 2011).

- For projects that require technological changes (e.g., electronic health records, remote video monitoring, physiological monitors), adopting an information systems feasibility tool may be appropriate. TELOS

(Technology and Systems, Economy, Legal, Operations, and Schedule) considerations address the organization's technological capabilities, analyze the cost benefit to the organization, weigh legal ramifications or regulatory risks, evaluate organizational expectations and alignment to organizational goals, and assess the viability of the timelines and availability of resources (McGonigle & Mastrian, 2018).

IDENTIFY PRACTICE SETTING-SPECIFIC RECOMMENDATIONS

After evaluating the characteristics of the evidence, risk, fit, feasibility, and acceptability, the team should record their organization-specific recommendations in the Translation Tool (Appendix I). This ensures they are on the same page and cements the proposals. It will also help plan communication with relevant impacted groups during the implementation phase.

There are various scenarios in which an EBP team will determine insufficient evidence to make a change, the risk is too high, or the best-evidence recommendations do not adequately meet the fit, feasibility, and acceptability requirements for implementation at the organization. If this is the case, the EBP team can wait for more information to become available, consider beginning a research project to fill the knowledge gap, or discontinue the project:

- Waiting for more information to become available: There are constant and consistent changes to the state of the healthcare literature. If their evidence is insufficient, an EBP team can decide to continue to monitor the available information on a topic to gauge if and when it would be worthwhile to restart the project. One way to help with this approach is using Google Scholar alerts or notifications from other biomedical databases. These sites allow users to set notices for specific authors, topics, or journals. This is an excellent strategy to stay updated with literature and be ready for changes in evidence.

- Considering a research project: Conducting a thorough evidence review and determining a gap in the literature is a strong foundation for building a research project. If an EBP team has a compelling question, yet they discover a lack of evidence on a topic, they can contribute to the state of the literature by conducting their own research. While this is meaningful to the EBP team and the science and profession of nursing, teams should not underestimate the time and effort needed to conduct meaningful research. Teams should consider contacting research experts to help advise on the next steps and guide more novice participants.

- Discontinuing the project: Insufficient evidence, high risk, or an organizational context that is not ready for change may lead a team to decide to terminate a project. Suppose a change is not made because of a lack of fit, feasibility, or acceptability. In that case, a team can continue to monitor organizational factors that may evolve and be more accommodating to a change. Additionally, they should disseminate their results because their findings may be helpful to others outside of their organization who may have a different context.

SUMMARY

Translation involves the examination of evidence criteria that may or may not result in recommendation(s) for implementation. If practice change is indicated, then organization-specific considerations such as safety risk, fit, feasibility, and acceptability are essential to evaluate. Translation of best evidence is prone to failure and wastes valuable time and resources if a proper organizational readiness assessment is not completed. The EBP project on the ICU nurse-managed discontinuation algorithm was determined to have good, mostly compelling, consistent evidence based primarily on evidence that provides moderate to strong support for decision-making with a low-to-medium safety risk. It was determined to be a reasonable certainty recommendation with a good fit, feasible, and an acceptable intervention to translate into practice. The next chapter will walk through the translation process using a framework to guide implementation.

REFERENCES

Aarons, G. A., Ehrhart, M. G., Farahnak, L. R., & Hurlburt, M. S. (2015). Leadership and organizational change for implementation (LOCI): A randomized mixed method pilot study of a leadership and organization development intervention for evidence-based practice implementation. *Implementation Science, 10*(11), 1–12. https://doi.org/10.1186/s13012-014-0192-y

Chan, L. K., & Wu, M. L. (2002). Quality function deployment: A literature review. *European Journal of Operational Research, 143*(3), 463–497.

Mazure, G. H. (2023). *Success by design—That's what QFD does!* QFD Institute. https://www.qfdi.org/how-qfd-works

McGonigle, D., & Mastrian, K. (2018). *Nursing informatics and the foundation of knowledge.* Jones & Bartlett.

Michie, S., Van Stralen, M. M., & West, R. (2011). The behavior change wheel: A new method for characterizing and designing behavior change interventions. *Implementation Science, 6*(1), 1–12.

Patel, P. K., Advani, S. D., Kofman, A. D., Lo, E., Maragakis, L. L., Pegues, D. A., Pettis, A. M., Saint, S., Trautner, B., Yokoe, E. S., & Meddings, J. (2023). Strategies to prevent catheter-associated urinary tract infections in acute-care hospitals: 2022 update. *Infection Control & Hospital Epidemiology, 44*(8), 1209–1231. https://doi.org/10.1017/ice.2023.137

Proctor, E., Silmere, H., Raghavan, R., Hovmand, P., Aarons, G., Bunger, A., Griffey, R., & Hensley, M. (2011). Outcomes for implementation research: Conceptual distinctions, measurement challenges, and research agenda. *Administration & Policy in Mental Health, 38*(2), 65–76. https://doi.org/10.1007/s10488-010-0319-7

Siminoff, L. A. (2013). Incorporating patient and family preferences into evidence-based medicine. *BMC Medical Informatics & Decision-Making, 13*(Suppl. 3), S6. https://doi.org/10.1186/1472-6947-13-S3-S6

Titler, M. G. (2018, May 31). Translation research in practice: An introduction. *Online Journal of Issues in Nursing, 23*(2). https://doi.org/10.3912/OJIN.Vol23No02Man01

Victor-Chmil, J. (2013). Critical thinking versus clinical reasoning versus clinical judgment: Differential diagnosis. *Nurse Educator, 38*(1), 34–36. https://doi.org/10.1097/NNE.0b013e318276dfbe

Warren, J. I., McLaughlin, M., Bardsley, J., Eich, J., Esche, C. A., Kropkowski, L., & Risch, S. (2016). The strengths and challenges of implementing EBP in healthcare systems. *Worldviews on Evidence-Based Nursing, 13*(1), 15–24. https://doi.org/10.1111/wvn.12149

Watson, A. K., Hernandez, B. F., Kolodny-Goetz, J., Walker, T. J., Lamont, A., Imm, P., Wandersman, A., & Fernandez, M. E. (2022, May 11). Using implementation mapping to build organizational readiness. *Frontiers in Public Health, 10*, 904652. https://doi.org/10.3389/fpubh.2022.904652

White, K. M., Dudley-Brown, S., & Terhaar, M. (2019). *Translation of evidence into nursing and healthcare* (3rd ed.). Springer.

Wisdom, J. P., Chor, K. H. B., Hoagwood, K. E., & Horwitz, S. M. (2013). Innovation adoption: A review of theories and constructs. *Administration & Policy in Mental Health, 41*(4), 480–502. https://doi.org/10.1007/s10488-013-0486-4

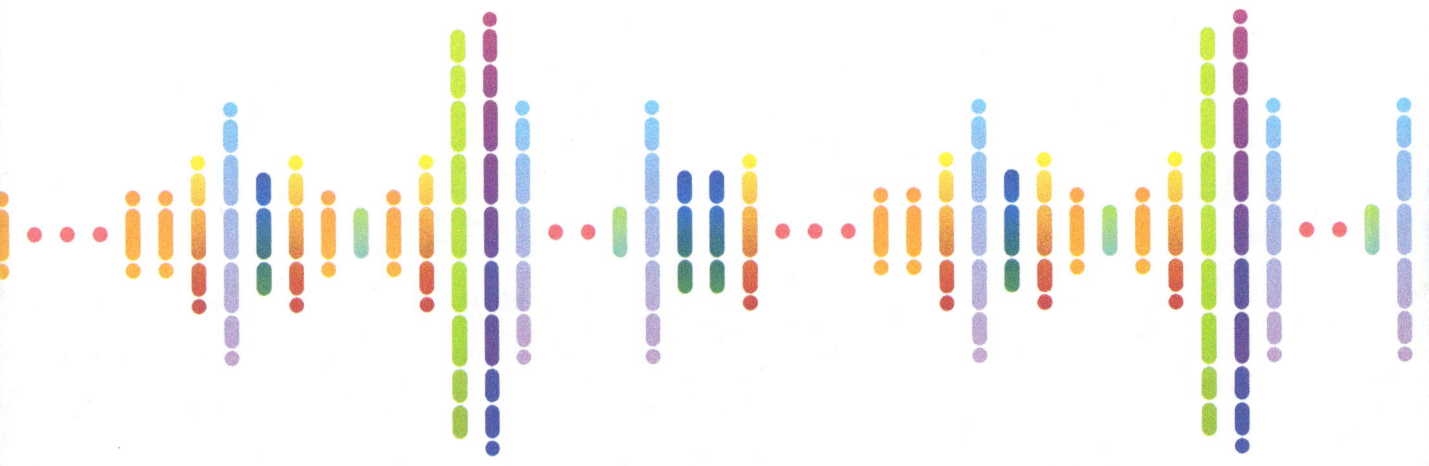

OBJECTIVES

- Discuss the importance of a well-planned and executed implementation strategy

- Describe project management tools

- Review the purpose of implementation frameworks and models

- Describe the Johns Hopkins Quality and Safety Research Group Translating Evidence Into Practice Model

- Discuss strategies for sustainability

11

TRANSLATION PHASE: IMPLEMENTATION

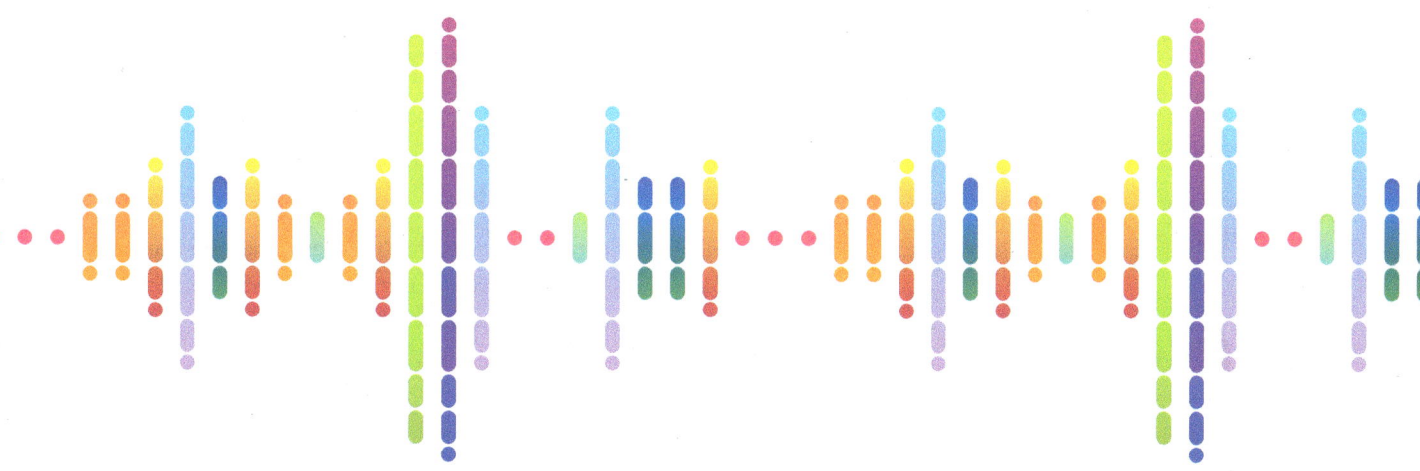

KEY POINTS

The translation phase contains six steps. This chapter provides an overview of the final steps (13–16) to implement any changes identified in Step 12 (see Box 11.1). Information in this chapter will assist the EBP team in completing the Johns Hopkins Evidence-Based Practice (JHEBP) Implementation and Action Planning (A3) Tool (Appendix J).

- Selecting the correct project management tools is crucial for successful EBP implementation.
    - The *A3 tool* is a project plan that consolidates the entire project implementation into one tool.
    - A detailed project timeline can be incorporated into the project's A3.
    - A *Gantt chart* is a high-level visual representation where a Work Breakdown Structure (WBS) tool is more granular in identifying specific tasks and when they need to be completed by.
- Identifying an implementation framework to help guide your project implementation can enhance the efficiency, effectiveness, and sustainability of your implementation.
- The *TRIP model* is an implementation framework that works well with the JHEBP model.
- A sustainability plan is imperative to ensure that project changes outlast the closure of the project.

> **BOX 11.1   STEPS IN THE TRANSLATION PHASE: THE T IN THE PET PROCESS**
>
> 11. Assess the risk, fit, feasibility, and acceptability of the best-evidence recommendations
> 12. Identify practice setting-specific recommendations
> 13. Identify an implementation framework
> 14. Create an implementation/action plan
> 15. Implement
> 16. Monitor sustainability and identify next steps

INTRODUCTION

After the EBP team has determined if a practice change is indicated and translated the best evidence to their practice setting, the next task is to implement the change. Implementation is one of the final steps of the EBP process and is essential to bring the best evidence to the bedside. To ensure not only success but also sustainability, the EBP team should be deliberate in the planning and execution of their intervention or innovation (White et al., 2024). Three keys to successful implementation are identifying an implementation framework or model with a timeline, selecting and using project management tools, and a sustainability plan. See Table 11.1 for definitions related to these components.

IDENTIFYING AN IMPLEMENTATION FRAMEWORK OR MODEL

Using an implementation framework to guide your EBP project offers several significant benefits: (Moulin et al., 2020):

- Structured approach: Provides a method for translating effective interventions and research evidence into practice.
- Identify influences: Helps analyze factors that influence implementation outcomes.
- Evaluate effectiveness: Offers tools for evaluating the success of your implementation.
- Consistency and replication: Ensures consistency, making it easier to replicate successful strategies in different settings.
- Sustainability: Helps ensure changes are effective and sustainable over the long term.

TABLE 11.1   Implementation Definitions

IMPLEMENTATION COMPONENTS	DEFINITION
Project management	*Project management* is the skillful coordination of a team to achieve successful project completion (Day & Colburn, 2024).
Framework	A *framework* is an organized structure, outline, or plan that categorizes various descriptive elements—such as concepts, constructs, or variables—and the relationships between them, which are believed to explain a phenomenon. Frameworks are not designed to offer explanations but rather to describe empirical phenomena by classifying them into categories (Nilsen, 2020).
Model	A *model* is a descriptive, simple representation of a phenomenon or theory (Nilsen, 2020).

Overall, implementation frameworks enhance the efficiency, effectiveness, and sustainability of your EBP project's implementation.

According to Milat and Li, there are 41 different frameworks and models to translate research evidence into policy and practice (2017). Implementation frameworks or models apply to many fields, such as health services research, public health, guideline development, and preventive medicine (Milat & Li, 2017).

See Table 11.2 for a list of some commonly used implementation frameworks with healthcare EBP project implementations. While many choices exist, the EBP team's specific problem and setting can inform their selection. In this chapter we cover the Johns Hopkins Quality and Safety Research Group Translating Evidence Into Practice (TRIP) Model and how it can be used within an EBP implementation.

TABLE 11.2 Implementation Models and Frameworks

MODEL OR FRAMEWORK	DESCRIPTION	BEST USED FOR
Model for Improvement (PDSA)	The Plan-Do-Study-Act (PDSA) cycle is a four-stage quality improvement model. PDSA approaches are simple, rapid-cycle quality improvement processes that provide a structured, data-driven learning approach that allows teams to assess whether a change leads to improvement in a particular setting and to make appropriate, timely adjustments (Donnelly & Kirk, 2015).	PDSA is used to translate the best evidence into practice. It uses a "test of change" approach to quickly troubleshoot issues and increase the scale and complexity of the translation to achieve the desired improvement.
Lean Six Sigma (DMAIC)	DMAIC (Define, Measure, Analyze, Improve, Control) is a systematic, data-driven improvement methodology used in process improvement and quality improvement implementation projects (Hessing, n.d.).	This methodology can benefit implementation projects involving changes in processes, systems, or organizational structures.
AHRQ: Knowledge Transfer	This model from the Agency for Healthcare Research and Quality (AHRQ) accelerates the transfer of research findings to organizations that can benefit from it. Includes three phases: 1) knowledge creation and distillation, 2) diffusion and dissemination, and 3) end-user adoption (Carpenter et al., 2005).	This framework helps develop tools and strategies to implement research findings, specifically for AHRQ grantees and healthcare providers engaged in direct patient care to improve care quality (Carpenter et al., 2005).

continues

TABLE 11.2 Implementation Models and Frameworks (cont.)

MODEL OR FRAMEWORK	DESCRIPTION	BEST USED FOR
Knowledge-to-Action	This integrates creation and application of knowledge. Knowledge creation includes knowledge inquiry, synthesis, and tools/products; knowledge becomes more refined as it moves through these three steps. Action includes identifying and appraising the problem and the known research, identifying barriers and successes, planning and executing, monitoring, evaluating, and adjusting (Graham et al., 2006).	This model facilitates using research knowledge by several impacted groups, such as practitioners, policymakers, patients, and the public (Graham et al., 2006).
PARIHS	The Promoting Action on Research Implementation in Health Services (PARIHS) framework examines the interactions between evidence, context, and facilitation to translate evidence into practice by placing equal importance on the setting, how the evidence is introduced into the setting, and the quality of the evidence itself (Kitson et al., 2008).	PARIHS is an organizing framework to specify determinants that act as barriers and enablers influencing implementation outcomes (Bergström et al., 2020).
QUERI Implementation Roadmap	The Quality Enhancement Research Initiative (QUERI) drives the adoption of high-value research innovations by empowering frontline providers, researchers, administrators, and health system leaders by focusing on developing practical products (e.g., an implementation playbook) and a data-driven evaluation plan (Stetler et al., 2008).	Based on quality improvement science, QUERI is distinctively suited for use in real-world settings to support further scale-up and spread of an effective practice (Stetler et al., 2008).

RE-AIM	RE-AIM is designed to enhance the quality, speed, and public health impact of efforts to translate research into practice in five steps: • Reach your intended target population • Efficacy (or effectiveness) • Adoption by target staff, settings, systems, or communities • Implementation consistency, costs, and adaptations made during delivery • Maintenance of intervention effects in individuals and settings over time (Glasgow et al., 1999)	RE-AIM helps determine public health impact, translate research into practice, plan programs and improve their chances of working in "real-world" settings, and understand the relative strengths and weaknesses of different approaches to health promotion and chronic disease self-management, such as in-person counseling, group education classes, telephone counseling, and internet resources (Glasgow et al., 1999).

The TRIP Model

The TRIP model was developed in 2008 to assist organizations in implementing change in a more extensive healthcare system with a collaborative team approach (Pronovost et al., 2008). There are four stages to this model, which are discussed in the following sections: 1) summarize the evidence, 2) identify local barriers to implementation, 3) measure performance, and 4) ensure all receive the intervention through the "four E's" of implementation (engage, educate, execute, and evaluate; White et al., 2016). The greatest strength of this model is the emphasis on adequate measurements of effectiveness. See Figure 11.1 for an overview of the TRIP model.

Stage 1: Summarize the Evidence Provide a summary of the evidence that will be translated into practice. This step was completed in the summary, synthesis, best evidence, and translation steps of the EBP model (Chapters 9 and 10).

Stage 2: Identify Barriers to Implementation When planning for a change, the team must proactively identify and plan for implementation barriers. This allows for risk mitigation using inherent strengths and resources. These risks may impact the project's success (risks to the patient, staff, or environment as assessed in Chapter 10). You may find specific challenges that will likely impact the ability to deliver on the action plan. Barriers to implementation may include inexperienced staff, competing priorities, illness surges (such as COVID-19 or RSV), and increased capacity or throughput. For example, if staff turnover poses a barrier to implementing the change, the clinical area may include onboarding new staff to the policy expectations as a part of their orientation to ensure sustainability of the new practice. Though these obstacles can get in the way, knowing about them upfront is helpful so that you can engage support and create a plan to move forward. When barriers occur during project implementation, the EBP team can review previously established mitigation strategies.

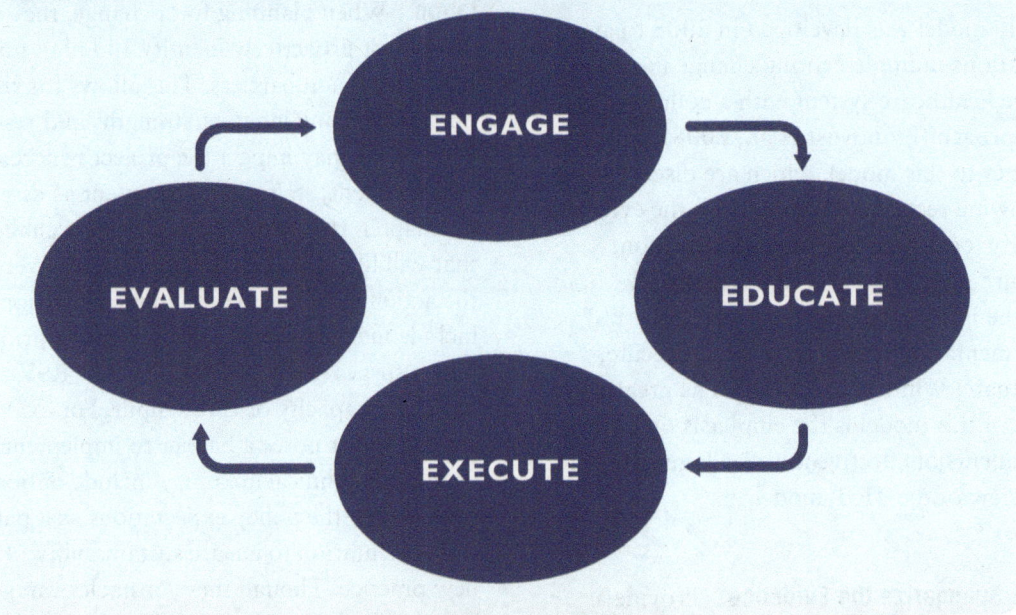

FIGURE 11.1 Overview of the TRIP model.

Stage 3: Measure Performance

Goal Setting   When defining project goals, record what the team hopes to accomplish by implementing the change(s). These can be high-level statements used to inform the measurement plan and implementation. The goal should reflect an improvement in the problem identified and address the broad strategic priority of the organization when available. Goal setting includes drafting aims using the SMART goal format (Leonard & Watts, 2024; see Table 11.3) and establishing measures to assess change.

Aims and Measures   Aims and measures contribute to the overall goal. Changes should result in an improvement in structures, processes, and outcomes in healthcare. Measurement is a critical part of testing and implementing changes. Measures inform the team if the change is effective and leads to improvement. Establish how the project can address the process measures and any patient outcomes identified in the initial problem statement. Donabedian (1966) developed methods to measure healthcare quality using structures, processes, and outcome metrics. Definitions of each measurement are in Table 11.4.

Your team can choose to examine just one critical metric, such as handwashing compliance rates, or it can choose to examine a couple of interrelated metrics, such as handwashing compliance rates and CLABSI rates.

TABLE 11.3   Definition of a SMART Goal

Specific	Goals should be straightforward and state what the team wants to happen. Be specific and define what the team is going to do. Use action words such as direct, organize, coordinate, lead, develop, plan, etc.
Measurable	If you cannot measure it, you cannot manage it. Choose goals with measurable progress and establish concrete criteria for measuring the success of your goal.
Achievable	Goals must be within the team's capacity to reach. Teams cannot commit to accomplishing goals if they are too far out of their reach. Goals need to stretch the group slightly but still be within reach, with a real commitment from the team. Success in reaching attainable goals keeps team members motivated.
Relevant	Goals should be relevant. Make sure each goal is consistent with other team goals and aligned with the goals of the unit, department, and organization.
Time-bound	Set a time frame for the goal: next week, in three months, at the end of the quarter. Putting an end point on each goal provides a clear target. Without a time limit, there is no urgency to act now.

TABLE 11.4 Measurements in Healthcare

MEASURE	DEFINITION	EXAMPLES
Structure	Measures the infrastructure, or the physical equipment and facilities	Organizational policies, risk assessment tools, huddle boards, electronic medical records, availability of hand sanitizer pumps
Process	Measures all the activities that revolve around improving an outcome of care, or the activity performed	Compliance with infection prevention bundles, handwashing compliance, occurrences of purposeful hourly rounding, fall prevention measures in place, compliance to protocol, stocking supplies differently
Outcome	Measures the impact on patients or staff with clear definitions of the final product/result	Falls with injury, central line–associated bloodstream infections (CLABSI), staff satisfaction, patient burns

Stage 4: Implement Using the 4 E's

Stage 4 of the TRIP model details Step 15 ("Implement") of the JHEBP PET process.

Engage The project leader and working group are responsible for identifying collaborating groups and impacted groups for the implementation. To engage with impacted groups and facilitate the buy-in of key personnel, the EBP team explains why the project is essential. The team seeks input from impacted groups and staff affected by the change and communicates the plan for effective implementation and evaluation. This communication can be an agenda item at a staff meeting, an inservice, a direct mailing, an email, a bulletin board, or a video. See Chapter 12 for more information about communication planning.

Educate The next step is educating impacted groups on the evidence supporting the intervention and the implementation of plans. Educational toolkits, defined as "an action-oriented compilation of related information, resources, or tools that together can guide users to conform to evidence-based recommendations" (White et al., 2016, p. 175), can be a helpful strategy to organize and disseminate details about a change in practice. A toolkit may be created to support implementations for all aspects of the project, including the description of the local problem, intervention evidence summary, specifics of the intervention, roles and responsibilities for all impacted groups, audit and tracking tools, and outcomes to monitor. A toolkit may include materials needed to facilitate the appropriate use of interventions. Many toolkits are available in paper format, such as a resource binder; electronic versions shared on an electronic platform are also an option. The audience for the toolkit should be the implementation unit staff to facilitate "the use of knowledge in practice to improve outcomes" (White et al., 2016, p. 175).

Execute Executing your implementation plan begins when the project plan, engagement, and education are complete. Impacted groups and staff must know who the project leader is, where to access needed information or supplies, and how to communicate issues to the project leader as they arise. Throughout execution, the project team should obtain staff input to identify and address problems immediately. During project execution, the team may monitor for barriers and risks to the project, perform data collection, highlight project toolkits, and set aside time to be present at huddles or staff meetings to keep the project moving.

Evaluate After implementing the change, the project team uses the measures identified in Stage 3 to evaluate its success. The team should compare baseline data to post-implementation data to determine whether the change met the project's aims and should be implemented on a broader scale. While there is no set length of time for collecting pre- and post-data, teams should allow enough time to detect any changes. Teams should also consider collecting pre- and post-data at similar times of the year, which may help control variability in population. For instance, if the pre-data is collected during a time of year when the inpatient census is high due to respiratory viral season, the team may also want to implement and collect post-data during a similar time of high respiratory viral admissions. Such measures assist the team in determining if the EBP intervention showed an improvement.

Figure 11.2 shows an example of the TRIP model for a project to reduce unassisted falls.

CREATE AN IMPLEMENTATION ACTION PLAN

Project management tools are an essential component of implementation/action planning. Selecting the correct project management tools is vital for the successful implementation of an EBP project for several reasons:

- Efficiency and organization: Proper tools streamline processes, ensuring tasks are completed efficiently and on time. They also provide a structured approach to project management, which is essential for maintaining high standards and meeting deadlines.

- Data management: EBP projects often require collecting and analyzing data. The appropriate tools facilitate accurate data collection, storage, and analysis, which are critical for making informed decisions and tracking progress.

- Collaboration and communication: Effective project management tools enhance communication and collaboration among team members. They ensure everyone is aligned, vital for coordinating efforts and achieving project goals.

- Problem-solving: Quality tools offer methodologies for identifying potential issues and implementing practical solutions. This systematic approach helps in maintaining the quality and success of the project.

- Monitoring and evaluation: These tools allow for continuous monitoring and evaluation of the project. They help identify areas for improvement and make necessary adjustments to stay on track.

Choosing the correct project management tools ensures your EBP project is well-organized, efficient, and successful.

A3s

The A3 is a valuable tool for consolidating an entire project into one document to facilitate communication on progress to teammates, peers, and leadership. Named for the type of paper it is printed on, an *A3* is a project management planning tool. The A3 summarizes a project and provides a standardized process for teams. However, it also encourages buy-in by including a section on alignment with organizational strategic priorities. Additionally, it can be modified to meet the team's needs. The EBP team completes the Implementation and Action Planning (A3) Tool (Appendix J) by filling in each section according to the prompt on the header.

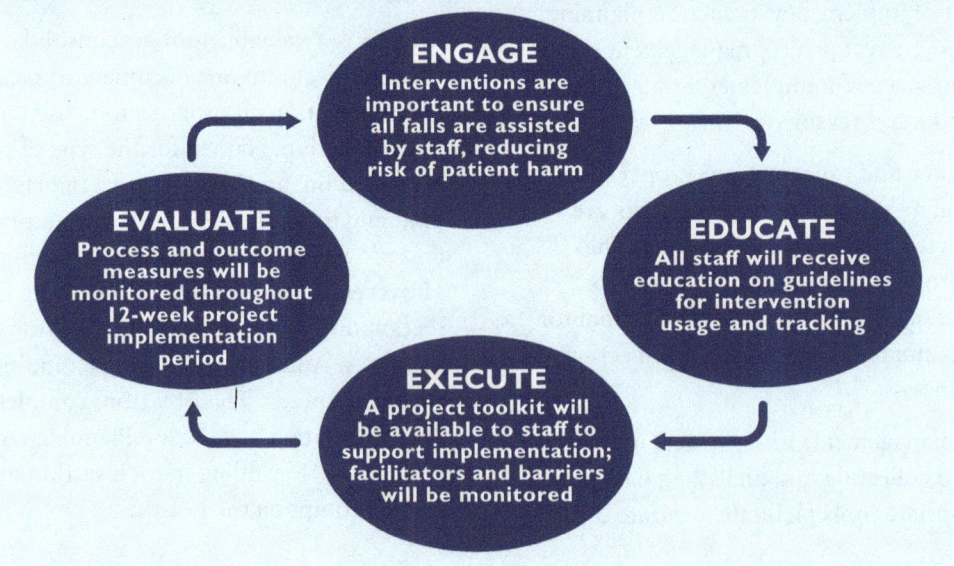

FIGURE 11.2 Example of the TRIP model to implement a project to reduce unassisted falls.

Project Timelines

Project management tools for mapping a timeline include the Gantt chart and Work Breakdown Structure. Templates can be found in the additional resources online (Hopkins.org/resources). To complete these tools, the team determines and records the anticipated implementation date and the outcomes data collection period needed to evaluate success. This can be updated throughout implementation to reflect adjustments to the timeline.

Gantt Chart A *Gantt chart* is a visual representation of a project's schedule, illustrating the planned start and finish dates for the various components of implementation. It is named after Henry L. Gantt, who introduced this type of chart in the early 20th century to illustrate a project's timeline. The Gantt chart gives a high-level overview of the work to be completed from conception to completion. Critical components of a Gantt chart include task bars, timelines, dependencies, milestones, and resources. Figure 11.3 provides an example of a Gantt chart illustrating the key components. The color coding on the Gantt chart of complete, in process, and planned tasks provides a visual status of work to be done.

> **TIP**
> **DO NOT START FROM SCRATCH**
>
> Gantt charts can be made with project management software, Google Forms, or Microsoft Excel. A Gantt chart specific to the JHEBP model can be found in the additional resources online (Hopkins.org/resources).

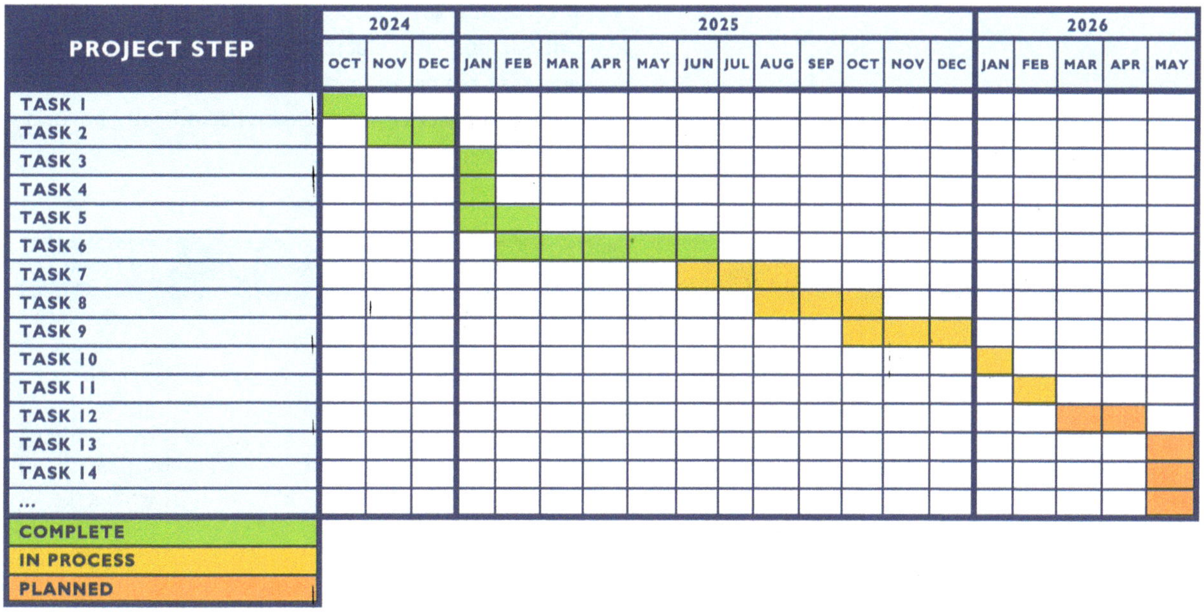

FIGURE 11.3 Gantt chart example.

Work Breakdown Structure From the Gantt chart, a more detailed description of project tasks and corresponding timelines may be visualized on a *Work Breakdown Structure* (WBS). The WBS (see Figure 11.4) is an essential tool in project management and is most often created at the beginning of the project during the planning phase. The WBS is usually presented in a graphical format, such as a tree structure where each level provides more detail about the implementation steps and sub-steps. The visual representation gives project managers and team members an understanding of the scope and dependencies between implementation tasks while aligning the project aims and translation framework. Benefits of using the WBS include clarification of the project's scope and components, estimation of time and cost of implementation, organization, planning of the project activities, and enhanced communication among team members and impacted groups.

MONITOR SUSTAINABILITY AND IDENTIFY NEXT STEPS

The TRIP model also addresses the final step in the JHEBP PET process, sustainability and next steps.

One limitation of the original TRIP model is the lack of a control phase that allows the implementation to sustain improvements (Hessing, n.d.). To address this gap, the Johns Hopkins Armstrong Institute suggested the addition of two E's: "endure" (e.g., include in organizational policy or new employee orientation) and "expand" (e.g., implement on a larger scale).

Enduring and expanding a project allows the implementation to thrive after a project team closes. Sustainability is essential to maintain the quality of healthcare. Additional strategies to sustain the project include incorporating the project into organizational policy, new employee onboarding, and electronic medical records. An accountable person or department may monitor data and practice compliance periodically beyond the project period.

Due Date	Task	Dependencies	Accountable Person(s)	Status	Planned Completion	Actual Completion	Resource
March 15, 2025	Survey built in REDCap	Permission to use the survey from the author	Jane Smith, EBP Team Leader	In progress	March 15, 2025	March 1, 2025	Reach out to unit-based clinical nurse specialist for support in writing the permission letter. REDCap specialist can offer support in building survey into the system.

FIGURE 11.4 Work Breakdown Structure example.

A final strategy for sustainability is through dissemination, which we discuss in the next chapter.

SUMMARY

This chapter reviewed how an implementation framework (TRIP model) may be used to translate the EBP team's evidence-based recommendations into practice. Goal setting, timelines, barrier mitigation, measurements, communications, and other strategies shared here may be easily used with other implementation frameworks. A sustainability plan is imperative to ensure that practice changes outlast the project closure. The next chapter discusses communication strategies both within and outside of the EBP team's organization.

REFERENCES

Bergstrom, A., Ehrenberg, A., Eldh, A. C., Graham, I. D., Gustafsson, K., Harvey, G., Hunter, S., Kitson, A., Rycroft-Malone, J., & Wallin, L. (2020). The use of the PARiHS framework in implementation research and practice—a citation analysis of the literature. *Implementation Science, 15*(1), 68.

Carpenter, D., Nieva, V., Albaghal, T., Sorra, J. (2005). Development of a planning tool to guide research dissemination. In K. Henriksen, J. B. Battles, E. S. Marks, & D. I. Lewin (Eds.), *Advances in patient safety: From research to implementation* (Volume 4: Programs, tools, and products). Agency for Healthcare Research and Quality. https://www.ncbi.nlm.nih.gov/books/NBK20594/

Day, B., & Colburn, B. (2024, Oct. 22). What is project management? Definitions, examples & more. *Forbes Advisor.* https://www.forbes.com/advisor/business/what-is-project-management/

Donabedian, A. (1966). Evaluating the quality of medical care. *The Milbank Memorial Fund Quarterly, 44*(3), 166–206.

Donnelly, P., & Kirk, P. (2015). Use the PDSA model for effective change management. *Education for Primary Care, 26*(4), 279–281. doi: 10.1080/14739879.2015.11494356

Glasgow, R. E., Vogt, T. M., & Boles, S. M. (1999.) Evaluating the public health impact of health promotion interventions: The RE-AIM framework. *American Journal of Public Health, 89,* 1322–1327. https://doi.org/10.2105/AJPH.89.9.1322

Graham, I. D., Logan, J., Harrison, M. B., Straus, S. E., Tetroe, J., Caswell, W., & Robinson, N. (2006). Lost in knowledge translation: Time for a map? *Journal of Continuing Education in the Health Professions, 26*(1), 13–24. doi: 10.1002/chp.47

Hessing, T. (n.d.). *Control phase (DMAIC).* Six Sigma Study Guide. https://sixsigmastudyguide.com/control-phase/

Kitson, A. L., Rycroft-Malone, J., Harvey, G., McCormack, B., Seers, K., & Titchen, A. (2008). Evaluating the successful implementation of evidence into practice using the PARiHS framework: Theoretical and practical challenges. *Implementation Science, 3,* 1. doi: 10.1186/1748-5908-3-1

Leonard, K., & Watts, R. (2024, July 9). The ultimate guide to S.M.A.R.T. goals. *Forbes Advisor.* https://www.forbes.com/advisor/business/smart-goals/

Milat, A. J., & Li, B. (2020). Narrative review of frameworks for translating research evidence into policy and practice. *Public Health Research and Practice, 27*(1), e2711704.

Moullin, J. C., Dickson, K. S., Stadnick, N. A., Albers, B., Nilsen, P., Broder-Fingert, S., Mukasa, B., & Aarons, G. A. (2020). Ten recommendations for using implementation frameworks in research and practice. *Implementation Science Communications, 1,* 42. https://doi.org/10.1186/s43058-020-00023-7

Nilsen, P. (2020). Making sense of implementation theories, models, and frameworks. *Implementation Science, 3*(0), 53–79.

Poe, S. S., Abbott, P., & Pronovost, P. (2011). Building nursing intellectual capital for safe use of information technology: A before-after study to test an evidence-based peer coach intervention. *Journal of Nursing Care Quality, 26*(2), 110–119. doi:10.1097/NCQ.0b013e31820b221d

Pronovost, P. J., Berenholtz, S. M., & Needham, D. M. (2008). Translating evidence into practice: A model for large scale knowledge translation. *BMJ, 337.* https://www.bmj.com/content/337/bmj.a1714

Stetler, C. B., McQueen, L., Demakis, J., & Mittman, B. S. (2008). An organizational framework and strategic implementation for system-level change to enhance research-based practice: QUERI series. *Implementation Science, 3,* 30. https://doi.org/10.1186/1748-5908-3-30

White, K. M., Dudley-Brown, S., & Terhaar, M. F. (Eds.). (2016). *Translation of evidence into nursing and health care* (2nd ed., pp. 47–49). Springer.

White, K. M., Dudley-Brown, S., & Terhaar, M. F. (Eds.). (2024). *Translation of evidence into nursing and healthcare* (4th ed.). Springer.

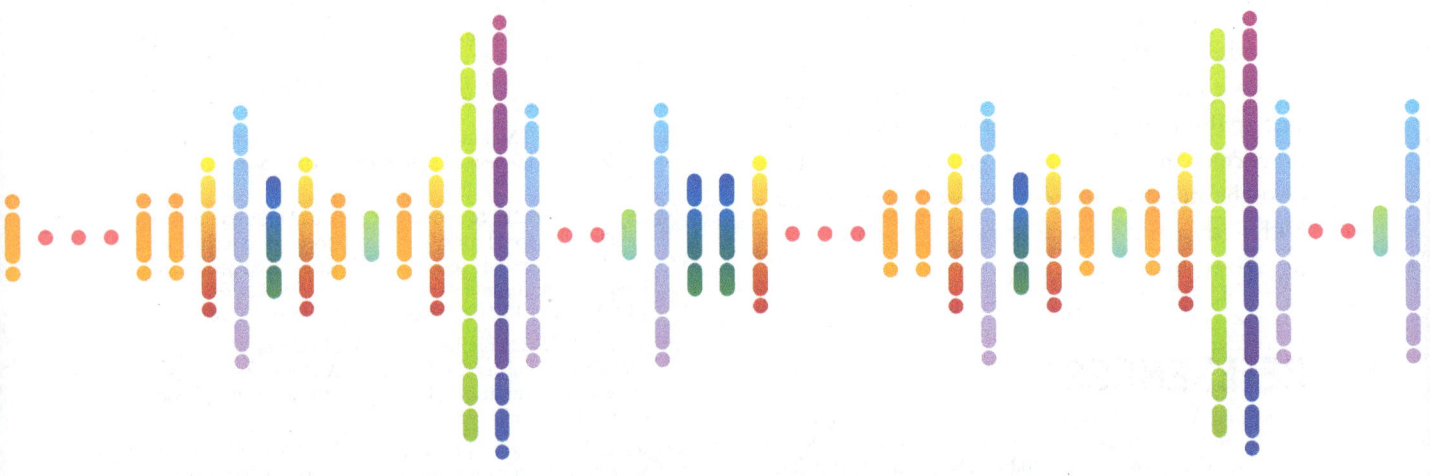

OBJECTIVES

- Describe the process of creating a dissemination plan
- Discuss strategies for disseminating the EBP project results to internal impacted groups
- Describe several processes for external dissemination, such as conferences and publications
- Compare and contrast the strengths and weaknesses of various dissemination strategies
- Discuss future directions for external dissemination strategies

12

ONGOING CONSIDERATIONS: COMMUNICATION AND DISSEMINATION

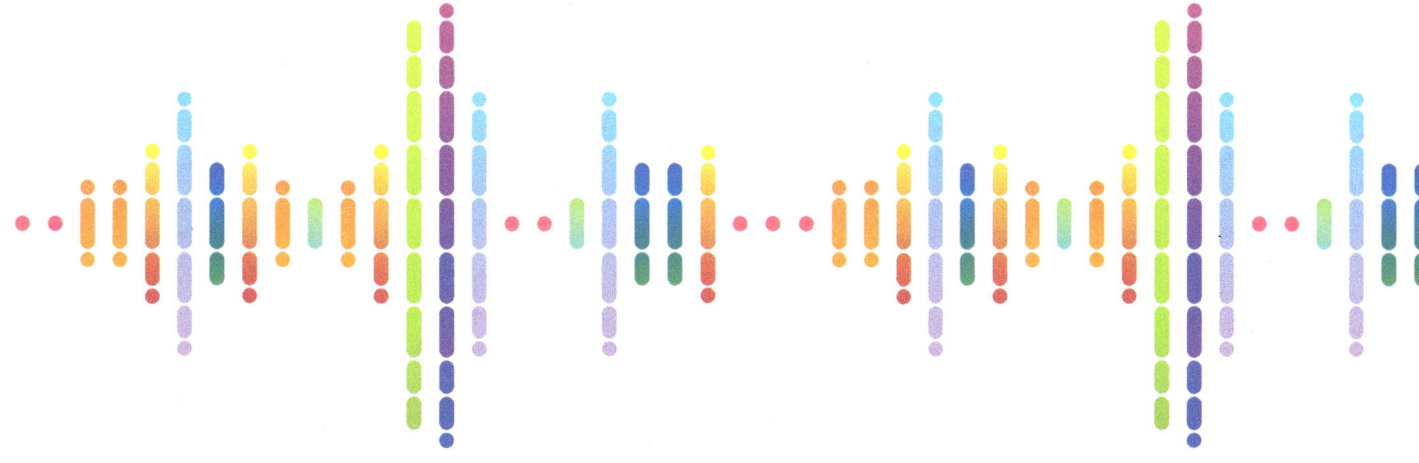

KEY POINTS

Dissemination can occur throughout the EBP project. Resources to facilitate the process include the Impacted Groups Analysis and Communication Resource and the EBP Reporting Guidelines provided in the additional resources online (Hopkins.org/resources).

- There are five components of an effective dissemination plan, including purpose, message, audience, timing, and method.

- *Internal dissemination* refers to sharing information with groups within a team's organization.

- Communication strategies should be tailored for unit-, departmental-, and organization-level groups. Executive summaries can be an effective communication strategy for executive leadership.

- *External dissemination* refers to sharing information outside a team's organization.

- Venues for external dissemination include conferences, peer-reviewed journals, and social media.

- Communication and dissemination are essential components of an EBP project. Not only are they mandates by healthcare organizations, such as the American Nurses Association, but they are also essential for improving care for patients and advancing the science of healthcare.

INTRODUCTION

Dissemination is one of the ongoing considerations throughout an evidence-based practice (EBP) project. Dissemination is an explicit process of sharing knowledge with a target audience to influence process or practice changes (Wilson et al., 2010). According to Serrat (2017), "At the simplest level, dissemination is best described as the delivery and receipt of a message, the engagement of an individual in a process, or the transfer of a process or product. Dissemination serves three broadly different purposes: awareness, understanding, and action" (p. 872). In the context of EBP, it means sharing information with people who need it, strengthening the literature on a topic, or implementing practice change (Sarver & McNett, 2020).

While completing an EBP project may have direct benefits to the EBP team's setting, successful dissemination can serve as the basis for evidence-based changes on a much broader scale. Formulating and following a dissemination plan, both within the team's organization and to an external audience, can ensure the highest impact of an EBP project. Efficient and effective dissemination can help to close the gap between establishing evidence and everyday practice change (Sarver & McNett, 2020).

HOW TO CREATE A DISSEMINATION PLAN

Creating a purposeful dissemination plan helps to ensure the findings of an EBP project result in impactful changes. When developing a plan, the team should consider the following elements: the purpose of the dissemination, the message to be disseminated, the audience, the timing, and the method (Agency for Healthcare Research and Quality [AHRQ], 2014). You may need to include additional team members who can provide expertise in messaging, marketing, and reaching intended audiences.

Here are the details on dissemination elements:

- **Purpose:** The purpose for dissemination will drive all other factors and can include raising awareness, informing, and promoting results (AHRQ, 2014).

- **Message:** Messages should be clear, targeted, actionable, and repeated (AHRQ, 2014; Scala et al., 2019).

- **Audience:** Previously identified impacted groups should inform decisions about the intended audience. While the overall purpose is the same, tailoring the message will depend on the intended recipients, their interests, and their backgrounds. Teams should adjust messaging accordingly (AHRQ, 2014).

- **Timing:** Timing is an important consideration and varies by the impacted group. For example, the start of the fiscal year might be an appropriate time to target leadership, or policy renewal windows may be a prime time to influence standards of practice. Additionally, topics can fall in and out of popularity, and the EBP team can capitalize on a focus from legislators or professional nursing organizations. Messages should also be repeated. The "Marketing Rule of Seven" suggests it may take up to seven contacts for a person to take a desired action (Goncalves, 2017).

- **Method:** There are numerous approaches to sharing information, from a staff email to a peer-reviewed publication. The method should match the intended reach of the message and be tailored to the specific audience. To reach the most people, the same idea should be spread through a variety of channels (AHRQ, 2014; Scala et al., 2019).

THE FOUR P'S

Managing transition can be challenging, and the EBP team may meet resistance to anticipated changes within their organization. The Bridges and Bridges (2017) model suggests using a strategy called "The Four P's" to encourage successful transitions. This gives those affected by the change time and opportunity to internalize the change and a forum to express their questions or concerns. Those who are outspoken about the change are often those who genuinely care about getting things right and can recognize the pitfalls and make great suggestions to improve the planning activities. The Four P's include:

Purpose: Why are you making the change? Share with others who are not involved in the planning why things are changing and what will happen if things stay the same.

Picture: What will it look like? Share what the desired outcome will look like; invite staff to co-create the picture with you. Paint a picture of how the outcome will look and feel.

Plan: What is the plan and path to the end point? Layout, step by step, the plan and path to the new state; invite staff to critique, contribute to, and change the path; make an idea list and a worry list.

Part: What part will staff have in creating the plan and end point? People own what they create, so let staff know what you need from them, what part they will have, and where they will have choices or input.

INTERNAL DISSEMINATION

Internal dissemination refers to information-sharing with impacted groups within the team's organization. It is important to share both the progress and results of the EBP project with internal audiences to create buy-in and foster support. Dissemination within the organization starts with developing an effective communication plan specific to the people who receive the information. This plan should ensure messaging occurs through multiple channels, is timely and frequent, is quickly and easily digestible, is personalized to the audience, is benefit-focused, and solicits action (Scala et al., 2019). Teams should consider if the population of interest should also receive communication regarding the results of the project and use applicable patient education and engagement strategies. EBP projects can spark small or large changes in an organization. These may be met with predictable or even unexpected challenges, and an effective internal dissemination plan is a powerful strategy to move forward with the team's desired change.

Communication Strategies for Unit-, Departmental-, and Organization-Level Groups

Once the EBP team has determined the purpose of disseminating their message, they must identify existing communication strategies within their organization. Standard communication venues include newsletters, internal websites, private social media groups, journal clubs, grand rounds, staff meetings, and unit-based inservices. More customized communication strategies might include simulation scenarios, the development of pocket cards, toolkits, focus groups, unit-based huddle boards, or lunch and learns. For maximum impact, the team should address each component of the dissemination plan listed above. Additionally, a key strategy for dissemination to internal impacted groups is to focus on addressing "what's in it for the staff?" by emphasizing how potential changes impact them and what role they will play in implementing this change (Scala et al., 2019). For example, in discussing education with nurses to promote safe patient mobility, the EBP team may want to focus on what this means for staff, including how safe patient handling equipment reduces the risk of musculoskeletal injuries to staff, what equipment is available, and how the practice change will be incorporated into their workflow. See Figure 12.1 for an example of a communication plan for frontline staff.

Communication Strategies for Executive Leadership

Leadership, such as executive or director-level groups, are also key for most EBP projects. Because of their limited time and focus on organizational priorities, they may require special considerations when drafting communications. One common approach is an executive summary. An *executive summary* is a document that "synthesizes complete data into a succinct and coherent whole that allows a decision-maker or general reader in a few minutes of reading to glean the problem, supporting evidence, and solutions" (Herman, 2012, para. 1). See Figure 12.2 for details on planning for internal dissemination for executive leadership. You may have also seen executive summaries accompanying large, commissioned reports, such as the Centers for Disease Control and Prevention Infection Control for Healthcare Personnel or the US Preventive Services Task Force Annual Report to Congress. They can be used as a supplement to a PowerPoint presentation and are typically a one- to two-page document that includes:

- Description of the current state of the problem within the organization/setting
- Why the change is needed
- Overview of the project that outlines how the project aligns with the strategic priorities and mission/vision of the organization
- Implementation process
- Evaluation metrics
- Project outcomes as they relate to specific metrics:
  - Financial
  - Patient satisfaction
  - Clinical
  - Other
- Sustainability plan
- Other organizational implications, such as future initiatives

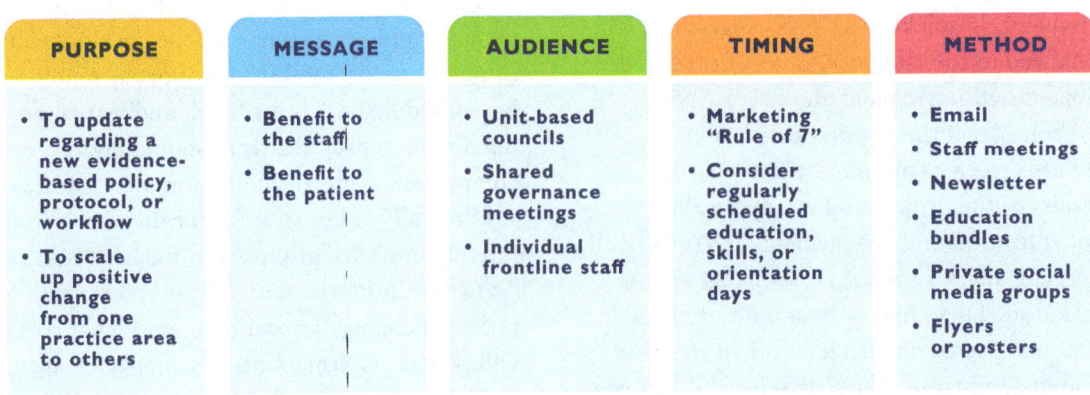

(Sarver & McNett, 2020; Scala et al., 2019)

FIGURE 12.1 Communication plan for frontline staff.

PURPOSE	MESSAGE	AUDIENCE	TIMING	METHOD
• To seek support or endorsement for evidence-based practice change • May be necessary for approval for next steps	• Benefit to the organization • Alignment with strategic priorities	• Directoral level leaders • Executive leadership • C-suite	• Regularly held operations or strategy meetings	• Executive summary presentation and Word document

FIGURE 12.2 Communication plan for executive leadership.

> **EXAMPLE**
>
> ### EXECUTIVE SUMMARY: EVIDENCE OF BEST PRACTICES FOR ENSURING SAFE PATIENT CARE BY TRAVELING CLINICAL STAFF
>
> **Description of the Current State**
>
> Nursing and allied health staffing shortages have increased widespread use of traveling clinical staff nationwide. Like other hospitals across the country, our hospital has been affected by this shortage and has experienced a large increase in traveling clinical staff since the start of the COVID-19 pandemic. With this change, leadership has raised concerns about patient safety events detailed in safety reports. These issues may be due to the unfamiliarity of hospital processes, variability of experience level, and lack of standardized orientation within hospitals. Anecdotally, there is also tension between permanent staff and their temporary counterparts. These dynamics can adversely affect patient safety, unit teamwork, and workflow. Adequate and competent staff are necessary to provide and ensure the highest quality of care. Traveling clinical staff, especially in current times, are an essential component to fulfilling staffing needs.
>
> **Why Change Is Needed**
>
> Our hospital has seen an increase in safety reports coinciding with an increase of employing traveling clinical staff. In order to prevent further safety events impacting patients and improve overall staff well-being, we need to address the problem with evidence-based solutions.
>
> **Project Overview and Recommendations**
>
> We completed a rigorous and replicable literature review focused on best practices for ensuring hospital-based traveling clinical staff provide safe patient care to reduce adverse safety events. We screened 2,697 articles and conducted a critical appraisal of 13 articles that met inclusion criteria. The evidence reveals a need for standardized onboarding, orientation, and improved teamwork and socialization between traveling clinical staff and permanent staff. Based on the evidence, we recommend that a workgroup be created to analyze recommendations from the literature, assess gaps, and implement necessary changes.

Best-evidence recommendations cover three phases of the onboarding process and include:

Pre-employment:

- Ensure experience matches needs through standardized interview process including targeted questions (Ferguson et al., 2020; Jooste & Prinsloo, 2013; Matlakala et al., 2015; Matlakala & Botha, 2016; Rispel & Moorman, 2015; Ronnie, 2020).

- Include physical access, passwords, and test-out options for training as part of pre-orientation requirements (Bethel et al., 2019; Tuttas, 2015).

Orientation and onboarding:

- Ensure good unit fit for travelers by using competency assessment (Mazurenko et al., 2015).

- Provide each traveler with a unit specific resource packet (Bethel et al., 2019; Birmingham et al., 2019; Matlakala et al., 2015; Mazurenko et al., 2015).

- Assign mentor for successful integration (Bethel et al., 2019; Jooste & Prinsloo, 2013; Matlakala et al., 2015; Ronnie, 2020; Senek et al., 2020; Tuttas, 2015).

Ongoing support and evaluation:

- Promote socialization of travelers using mentorship to create a welcoming environment and foster teamwork (Birmingham et al., 2019; Gan, 2020; Mazurenko et al., 2015; Ronnie, 2020; Senek et al., 2020; Shuldham, 2016).

- Create a formalized feedback structure between managers and travelers; formalized feedback about travelers from permanent staff (Bethel et al., 2019; Rispel & Moorman, 2015).

- Provide travelers with professional development opportunities (Birmingham et al., 2019; Mazurenko et al., 2015; Shuldham, 2016).

Alignment With the Strategic Plan

This proposal aligns with the goal in the Hospital Strategic Plan of *Ensuring High Quality Healthcare* by ensuring that traveling clinical staff have an adequate orientation. This will prepare them to provide safe patient care and maximize value for the patients we serve with an intense focus on quality, safety, and efficiency. In addition, creating education targeted to travelers aligns with the strategic plan to *Help Staff Grow*. Although these members of the team are temporary, their influence on outcomes and the clinical environment is enduring and important to support.

Implementation Process

We propose creating a workgroup to develop/revise a Clinical Traveler Onboarding Program that includes staff pre-employment screening, unit-specific orientation plan, and ongoing support. Membership of the workgroup, at a minimum, should include education specialists, nursing leadership, traveling clinical staff, and preceptors.

Evaluation Metrics

Safety reports: Decrease in safety reports related to safety errors involving travel staff

Apparent cause analysis findings: Decrease in preventable harm events related to hospital acquired conditions involving travel staff

Auditing data: Overall decrease in non-compliant elements on audits related to high travel staff volume

Evaluations: Increased satisfaction from program evaluation survey from travelers; increased satisfaction from travel staff evaluations from peers

Project Outcomes as They Relate to Specific Metrics

Implementing the above recommendations will benefit traveling clinical staff and permanent staff satisfaction, patient safety, and teamwork. Enhanced onboarding practices will better equip traveling clinical staff to provide safe patient care and improve traveling clinical staff satisfaction. Unit-specific competency lists and skills assessments will ensure agency staff are qualified to provide safe care for their unit's patient population, resulting in a reduction in safety events. Mentorship of traveling clinical staff and promotion of a welcoming culture will improve teamwork and satisfaction of traveling clinical staff and permanent staff. These practices may prevent patient harm and show financial benefits by reducing the costs associated with adverse events.

Sustainability Plan

Following implementation of the changes made to onboarding and orientation, sustainability can be established through the creation of a traveling clinical staff advisory group. This group would meet periodically to evaluate program success, discuss challenges, and plan necessary revisions in order to guarantee that this initiative remains successful.

Ensuring that each traveling clinical staff is trained appropriately for the unit and having ongoing support from designated staff is crucial to the success and decrease in safety events. This is a system-wide approach to improve the onboarding practice of traveling clinical staff and improve effective communication between permanent staff and traveling clinical staff. It is our responsibility to practice quality and evidence-based practices. With the increases in traveling clinical staff across the nation it is critical we restructure the onboarding process. Having the support and guidance from nursing leadership, educators, and staff for better patient care and safety is needed to make this change.

EXTERNAL DISSEMINATION

External dissemination is the process of sharing information with groups outside of the team's organization. This can occur on a local, regional, national, or international level. Methods can include conference presentations, webinars, social media posts, podcasts, manuscript publications, and more. See Figure 12.3 to explore the components of external dissemination planning. Because the EBP process involves many steps, the team has several opportunities to share the project throughout its life cycle. Keep in mind that many organizations have policies or protocols for sharing information with outside audiences. Be sure to verify the process with your local leadership.

The following sections review methods for external dissemination. When selecting the method and venue for external dissemination, the EBP team should consider the intended audience, the team's bandwidth for writing or presenting, and associated costs (e.g., conference fees and travel; Sarver & NcNett, 2020). Additionally, the role and order of authors should be agreed upon before beginning external dissemination efforts.

See Table 12.1 for a description of each author's role.

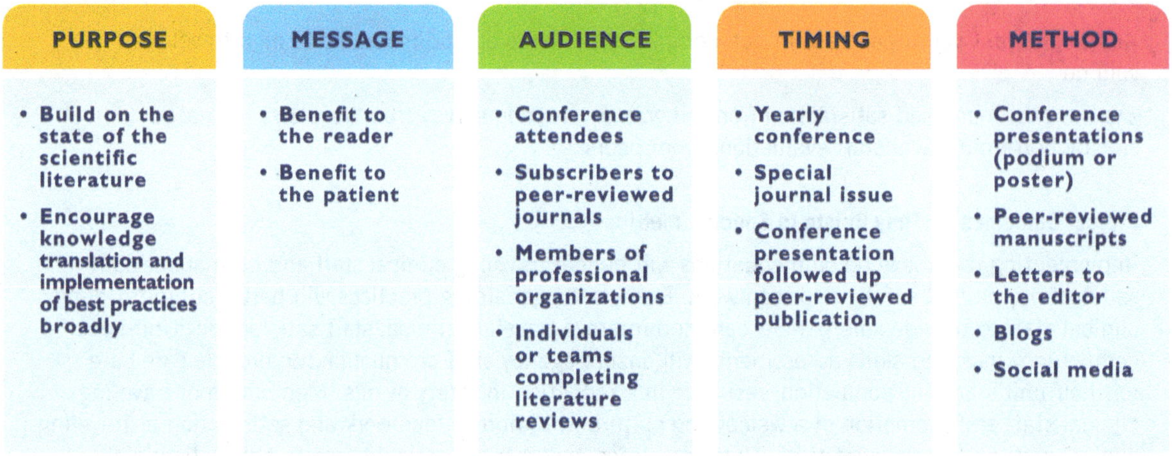

PURPOSE	MESSAGE	AUDIENCE	TIMING	METHOD
• Build on the state of the scientific literature • Encourage knowledge translation and implementation of best practices broadly	• Benefit to the reader • Benefit to the patient	• Conference attendees • Subscribers to peer-reviewed journals • Members of professional organizations • Individuals or teams completing literature reviews	• Yearly conference • Special journal issue • Conference presentation followed up peer-reviewed publication	• Conference presentations (podium or poster) • Peer-reviewed manuscripts • Letters to the editor • Blogs • Social media

FIGURE 12.3 Communication plan for external dissemination.

TABLE 12.1 Authorship Roles

ROLE	DESCRIPTION
Primary author	The person who made the most significant contribution. This person should be listed first.
Contributor author or co-author	Assume responsibility for their assigned section or task as well as ownership of the manuscript as a whole and responding to requests by the first author. Are required to provide review and approval of final drafts.
Senior author (last author)	The most experienced or senior member of the team. It is customary to list this person last.
Corresponding author	The person who is the point of contact regarding the submission. This person is responsible for communicating with the journal editors or conference planners and notifying all authors of acceptance or rejection. Is frequently the primary author.
Presenting author (for conferences)	The person(s) who will be physically present at the conference. Oftentimes this person is also the primary author.

> **TIP**
>
> ### CITING AUTHORS
>
> Authorship is an important part of external dissemination. According to the International Committee of Medical Journal Editors (2021), authorship should be based on four criteria:
>
> 1. Substantial contributions to the conception or design of the work; or the acquisition, analysis, or interpretation of data for the work; AND
> 2. Drafting the work or revising it critically for important intellectual content; AND
> 3. Final approval of the version to be published; AND
> 4. Agreement to be accountable for all aspects of the work in ensuring that questions related to the accuracy or integrity of any part of the work are appropriately investigated and resolved
>
> It is important to establish an authorship plan and expectations at the beginning of a project. Further guidance can be found at http://www.icmje.org/recommendations/browse/roles-and-responsibilities/.

Conferences

Generally, professional organizations host scientific conferences that act as a platform for learning and networking. They can take place at the local, state, regional, national, and international levels. To provide relevant content, conference organizers typically solicit applications for poster or podium presentations to take place during the event. Most conferences have themes, and depending on the size, may have specific categories or tracks for content. For example, the 2024 National Teaching Institute and Critical Care Exposition's theme was "Rising Together" and contains tracks such as "Beacon," "Chapter Best Practices," "Clinical Scene Investigator Academy," "Evidence-based Solutions," and "Research." In 2023, the American Physical Therapy Association's Combined Section Meeting theme was "Defining Physical Therapy's Value as a Profession and Breaking Away from Classical Tropes."

Each conference is unique in its requirements, but the center of most presentation applications is an abstract. This provides a short, high-level summary for the organizers to guide their decision on both the quality and the fit of the content for their program. When planning to submit to a conference, presenters should reference the event website, which usually provides details on the specific elements required (e.g., references, objectives, relevance to the field). Visit your profession's general and specialty organization websites for potential conference submissions.

> **TIP**
>
> ### PUBLISHING CONFERENCE PRESENTATIONS
>
> Many professional organizations that host conferences also publish the accepted abstracts in their associated journal. For examples of high-quality submissions that were accepted by the organization, review recent publications that feature conference content.

Poster presentations

Posters can be a physical printout or a digital display of a team's work, typically contained on a single, albeit large page. The benefits of these presentations are that they can be easy to read, encourage networking with colleagues, and have a much quicker turn-around time than writing and editing a manuscript (Edwards, 2015; Serrat, 2017). One major drawback is the abbreviated nature of the content because it is difficult to convey the depth and rigor of a project in a 3 x 4-foot visual display (Edwards, 2015; Serrat, 2017).

> **TIP**
> ### MAKING AN EFFECTIVE POSTER
> - Templates are often available to guide the design. The team's organization and/or the conference may provide blank prototypes in PowerPoint for the authors to customize with their project information.
>
> - Pictures, figures, and graphs make data not only visually appealing but also digestible. When possible, consider displaying information as an image.
>
> - Most people will be reading a poster from several feet away. Make sure all content is readable at that distance. For reference, on a printed 3 x 4-foot poster, the 40-point font will stand 1 inch tall.
>
> - While the inclination can be to share as much information as possible, white space is important and can make a poster much more visually appealing as well as readable for someone passing by.

Of note, in recent years there has been a re-evaluation of the traditional poster design, and newer approaches have emerged to take full advantage of data visualization tools and knowledge from the user experience (UX) field. These include Better Poster, Butter Poster, and "L" poster. The new designs better incorporate graphic design principles, large text, bright colors, and key points in an attempt to increase audience engagement. Gray and colleagues provide a detailed explanation of these poster approaches, including examples and benefits and drawbacks of each (Gray, 2022).

Podium Presentations

Podium presentations allow the presenter an opportunity to share their work in an oral format, usually with slides as a visual aid. Presentation formats include individual presenters, teams, or groups of panelists. Podium presentations have the advantages of being engaging for the audience and allowing time for in-depth explanation, and often include question and answer sessions. On the downside, they are typically only available to those in attendance and have a limited reach; however, the abundance of virtual and hybrid events since the COVID-19 pandemic has extended their reach. Additionally, the effectiveness of the presentation can rely heavily on the skills of the presenters (Foulkes, 2015; Serrat, 2017). A 2017 systematic review of expert opinions on giving a medical research presentation identified 29 frequent recommendations (in at least 20% of the articles). The top five tips are to keep slides simple, know the audience, make eye contact, rehearse, and do not read from the slides or manuscript (Blome et al., 2017). To create and deliver an effective and engaging podium presentation:

- Determine the key takeaway for the audience before opening your presentation software (Grech, 2018).

- Tailor both the content and the pace of your presentation to your audience (Alpert, 2019; Grech, 2018).

- Ensure you can present the information within the allotted time. As a rule of thumb, presentation time should be calculated at no more than one slide per minute (Grech, 2018).

- People can read or they can listen; it is hard to do both. Use text sparingly and in short phrases. Some people employ the "Rule of Seven" (not to be confused with the "Marketing Rule of Seven"). Do not use more than seven words per line and no more than seven lines per slide (Alpert, 2019; Brown, 2023; Foulkes, 2015).

- Slides should serve as an outline, or talking points, not a script. Do not read directly from the slides. A good rule to follow is the presenter should still be able to give the presentation even if the equipment fails (Grech, 2018).

- Use graphics liberally to augment the message you want to convey (Alpert, 2019; Grech, 2018).

- Color variation can be helpful, but ensure that it does not distract from the messaging (Alpert, 2019). You may want to select a small color palette to work from. Some organization's branding departments may have these pre-selected for you. Also remember some members of the audience may be color-blind (Grech, 2018).

- When using colored text or backgrounds, ensure all text is easily readable and in a legible font from a distance. Keep in mind that color slides may be printed in grayscale. Fonts should be consistent across all slides unless used for emphasis (Duarte, 2008).

- Content may be shared both virtually and in person. All data should be easy to read from a distance or on a smaller screen (Brown, 2023). Also, ensure you are speaking into the microphone as some content may be live-streamed or recorded for later.

Peer-Reviewed Journal Articles

Not only is the EBP process dependent on scientific literature availability, but the completion of an EBP project can add to available knowledge on a topic through the peer-reviewed publication process. While the publication process can be time-intensive, it has the benefits of being a well-established and thorough method to ensure the information being shared meets the standards of the journal and by extension the scientific community. Once published, the information shared in the article is not limited to people in attendance at a conference and can have a wide reach (Serrat, 2017). Figure 12.4 represents an overview of the typical article publication process. Other important elements when preparing a manuscript include identifying an appropriate target journal as well as adhering to relevant publication standards and reporting guidelines.

Selecting a suitable journal for a manuscript submission involves several factors. The process begins by reviewing the journal's website to determine the types of submissions they accept and their target audience. Additionally, reviewing recent publications will provide insights into the journal's areas of interest. The EBP team's submission should be a good fit for the scope of the journal and also fill a gap in their published content. For example, if the journal recently published an article on a similar topic, they may be more reticent to publish duplicative material. Journals also frequently distribute calls for papers for upcoming special issues (e.g., staff well-being, workplace violence, COVID-19, implementation science). This offers an opportunity for a team to submit their work to a journal that has already expressed interest in a topic. Other factors to consider are the journal's acceptance rate and *impact factor* (a calculation often used as an indicator of the reach or importance of the journal; Lariviere & Sugimoto, 2019). In the early stages of the publication process, the EBP team can also query a journal's editor to gauge interest in a potential submission. This might provide important feedback that would not be gleaned from the webpage alone.

To find potential journals, the EBP team can explore a variety of websites that act as a repository of potential journals. See Table 12.2 for a list of organizations and their associated web address. Additionally, many professional healthcare organizations have an associated journal that may be a good fit in the team's given field. Finally, the authors should be aware of predatory publishing. There is no standardized definition of a "predatory journal," but the term includes characteristics such as deceptiveness or lack of transparency, unethical practices, persuasive language, poor quality standards, and large or hidden article processing fees (Cobey et al., 2018; McLeod et al., 2018). Elmore and Weston discuss predatory journals and how to identify them in their 2020 paper published in *Toxicology Pathology*.

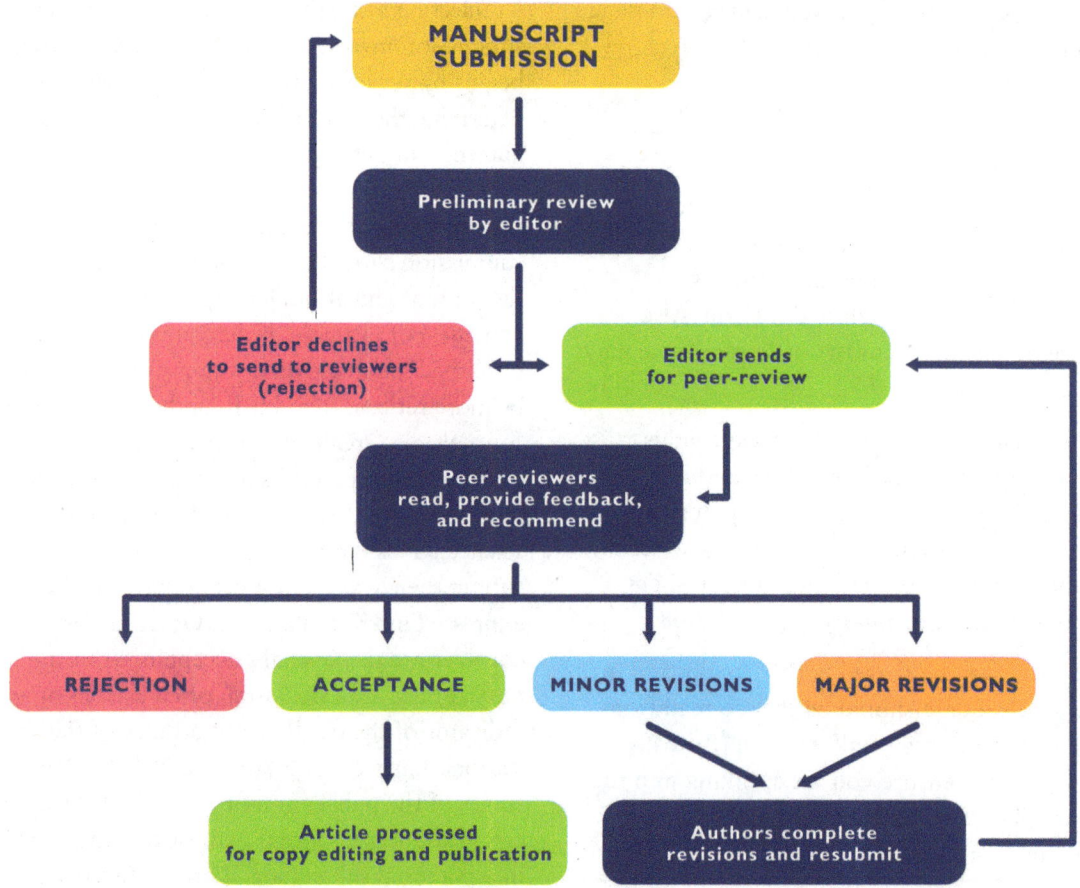

FIGURE 12.4 Manuscript pathway from submission to publication.

TABLE 12.2 Journal Repository Websites

ORGANIZATION	URL
International Academy of Nursing Editors (INANE)	https://nursingeditors.com/
Journal/Author Name Estimator (Jane)	https://jane.biosemantics.org/
InCites Journal Citation Reports	https://jcr.clarivate.com
Occupational Therapy Potential	https://otpotential.com/blog/list-of-ot-journals
American Physical Therapy Association	https://www.apta.org/patient-care/evidence-based-practice-resources/apta-section-and-academy-journals

After selecting a target journal, it is important to review the author guidelines carefully. There, the team will find specific journal requirements and references to publication standards and reporting guidelines. A *reporting guideline* is a simple, structured tool for the team to use while writing manuscripts and includes a "checklist, flow diagram, or structured text to guide authors in reporting a specific type of research, developed using explicit methodology" (EQUATOR Network, n.d., para. 4). The appropriate standards depend on the type of project (e.g., quality improvement, randomized control trial, systematic reviews), but all manuscripts will include some basic elements displayed in Table 12.3. Other common components include conflict of interest statements, attestation of authorship, reporting standard checklists, keywords, and important highlights or takeaways.

A list of reporting standards can be found on the Enhancing the QUAlity and Transparency Of health Research (EQUATOR) Network website (https://www.equator-network.org/contact/contact/). Based on a recent Delphi study to determine consensus among subject matter experts on the necessary components for high-quality reporting of an EBP project, there are now reporting guidelines for EBP projects (Whalen et al., 2024). They can be accessed on the Institute for Johns Hopkins Nursing website (Hopkins.org/resources). These reporting guidelines were published in 2024, and uptake among nursing journals varies, so it is important to continue to check the author guidelines for each journal prior to preparing a submission.

TABLE 12.3 Primary Components of a Manuscript Submission

PARTS OF A MANUSCRIPT SUBMISSION	DESCRIPTION
Cover letter	A letter written to the publisher of a journal briefly describing the intent of the submission and why it is of interest to the journal.
Title page	A separate document that contains the names, affiliations, and credentials of the authors to maintain anonymity in the manuscript itself.
Introduction	A brief description of the problem, available knowledge on the subject, and the question the study is attempting to address.
Methods	A description of the study's design, including what was done and how it was evaluated. This section should read as a guide or manual on the process.
Results	An overall description of the major findings and the data itself. The results section does not include commentary or discussion, just facts and figures.
Discussion	A summary of findings and how the findings compare to the current state of the science on the topic. It also should include any limitations, implications, or future directions of the work.

(Hall, 2012)

> **TIP**
>
> **HINTS FOR EXTERNAL DISSEMINATION**
> - When writing a manuscript, write the abstract last.
> - When preparing a poster or podium presentation, write the abstract first.
> - You can only submit to one journal at a time.
> - For conferences, scoring rubrics are usually used to select a certain number per track, not the total, so some tracks may be less competitive than others.
> - For online conference submissions, write (and save) the submission in a separate document first. Many online submission systems do not have word counters, spell check, etc.
> - Conferences can solicit submissions sometimes up to a year in advance, so be sure to keep an eye on anything of interest.
>
> More writing resources can be found at http://oedb.org/ilibrarian/150-writing-resources

Other Types of Dissemination

While conference presentations and peer-reviewed manuscripts are the most traditional external dissemination routes, there are other avenues to share scientific knowledge. These can still include publication-based pieces such as articles in professional journals or magazines (non-peer-reviewed), book chapters, opinion pieces, newsletters, interviews, video abstracts, podcasts, and letters to the editor. These options provide an outlet to share perspectives and communicate more readily with an intended audience (Saver, 2021).

Additionally, more social media–based alternatives such as blogs, X (previously known as Twitter), Facebook, LinkedIn, and YouTube are becoming ever more popular and have been proven effective in reaching a broader audience (Gates et al., 2018; Hoang et al., 2015; Konkiel et al., 2016; Markham et al., 2017; Ryan & Sfar-Gandoura, 2018). These platforms can be used to promote published articles to increase attention and share unique content with targeted messaging. One study found a blog post summarizing two articles was viewed approximately tenfold more than either article itself (Hoang et al., 2015). Another study found a disease-specific Facebook group effectively engaged members in the findings of clinical research (Ryan & Sfar-Gandoura, 2018). X is also a powerful tool to bring messages directly to decision-makers and policymakers by circumventing traditional barriers (Ryan & Sfar-Gandoura, 2018). Large organizations such as the Centers for Disease Control and Prevention and the World Health Organization provide excellent examples of using social media to convey messages to a wider readership (Breland et al., 2017).

These alternative types of dissemination may be a good starting point for people new to the scientific writing process. Additionally, research shows evidence-based practices have slow and incomplete uptake. Engaging in alternate forms of dissemination is one approach to ensuring information reaches clinicians and patients (Gates et al., 2018; Gregory & Twells, 2015).

FUTURE CONSIDERATIONS

In the rapidly evolving landscape of technology, the emergence of artificial intelligence (AI) stands out as a pivotal development, particularly in the realms of healthcare and scientific dissemination. AI in general refers to the ability of a machine to learn from experience. In the context of dissemination, we are referring specifically to interactive user interfaces that produce AI-generated responses based on information mined from thousands of internet sources, such as ChatGPT (Duan et al., 2019; Liebrenz et al., 2023). The integration of AI in these fields is multifaceted, offering a range of benefits while also presenting unique challenges that warrant caution. AI holds the potential to improve the dissemination of evidence-based practices by efficiently processing and analyzing large quantities of data and content. It also aids in the composition of results and conclusions, further streamlining the overall process and expediting the transition from research to practice. Additionally, it may further democratize the production and consumption of scientific literature by producing copies in multiple languages (Liebrenz et al., 2023).

On the other hand, there are concerns regarding the ethical use of AI, such as issues related to data privacy, the potential for compounding biases already built into the reference material, and the need for transparent and explainable AI systems (Solomon et al., 2023). Moreover, the reliability of AI-driven decisions in complex scenarios remains a topic of ongoing research. As such, while AI offers promising avenues for advancing evidence-based practices, its application in healthcare and scientific publishing must be approached with a balanced view, considering both its potential benefits and limitations.

As these tools continue to evolve, the healthcare scientific community is tasked with the critical responsibility of navigating these technological advancements prudently, ensuring that their adoption enhances, rather than compromises, the quality and integrity of scientific inquiry and dissemination. Both the International Committee of Medical Journal Editors (ICMJE) and the International Association of Scientific, Technical, and Medical Publishers (STM) have produced recommendations on the use of AI in editorial decision-making (Duan et al., 2019; STM, 2021; ICMJE, 2024).

SUMMARY

Dissemination of EBP projects can take various forms and is an essential step in the EBP process. As members of the healthcare community, the EBP team can improve knowledge accessibility, enhance the state of science on a given topic, and catalyze change. The importance of dissemination cannot be discounted and has even been included in healthcare providers' Codes of Ethics, including the American Nurses Association (ANA) and the American Medical Association (AMA). These documents call for the advancement of the profession through various scientific approaches including research development, evaluation, prompt dissemination, and application to practice (AMA, 2016; ANA, 2015). Clinically practicing healthcare providers completing an EBP project are in the unique position to provide firsthand knowledge of patient care coupled with best-practice evidence and realistic recommendations. Dissemination is a tool to advocate for patients, staff, and populations and is an opportunity for the EBP team to translate evidence into clinical practice and promote science and healthcare professions.

REFERENCES

Agency for Healthcare Research and Quality. (2014, June). *Quick-start guide to dissemination for practice-based research networks*. https://www.ahrq.gov/sites/default/files/wysiwyg/ncepcr/resources/dissemination-quick-start-guide.pdf

Alpert, J. S. (2019, May). So, you have to give a lecture—are you anxious? [Editorial]. *The American Journal of Medicine, 132*(5), 545–546. https://doi.org/10.1016/j.amjmed.2018.11.024

American Medical Association. (2016). *AMA principles of medical ethics*. https://www.ama-assn.org/delivering-care/ama-principles-medical-ethics

American Nurses Association. (2015). *Code of ethics for nurses with interpretative statements*. https://www.nursingworld.org/practice-policy/nursing-excellence/ethics/code-of-ethics-for-nurses/coe-view-only/

Bethel, C., Olson, S., Bay, C., Uyeda, T., & Johnson, K. (2019, September). Travel nurse onboarding: Current trends and identified needs. *JONA: The Journal of Nursing Administration, 49*(9), 436–440. https://doi.org/10.1097/nna.0000000000000781

Birmingham, C., van de Mortel, T., Needham, J., & Latimer, S. (2019, November). The experiences of the agency registered nurse: An integrative literature review. *Journal of Nursing Management, 27*(8), 1580–1587. https://doi.org/10.1111/jonm.12850

Blome, C., Sondermann, H., & Augustin, M. (2017, Feb. 15). Accepted standards on how to give a medical research presentation: A systematic review of expert opinion papers. *GMS Journal for Medical Education, 34*(1), doc. 11. https://doi.org/10.3205/zma001088

Breland, J. Y., Quintiliani, L. M., Schneider, K. L., May, C. N., & Pagoto, S. (2017, December). Social media as a tool to increase the impact of public health research. *American Journal of Public Health, 107*(12), 1890–1891. https://doi.org/10.2105%2FAJPH.2017.304098

Bridges, W., & Bridges, S. M. (2017). *Managing transitions: Making the most of change* (4th ed.). Da Capo.

Brown, J. D. (2023). I hear you, but I can't read your slides: Tips for creating a basic PowerPoint presentation. *The American Journal of Medicine, 136*(4), 341–342. https://doi.org/10.1016/j.amjmed.2022.12.005

Cobey, K. D., Lalu, M. M., Skidmore, B., Ahmadzai, N., Grudniewicz, A., & Moher, D. (2018). What is a predatory journal? A scoping review. *F1000Research, 7*, 1001. https://doi.org/10.12688/f1000research.15256.2

Duan, Y., Edwards, J. S., & Dwivedi, Y. K. (2019, October). Artificial intelligence for decision-making in the era of big data—Evolution, challenges, and research agenda. *International Journal of Information Management, 48*, 63–71. https://doi.org/10.1016/j.ijinfomgt.2019.01.021

Duarte, N. (2008). *slide:ology: The art and science of creating great presentations*. O'Reilly Media.

Edwards, D. J. (2015). Dissemination of research results: On the path to practice change. *The Canadian Journal of Hospital Pharmacy, 68*(6), 465–469. https://doi.org/10.4212/cjhp.v68i6.1503

Elmore, S. A., & Weston, E. H. (2020, June). Predatory journals: What they are and how to avoid them. *Toxicologic Pathology, 48*(4), 607–610. https://doi.org/10.1177/0192623320920209

EQUATOR Network. (n.d.). *What is a reporting guideline?* University of Oxford. https://www.equator-network.org/about-us/what-is-a-reporting-guideline/#:~:text=Reporting%20guidelines%20for%20main%20study,Search

Ferguson, A., Bradywood, A., Williams, B., & Blackmore, C. C. (2020, September). Association of use of contract nurses with hospitalized patient pressure injuries and falls. *Journal of Nursing Scholarship, 52*(5), 527–535. https://doi.org/10.1111/jnu.12572

Foulkes, M. (2015, Feb. 20). Presentation skills for nurses. *Nursing Standard, 29*(25), 52–58. https://doi.org/10.7748/ns.29.25.52.e9488

Gan, I. (2020, March). Social comparison and perceived envy-motivated communication involving travel nurses: A qualitative study. *Journal of Nursing Management, 28*(2), 377–384. https://doi.org/10.1111/jonm.12939

Gates, A., Featherstone, R., Shave, K., Scott, S. D., & Hartling, L. (2018). Dissemination of evidence in paediatric emergency medicine: A quantitative descriptive evaluation of a 16-week social media promotion. *BMJ Open, 8*(6), e022298. https://doi.org/10.1136/bmjopen-2018-022298

Goncalves, P. (2017, August). Want successful employee communications? Think like a marketer. *Strategic HR Review, 16*(5), 0. http://dx.doi.org/10.1108/SHR-07-2017-0038

Gray, A. L., Curtis, C. W., Young, M. R., & Bryson, K. K. (2022, April 1). Innovative poster designs: A shift toward visual representation of data. *American Journal of Health-System Pharmacy, 79*(8), 625–628. https://doi.org/10.1093/ajhp/zxac002

Grech, V. (2018, October). WASP (Write a scientific paper): Optimisation of PowerPoint presentations and skills. *Early Human Development, 125*, 53–56. https://doi.org/10.1016/j.earlhumdev.2018.06.006

Gregory, D. M., & Twells, L. K. (2015). Evidence-based decision-making 5: Translational research. In P. S. Parfrey & B. J. Barrett (Eds.), *Clinical epidemiology* (pp. 455–468). Humana Press.

Hall, G. M. (Ed.). (2012). *How to write a paper*. Wiley.

Herman, L. (2012). *Executive summary guidelines*. Harvard Kenney School. https://projects.iq.harvard.edu/files/hks-communications-program/files/ho_herman-exec-summary_2-14-13_0.pdf

Hoang, J. K., McCall, J., Dixon, A. F., Fitzgerald, R. T., & Gaillard, F. (2015, July). Using social media to share your radiology research: How effective is a blog post? *Journal of the American College of Radiology, 12*(7), 760–765. https://doi.org/10.1016/j.jacr.2015.03.048

International Association of Scientific, Technical, & Medical Publishers. (2021). *AI ethics in scholarly communication: STM best practice principals for ethical, trustworthy and human-centric AI*. https://www.stm-assoc.org/2021_05_11_STM_AI_White_Paper_April2021.pdf

International Committee of Medical Journal Editors. (2024). *Defining the role of authors & contributors*. https://www.icmje.org/recommendations/browse/roles-and-responsibilities/defining-the-role-of-authors-and-contributors.html

Jooste, K., & Prinsloo, C. (2013, March 13). Factors that guide nurse managers regarding the staffing of agency nurses in intensive care units at private hospitals in Pretoria. *Curationis, 36*(1), E1–10. https://doi.org/10.4102/curationis.v36i1.115

Konkiel, S., Madjarevic, N., & Lightfoot, A. (2016, January). *Altmetrics for librarians: 100+ tips, tricks, and examples*. https://figshare.com/articles/journal_contribution/Altmetrics_for_librarians_100_tips_tricks_and_examples/3749838/1?file=6035787

Lariviere, V., & Sugimoto, C. R. (2019). The journal impact factor: A brief history, critique, and discussion of adverse effects. In W. Glänzel, H. F. Moed, U. Schmoch, & M. Thelwall (Eds.), *Springer handbook of science and technology indicators* (pp. 3–24). Springer.

Liebrenz, M., Schleifer, R., Buadze, A., Bhugra, D., & Smith, A. (2023, March). Generating scholarly content with ChatGPT: Ethical challenges for medical publishing. *The Lancet Digital Health, 5*(3), e105–e106. https://doi.org/10.1016/S2589-7500(23)00019-5

Markham, M. J., Gentile, D., & Graham, D. L. (2017). Social media for networking, professional development, and patient engagement. *American Society of Clinical Oncology Educational Book, 37*, 782–787. https://doi.org/10.1200/EDBK_180077

Matlakala, M. C., Bezuidenhout, M. C., & Botha, A. D. H. (2015, October). Strategies to address management challenges in larger intensive care units. *Journal of Nursing Management, 23*(7), 945–953. https://doi.org/10.1111/jonm.12240

Matlakala, M. C., & Botha, A. D. (2016, February). Intensive care unit nurse managers' views regarding nurse staffing in their units in South Africa. *Intensive and Critical Care Nursing, 32*, 49–57. https://doi.org/10.1016/j.iccn.2015.07.006

Mazurenko, O., Liu, D., & Perna, C. (2015, August). Patient care outcomes and temporary nurses. *Nursing Management, 46*(8), 32–38. https://doi.org/10.1097/01.numa.0000469351.33893.61

McLeod, A., Savage, A., & Simkin, M. G. (2018). The ethics of predatory journals. *Journal of Business Ethics, 153*(1), 121–131. https://doi.org/10.1007/s10551-016-3419-9

Rispel, L. C., & Moorman, J. (2015, May 11). The indirect costs of agency nurses in South Africa: A case study in two public sector hospitals. *Global Health Action, 8*(1), 26494. https://doi.org/10.3402%2Fgha.v8.26494

Ronnie, L. (2020, February). Us and them: Experiences of agency nurses in intensive care units. *Intensive and Critical Care Nursing, 56*, 102764. https://doi.org/10.1016/j.iccn.2019.102764

Ryan, G., & Sfar-Gandoura, H. (2018, May 2). Disseminating research information through Facebook and Twitter (DRIFT): Presenting an evidence-based framework. *Nurse Researcher, 26*(1). https://doi.org/10.7748/nr.2018.e1562

Sarver, W., & McNett, M. (2020). Determining the dissemination plan: Internal and external considerations. In M. McNett (Ed.), *Data for Nurses: Understanding and using data to optimize care delivery in hospitals* (pp. 101–110). Academic Press.

Saver, Cynthia. (2021). *Anatomy of writing for publication for nurses* (4th ed.). Sigma Theta Tau International.

Scala, E., Whalen, M., Parks, J., Ascenzi, J., & Pandian, V. (2019, December). Increasing nursing research program visibility: A systematic review and implementation of the evidence. *The Journal of Nursing Administration, 49*(12), 617–623. https://doi.org/10.1097/nna.0000000000000825

Senek, M., Robertson, S., Ryan, T., King, R., Wood, E., & Tod, A. (2020, July 10). The association between care left undone and temporary nursing staff ratios in acute settings: A cross-sectional survey of registered nurses. *BMC Health Services Research, 20*(637), 1–8. https://doi.org/10.1186/s12913-020-05493-y

Serrat, O. (2017). Disseminating knowledge products. In O. Serrat (Ed.), *Knowledge solutions* (pp. 871–878). Springer.

Shuldham, C. (2016, Aug. 31). Get the best from agency nurses. *Nursing Standard, 31*(1), 29. https://doi.org/10.7748/ns.31.1.29.s28

Solomon, D. H., Allen, K. D., Katz, P., Sawalha, A. H., & Yelin, E. (2023, June). ChatGPT, et al... Artificial intelligence, authorship, and medical publishing. *Arthritis & Rheumatology, 75*(6), 867–868. https://doi.org/10.1002/art.42497

Tuttas, C. A. (2015, January/March). Job integration factors as predictors of travel nurse job performance: A mixed-methods study. *Journal of Nursing Care Quality, 30*(1), 44–52. https://doi.org/10.1097/ncq.0000000000000070

Whalen, M., Bissett, K., Ascenzi, J., & Budhathoki, C. (2024, Oct. 4). Reporting guidelines for evidence-based practice projects: A Delphi study and publication checklist. *Worldviews on Evidence-Based Nursing,* online ahead of print. doi:10.1111/wvn.12748

Wilson, P. M., Petticrew, M., Calnan, M. W., & Nazareth, I. (2010, Nov. 22). Disseminating research findings: What should researchers do? A systematic scoping review of conceptual frameworks. *Implementation Science, 5*(1), 91. https://doi.org/10.1186%2F1748-5908-5-91

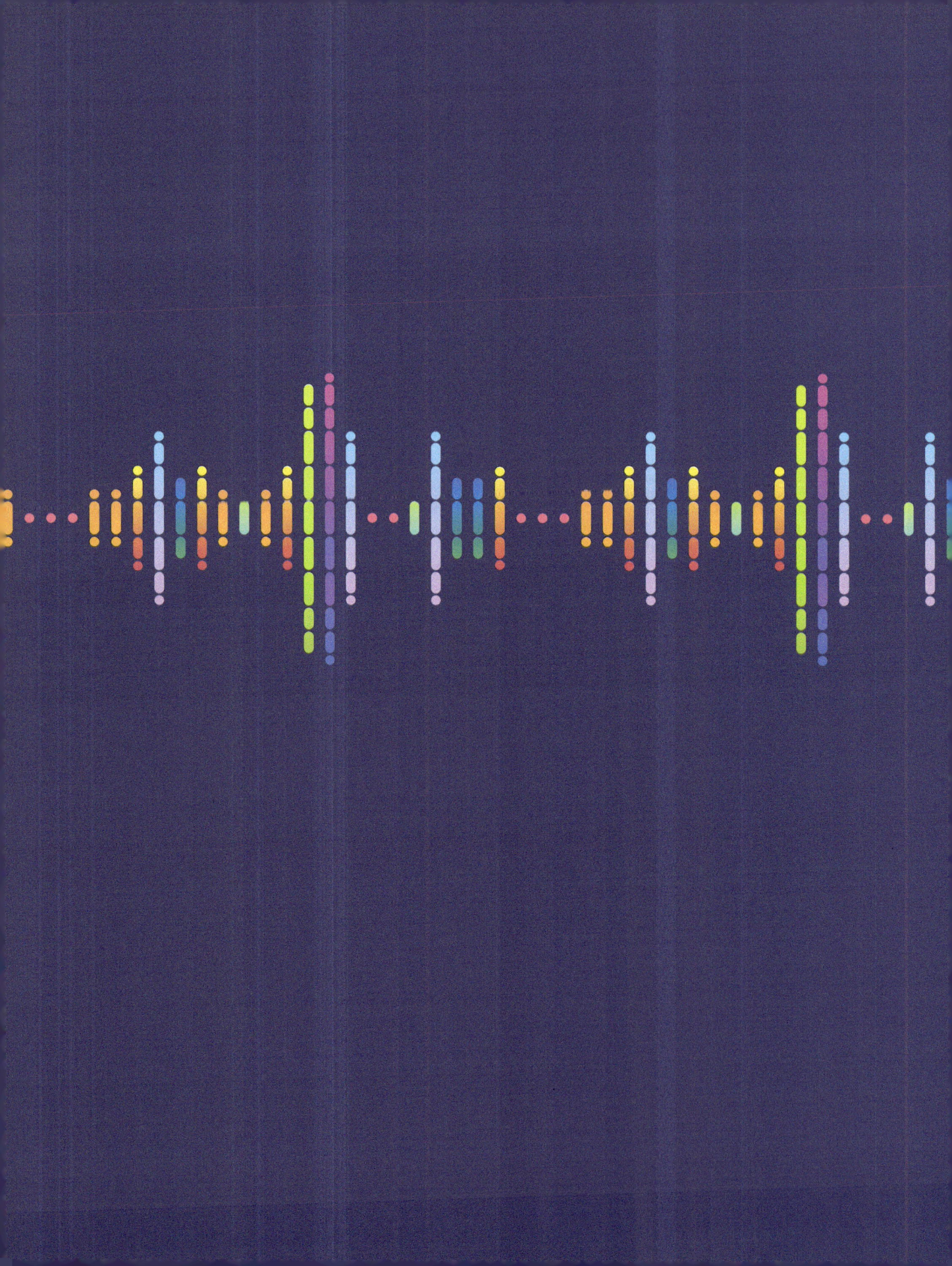

PART III

EXEMPLARS

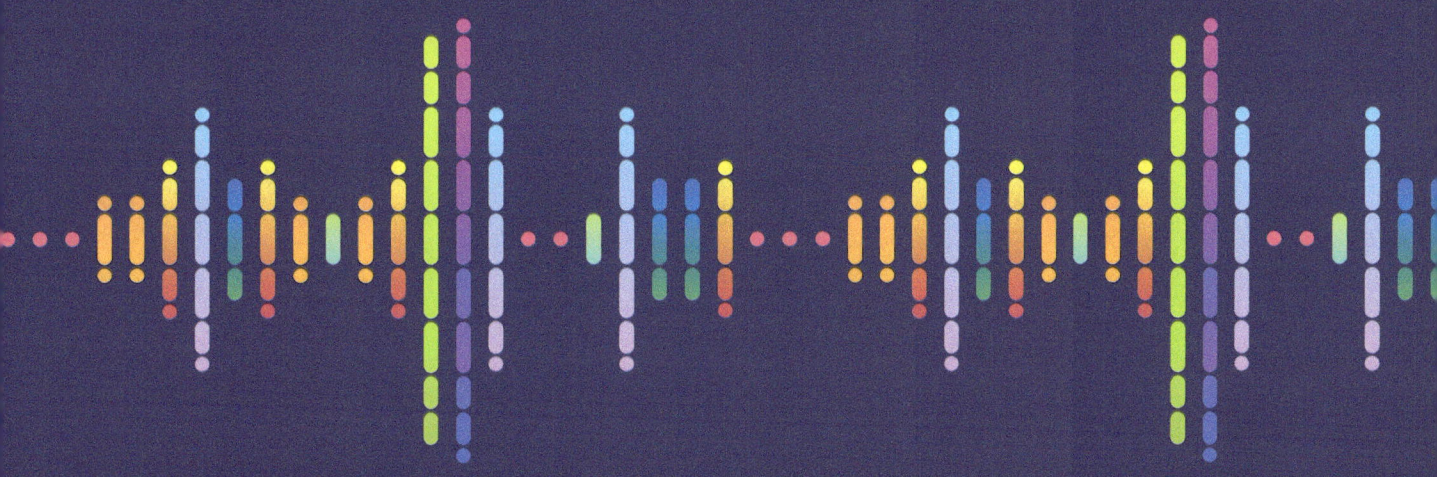

13   Exemplars.........................190

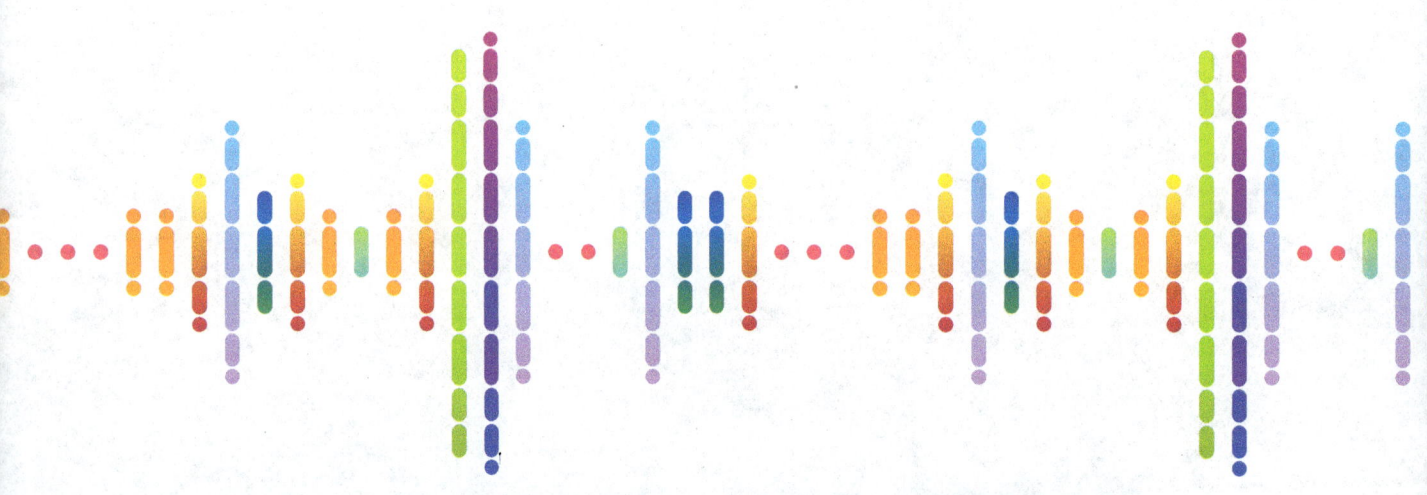

OBJECTIVES

- Highlight the use of the Johns Hopkins Evidence-Based Practice (JHEBP) model in real-world EBP projects

- Provide an example of one way to document an EBP project

13
EXEMPLARS

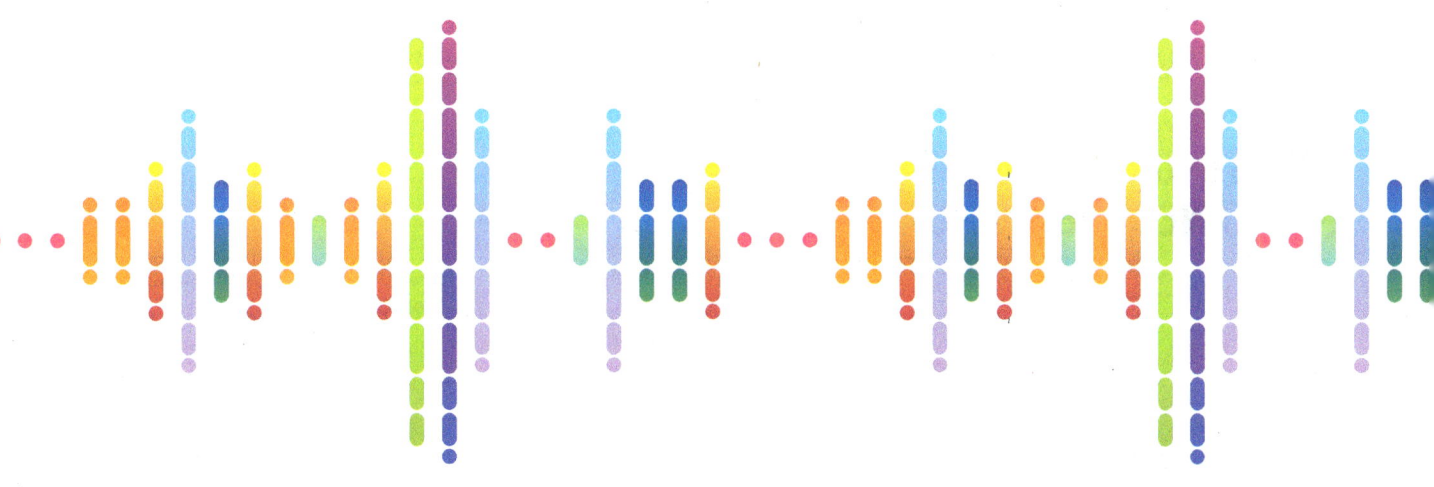

INTRODUCTION

The following exemplars were created from projects using the fourth edition of *Johns Hopkins Evidence-Based Practice for Nurses and Healthcare Professionals: Model & Guidelines*. While these good examples of the JHEBP model do not include the new tools and terminology changes for the new edition, the overall process remains the same.

STRATEGIES IN PROMOTING AND INCREASING CERTIFICATION AMONG PERIANESTHESIA NURSES

Marie Graziela F. Bautista, MSN, RN, CPAN, CAPA
Autumn L. Forester, MS, RN-BC
Mercy Medical Center
Baltimore, MD, USA

Practice Question

Health consumers are more knowledgeable than ever about safety and quality of healthcare. Above all, they want expert nursing and medical care. Certification is one way that nurses show to patients, employers, and colleagues that they possess advanced nursing knowledge, experience, expertise, and competence in their specialty field of nursing practice. Certification is encouraged and supported by the American Nurses Credentialing Center. The Magnet Recognition Program® recognizes nursing excellence in hospitals. For an organization to achieve Magnet® status, one requirement is focused on professional development and promoting certification in both clinical and administrative nursing roles. One strategic goal in our institution, under the Professional Growth and Development component of our hospital's nursing Professional Practice Model, is to increase the number of certified nurses. In our Orthopedic Surgical Center (Crane Preop/PACU), only 25% of nurses are certified, of which only one nurse (5%) is certified in the specialty of perianesthesia nursing.

The benefits of professional nursing certification have been widely supported and published; however, there is a recognized need to explore the nurses' perceived values of certification, determine the barriers in obtaining certification, and identify strategies that will promote certification among perianesthesia nurses in our unit/department. The EBP question to be evaluated was, "What are the best strategies in promoting and increasing certification among perianesthesia nurses?"

Evidence

To gather evidence on best strategies to promote certification, a literature search was conducted using the CINAHL and PubMed databases. A final selection of 16 articles was reviewed using the Johns Hopkins Evidence Based Practice (JHEBP) appraisal tools. Of the 16 articles, there were two Level II research studies. One study provided high quality (A) results to identify barriers and motivators to certification. The other study provided good quality (B) results to identify strategies to increase participation in certification. Many articles were descriptive quantitative/qualitative research, integrative review of literature, and program evaluation, graded at high (A) and good (B) quality. Level III articles ($n = 4$) were descriptive quantitative/qualitative studies that identified nurses' perceived values of certification, barriers to obtaining certification, and strategies to promote certification. The articles also discussed attributes that nurses and hospitals must have to promote and increase certification rates. Some Level V articles ($n = 7$) were integrative reviews of literature that reported the benefits of certification to patients, nurses, organizations, facilitators to certification, and strategies to promote and increase certification rate. Other Level V articles were program evaluations ($n = 3$) that reported strategies used to remove barriers and increase certification rates. The literature emphasizes the importance of recognizing obstacles to obtaining certification and recommends hospital institutions support their nurses in their journey toward achieving certification. Evidence synthesis revealed that:

- Certification improves patient outcomes and nursing sensitive indicators. Patients and families are more satisfied with care provided by certified nurses. Specialty certification is associated with better patient outcomes and nurse and organizational outcomes.

- Organizations supporting certification have a direct impact on success and outcomes.

- Nurses perceived and identified values of certification that are categorized into intrinsic (increased sense of professional growth, accountability, autonomy, confidence in clinical abilities) and extrinsic (recognition by peers and organization, financial incentives, increased marketability) benefits.

- The identified barriers to obtaining certification are cost of the examination, cost of review courses, lack of time to study, lack of access to resources to prepare for the examination, test-taking anxiety, fear of failure, lack of financial and leadership support from their institution, and inadequate recognition from nurse and hospital leadership.

- The identified facilitators to certification are reimbursement of examination costs, providing exam prep and review materials, in-house review courses, innovative educational delivery methods, and institutional support and recognition.

- In reviewing the evidence for this project, efforts should focus on certification campaigns on the intrinsic and extrinsic rewards of certification as well as developing strategies to remove identified barriers to certification.

Translation

A pre- and post-intervention survey was conducted to identify awareness, values, barriers, and facilitators to certification. Pre-intervention survey results were congruent with what the literature reported on the perceived values, barriers, and facilitators to certification. Strategies were implemented to address the barriers identified. Interventions were focused on awareness of the perianesthesia specialty certifications—Certified Post Anesthesia Nurse (CPAN) and Certified Ambulatory Perianesthesia Nurse (CAPA)—availability of a certification coach, easy access to review exam prep materials, coverage of exam fees, and free review courses. This was done via staff education, the selection of a nurse certification champion, and the creation of a certification station outfitted with review and exam preparation materials. After the intervention, there was a notable increase in awareness on perianesthesia specialty certification from 40% to 100%. The nurses' likelihood of taking the CPAN or CAPA exams increased from 20% to 85%. Nurses from the unit started utilizing resources from the certification station, sought the assistance of the nurse certification champion, and created study groups to review for the exams. From this, nursing leadership buy-in expanded, resulting in the purchase of exam vouchers with test assured programs and reimbursement of fees from review courses. To date, 45% of eligible nurses are scheduled to take the CPAN or CAPA certification exams within the year.

Summary

Providing resources and removing barriers to certification increases the likelihood for the nurses to prepare and take the exams. Organizations must facilitate and support their nurses' journey toward certification. Other units and departments in the institution seeking to increase certification rates could implement similar strategies and initiatives to increase the likelihood of success.

MANILA DOCTORS HOSPITAL EVIDENCE-BASED CULTURE OF NURSE RETENTION

Nicolo Martin A. Bello, BSN, RN
Aikee Millicent F. Salagoste, BSN, RN
Khristian D. Alfon, BSN, RN
Marcia C. Macaranas, BSN, RN
Dona-lee V. Espina, MAN, BSN, RN
Joy Carmel G. Gorospe, PhD, MAN, BSN, RN
Rodolfo C. Borromeo, EdD, MAN, BSN, RN, FFCHA
Manila Doctors Hospital
Manila, Philippines

Practice Question

Critical nursing workforce shortages have been reported in 57 countries, including the Philippines. In the Philippines, turnover is more common among nurses employed in private hospitals than in government hospitals, which also impacts nurse retention. This poses a challenge that may lead to substantial financial and quality loss and many severe organizational consequences. In 2019, 216 clinical nurses were hired at Manila Doctors Hospital (MDH), 107 (50%) of whom resigned. The average turnover rate of clinical nurses in MDH for the year 2019 was 31%, with the highest rates noted among critical care units. Average retention rate of clinical nurses in MDH for the year 2019 was 80%. As of August 2020, mean average years of retention of clinical nurses in MDH was 6.94 years. With the aim of synthesizing available literature to identify the factors affecting nurse retention and development of a culture of nurse retention supported by evidence-based programs/strategies, the team formulated the foreground EBP question, "Does development of a culture of retention supported by evidence-based practice strategies improve patient, nurse clinical, and process outcomes among clinical nurses?"

Evidence

Guided practice is an educational instruction approach based on the sociocultural theory of learning and teaching and is essential in building a culture. In this regard, the team applied the Johns Hopkins Evidence-Based Practice (JHEBP) model together with guided practice from its external partner, Mercy Medical Center. CINAHL, CINAHL PLUS, PubMed, EBSCO, and Joanna Briggs were the databases utilized for the literature search. The search yielded 103 articles, 53 of which were appraised, and of these, 37 were included for summary and synthesis.

There were no Level I and Level II articles determined eligible for summary and synthesis. The Level III evidence of A/B quality rating found that nurse retention is improved where there is a presence of authentic leadership encouraged through examples of leader-member exchange, leader's behavioral integrity, and provision of leadership programs. These articles also revealed that organizational commitment can be achieved by providing a supportive work environment through self-care workshops, coaching and mentoring, and a spiritual climate that encourages nurse autonomy, resiliency, flexibility, and self-efficacy. Findings also indicated that a nurse residency program that values the quality of orientation and proper conflict resolution through communication and listening skills can help in championing the nurse. Level IV evidence found that promoting autonomy, providing rewards and recognition, and encouraging open communication through a leadership framework can improve nurse retention. Level V evidence found that nurse retention is improved where there is effective leadership that promotes leader-staff communication, shared accountability, and adequate resources and staffing to the workforce. The implementation of a Nurse

Residency Program—which can maintain staff wellness through education, encouraging positive personality traits, and improving emotional intelligence–is also effective for nurse retention.

Based on the findings, the team created and implemented an evidence-based Culture of Nurse Retention program inclusive of the following themes:

1. Professional development
2. Communication/relationships
3. Culture and work environment
4. Organizational structure and support

Based on good and consistent evidence, the team recommends a pilot of change or further investigation. The team recommends measuring indicators of monthly patient satisfaction, quarterly nurse satisfaction, quarterly average nurse turnover rate, annual average nurse retention rate, and annual conducive work environment index to track the impact of EBP on the nurse retention in MDH.

Translation

Findings of this project led to the formulation of several programs on the identified themes. To support the professional development theme, the Nourish to Flourish program was established, which provides support to nurses for both horizontal and vertical advancement.

The communication and relationships theme is being addressed through programs developed and supported by the Human Resources Directorate and the Psychosocial Enriching Team Support. These programs support nurses by offering wellness programs and opportunities to meet in a casual environment to exchange ideas and concerns with leadership. To address the culture and work environment theme, new programs were developed on cultivating imperatives of organizational values. Camaraderie among nurses was supported with activities ranging from presentations on core values, personality enhancement, health enhancement, and socialization through group exercise and activities. The directorate also spearheaded a Workplace Incivility Prevention program to address workplace incivility. Lastly, the Nursing Service Directorate continued to reach out to its nursing staff to address the organizational structure and support theme with gestures such as providing rewards and recognition efforts, leadership seminars, and a quarterly Kumusta Ka Na? (How Are You?) survey to assess the nursing staff status on retention and status and to hear their thoughts and perspectives on how the nursing leaders can further improve our relationships and support to the whole directorate.

Summary

The development and implementation of multiple nurse engagement programs have begun to support improved MDH nurse retention. Continuous monitoring of nurse retention indicators is ongoing, although external factors such as the COVID-19 pandemic have affected the patient, nurse clinical, and process outcomes. The programs are continuously being improved through collaborative engagement with the institution's nursing leaders, who support the program. As a result, the retention rate increased from 50% (2020) to 57% (2023), and the conducive work environment index increased from 3.04/4 (2020) to 3.16/4 (2023).

RN-DRIVEN HIGH FLOW NASAL CANNULA GUIDELINES: USING EVIDENCE TO CHANGE PRACTICE MANAGEMENT

Mara M. Ceruto, DNP, APRN, CPNP-PC
Kaitlin Kobaitri, DO, FAAP
Kristen Lopenz, MSN, APRN, FNP-BC
Michelle Parmenter, MSN, APRN, FNP-BC
Monique Tarrou-Davis, MSN, APRN, FNP-BC, CPN
Nicklaus Children's Hospital
Miami, Florida, USA

Practice Question

Acute respiratory distress and bronchiolitis are the most common causes of admission into the pediatric intensive care unit (PICU). High-flow nasal cannula (HFNC) has become a prevalent mode of noninvasive respiratory support in the pediatric population, especially among infants and children inside and outside of the ICUs. When providing proper HFNC therapy, decreased intubation rates and improved airway resistance and lung compliance are noted.

The PICU team at Nicklaus Children's Hospital identified concerns with the current management of patients on HFNC. These concerns included gaps in RN education regarding effective HFNC settings, lack of appropriate weaning guidelines, and extended length of stay (LOS) for patients receiving HFNC therapy. These concerns also supported the need for HFNC guidelines to safely and effectively wean patients needing HFNC support. The background EBP question was, "What are best practices for implementing HFNC weaning guidelines in the PICU, and do they contribute to decreased LOS?"

Evidence

To gather evidence on HFNC guidelines, a literature search was conducted using key terms utilizing CINAHL, PubMed, and Google Scholar databases. A final selection of six articles was independently appraised by team members using the Johns Hopkins Evidence-Based Practice (JHEBP) Appendices E and F. Two articles were identified as a Level I and evaluated to be good quality. Level III ($n = 2$), Level IV ($n = 1$), and Level V ($n = 1$) articles provided evidence of a decrease in LOS while using a weaning protocol of between 10 and 24 hours. The literature emphasized the importance of implementing a standardized weaning guideline to shorten overall treatment time and hospital LOS. Evidence synthesis revealed that:

- Average HFNC duration per patient dropped from 2.5 days to 1.8 days with the use of a respiratory assessment score and protocol.

- PICU LOS decreased from 2.6 days to 2.1 days. Total hospital LOS dropped from 5.7 days to 4.7 days.

- Post-protocol patients had a lower HFNC failure rate, thus decreasing the number of intubations.

- The average time that the patients were on high-flow without a weaning protocol was 26 hours compared to 15 hours with the protocol.

In reviewing the evidence for this project, there was a clear association between the use of a weaning guideline, decreased length of treatment time, and a decrease in LOS.

Translation

The guideline was developed to decrease the gap in bedside RN education regarding safe HFNC weaning due to a lack of appropriate weaning guidelines in the PICU, which was causing an increase in the hospital LOS. A pilot was implemented in which age-specific weaning guidelines were included in the comment section of the HFNC order. The bedside RNs and respiratory therapists were educated on protocol and their role through inservices. Compliance with the guideline recommendations was monitored through daily random chart audits to identify barriers. Once the guidelines were utilized and 90% compliance was achieved, a need for a PICU-specific Power Plan was recommended to improve continuity among providers and efficiency when initiating orders.

Summary

Implementing an HFNC guideline in the PICU has helped to significantly decrease treatment time by almost 24 hours, PICU LOS by 24 hours, and overall hospital LOS by two days. Furthermore, implementation of the PICU HFNC Power Plan allows bedside nurses and respiratory therapists to drive the weaning process for their patients on HFNC through the instruction of age-specific guidelines when initiating HFNC. Such autonomy contributes to successful and safe weaning, decreased treatment days, and decreased days spent in the hospital.

SET SAIL FOR HOME: A NURSE-DRIVEN INITIATIVE PROMOTING EARLY AMBULATION IN POST-OPERATIVE NEUROSURGICAL PATIENTS

Jenna Lang, MSN, RN, CPN
Stephanie Ferrare, MSN, APRN, FNP-BC
Evelyn Garcia, BSN, RN
Nicklaus Children's Hospital
Maimi, Florida, USA

Practice Question

Early mobilization promotes a decrease in length of stay (LOS) and has been shown to prevent functional decline and hospital-acquired conditions. An inpatient neurology and neurosurgery unit identified a gap in which post-operative neurosurgical patients are experiencing a delay in discharge for reasons that can be remedied through ambulation. Ambulation is key to help promote bodily functions and improve overall patient wellness. Currently, there is no standardized process to ambulate post-operative neurosurgical patients. The project's purpose was to implement a standardized process to ambulate post-operative neurosurgical patients to prevent delay in discharge, decreasing stay length. The foreground PICO EBP question evaluated was, "In pediatric postoperative neurosurgical patients (P), does early ambulation (I) compared to our standard of care (C) impact length of stay (O)?"

Evidence

To gather evidence on initiating early mobilization programs for post-operative neurosurgical patients, a literature review was conducted using the search terms early mobilization/ambulation AND neurosurgery, early mobilization/ambulation AND pediatrics, and early mobilization/ambulation AND neurosurgery AND pediatrics. Our team searched for the most relevant articles using PubMed, CINAHL, and Google Scholar. Nine total articles met criteria through screening. Two individual team members independently appraised each of the articles using the Johns Hopkins Evidence-Based Practice (JHEBP) Appendices E and F. The articles were then graded for level and quality of evidence. Three articles were Level I studies with good quality evidence, and three quasi-experimental studies were graded Level II with high-quality evidence. All Level I and Level II studies demonstrated that implementing an early mobilization program versus standard practice decreased LOS in different patient populations including PICU and post-operative patients. One Level III and two Level V high-quality studies were included that found the use of early mobilization helps with restoration of normal bowel function and prevention of hospital-acquired conditions. Evidence synthesis revealed that:

- Early mobilization not only promotes a decreased LOS but also prevents loss of muscle mass, reduces readmission rates, improves quality of life, decreases opioid use, and successfully leads to a faster return to performing activities of daily living.

- Successful collaboration with physical therapists, occupational therapists, speech language pathologists, providers, and nurses improved outcomes by helping patients follow early mobilization interventions.

- Initiating early mobilization for post-operative neurosurgical patients such as those admitted for external ventricular drains, subarachnoid hemorrhages, and Chiari decompressions is both safe and feasible, leading to a decreased LOS.

Translation

After evaluating and synthesizing the evidence, our team determined that establishing a standard protocol and safety checklist when implementing early mobilization programs was key to shortening average LOS. A standardized education sheet, titled "Set Sail for Home," was created in collaboration with neurosurgery providers, advanced practice nurses, and the Child Life team to promote ambulation three times a day. Different methods of ambulation practices such as playing, dancing, and walking were presented on the sheet to help engage patients. All nurses and care assistants were first educated on this standardized education sheet so they could better educate parents and patients about the importance of early ambulation for post-operative neurosurgical procedures. Nurses were empowered to initiate the "Set Sail for Home" education once patients were cleared to ambulate by neurosurgery providers. Nurses would then monitor these patients to ensure they were compliant with ambulation. A post survey for parents and patients was created using Survey Monkey. This survey was to be completed prior to discharge to assess knowledge and satisfaction on the standardized education sheet. After implementation, all patients and families who received the education commented that it was a great way to get patients moving and understanding its importance. All patients met the goal of ambulating three times a day.

Summary

A standardized process to ambulate post-operative neurosurgical patients was implemented to decrease LOS. By conducting a thorough literature review, it was evident that empowering nurses to educate patients and their parents to engage in ambulating at least three times a day post-operatively improves mobility function and results in decreased hospital LOS. The results were favorable and will continue to be utilized to aid in decreasing LOS. Future implications include a plan to add an ambulation task in the electronic health record to remind nurses to set an ambulation goal for this patient population. Plans are in place to provide patient education in languages other than English. Having a standardized process for ambulation of post-operative patients has proven effective in positive patient outcomes and decreasing LOS.

REDUCING NURSE BURDEN RELATED TO LIMITED CARE PARTNER VISITATION

Chana Peele, BSN, RN
Sara Zachmann, BSN, RN, BMT-CN
Katelin Santhin, BSN, RN, RN-C
Anna Alisch, BSN, RN
Michael Mannello, BSN, RN
Carinna Emilio, BSN, RN, RN-CEFM
Madeleine Whalen, MSN/MPH, RN, CEN, NPD-BC
The Johns Hopkins Hospital
Baltimore, MD, USA

Practice Question

The COVID-19 virus presented unique challenges to inpatient bedside nurses and visiting care partners. Hospitals across the nation implemented visitor restrictions to mitigate the spread of the respiratory disease. This inadvertently added additional stress to the bedside nurse's workload, as family and friends of the patient could either no longer, or for a minimal amount of time, visit their loved ones. With open visitation policies, care partners can and are encouraged to visit patients, provide emotional support, and assist with the patient's daily plan of care. The removal of this healthcare partner role increased the bedside nurse's workload, diminished communication with care partners, and involuntarily left nurses as visitor restriction enforcers due to a lack of comprehensive policies. This strained work environment ultimately increased work dissatisfaction and decreased productivity. Given these drawbacks, a team of nurses across different specialties from the Johns Hopkins Hospital conducted an evidenced-based practice (EBP) project to address the question, "What are best practices to reduce undue burden on nurses related to limited care partner visitation in the hospital setting?"

Evidence

Databases including PubMed, Embase, CINAHL, and PsycInfo were used to identify articles that answered the EBP question. The team used the Johns Hopkins Evidence-Based Practice (JHEBP) model for evidence appraisal, synthesis, and translation. During article screening and appraisal, two team members independently assessed its relevancy and ability to answer the practice question. Ultimately, 11 articles were included in the review. Eight were Level III, and three were Level V evidence. The Level III studies were comprised of four qualitative studies, three quantitative studies, and one mixed-methods design. The three Level V articles consisted of two expert opinions and one integrative review. All articles included in this review were assigned A or B quality. Overall synthesis generated good and consistent evidence that supported four main themes: policy improvement ($n = 7$), use of technology to facilitate communication ($n = 6$), use of a dedicated communication liaison role or team ($n = 5$), and providing nurses with communication skills training ($n = 7$).

Translation

Nurses experienced increased workload and anxiety from navigating, communicating, and enforcing frequently changing policies. Mitigation of nurse distress during restricted visitation requires visiting policies that are easily understandable, leaving limited room for interpretation and minimizing policy changes. Using smart devices to aid in communication between patients and loved ones virtually demonstrated less emotional exhaustion in nurses compared to those who did not. Findings of one institution's use of nurse liaisons discovered that moral distress and workflow hurdles were reduced on the ICUs where this role was piloted. Furthermore, ICU nurses were relieved that care partners' needs were being attended to even if they were unable to provide support themselves. Providing communication skills training to bedside nurses is a recommended strategy to support nurses through the challenges of restricted visitation. One study found that clinicians with communication training felt less of a time strain when dealing with care partners compared to those without.

Summary

Recommendations include the application of evidence-based policies, expansion and thoughtful use of communication technology, development of a family support team or nurse liaison role, and providing communication skills training to nurses. Although currently still amid COVID-19 pandemic challenges, other global health issues are possible in the future, and preparation with the proper interventions can help mitigate the disadvantages of visitor restrictions. Next steps include submission of our manuscript to *The Journal of Nursing Administration* for publication.

TRANSFORMING THE LANDSCAPE OF GENDER-AFFIRMING CARE FOR TRANSGENDER YOUTH THROUGH ACUTE REHABILITATION PROVIDER EMPOWERMENT

Melissa Radlein, DPT, PT, PCS
Priya Meyer, DNP, RN, NEA-BC, NPD-BC, PCNS-BC
Children's Hospital Los Angeles
Los Angeles, CA, USA

Problem Description and Practice Question

Transgender and gender-diverse (TGD) individuals are at higher risk for mortality, medical morbidities, and poor psychosocial outcomes, and they experience significant barriers to accessing healthcare. These barriers often stem from existing provider bias, knowledge deficit, and/or lack of skills in the provision of gender-affirming care. Graduate-level clinical training and continued education have failed to keep up with the increasingly complex needs of this vulnerable population, resulting in a lack of foundational knowledge and self-efficacy among clinicians providing care today.

At a freestanding children's hospital on the West Coast, the gender affirmation (GA) team provides specialty surgical services for TGD youth as one of only eight pediatric programs in the nation. The interprofessional GA team includes acute rehabilitation (AR) providers, who provide care at a pivotal moment in these patients' GA journey and are thereby uniquely positioned to influence an affirming environment for this vulnerable population.

Cultural humility (CH) training is offered during employee orientation, but content is generalized to all patient care services.

The evidence-based practice (EBP) question to be evaluated was, "For AR providers, what are best practices for improving CH and self-efficacy in the care of TGD patients?"

Evidence

An interprofessional team of providers representing physical therapy, occupational therapy, social work, and nursing collaborated to initiate an EBP project to address the gender-affirming needs of inpatient TGD youth. A literature search was completed using the following databases: CINAHL Complete, EBSCO Research Databases, ERIC, Health Business Elite, LGBTQ+ Source, MEDLINE, Nursing & Allied Health Database (ProQuest), PsycARTICLES, PsycINFO, Psychology and Behavioral Sciences Collection, PubMed@CHLA, and SocIndex with Full Text. The search produced 54 articles. After screening and reviewing full-text articles for eligibility, nine articles were included. The evidence was graded for strength and quality using the JHEBP model. Of the nine articles included, one article was rated Level III, and the other eight articles were rated Level V evidence. All articles were graded high quality.

The search yielded a paucity of research and clinical evidence specifically related to rehabilitation providers and the care of TGD individuals. However, there was consistent compelling research and clinical evidence that supported transgender-specific CH training for providers. Summary and synthesis also consistently supported multimodal training as having positive impacts on clinician knowledge, self-efficacy, and attitudes related to the provision of care for TGD individuals.

Translation

A three-part, multimodal, experiential, educational intervention was designed with input from impacted groups to meet the specific needs of AR providers. The curriculum covered CH foundational knowledge, gender-affirming surgical information, AR considerations, and gender-inclusive communication strategies.

Instructors were clinical experts in their respective fields (e.g., nursing, rehabilitation, and social work). Education was open to all AR providers including rehabilitation aides, occupational therapists, physical therapists, and speech language pathologists. The pilot program was launched in the AR department in August 2023.

A pre-post survey design was used to determine the effectiveness of the intervention. Data collected included: 1) demographic information; 2) scores from the validated tool Lesbian Gay Bisexual and Transgender Development of Clinical Skills Scale, which assessed changes in provider knowledge, self-efficacy, and bias; and 3) course evaluation information. A two-tailed paired t-test was used for analysis with an α set to 0.05.

Summary

Forty-nine of 55 eligible participants engaged in one or more of the three-part education program (20% one part, 36% two parts, and 33% all three parts). Data was matched for 28 (51%) staff when comparing both pre- and post-education surveys. There was a statistically significant improvement in provider self- efficacy ($p = < 0.001$) and knowledge ($p < 0.05$) in pre-to-post education implementation. There was no significant change in provider attitudes ($p > 0.50$).

Multimodal, experiential, rehabilitation-specific CH training related to the acute post-operative needs of TGD patients effectively translates to improvements in provider knowledge and self-efficacy. These findings have been disseminated at the institutional level. Next steps include translation of this program to additional work areas and disciplines at our institution and sustainability planning/standard setting of education for future providers. Future research with rigorous methodology is needed, particularly to inform the needs of TGD patients immediately post-operative from GA surgeries to ensure that consistent, skilled, respectful care is provided in an affirming environment.

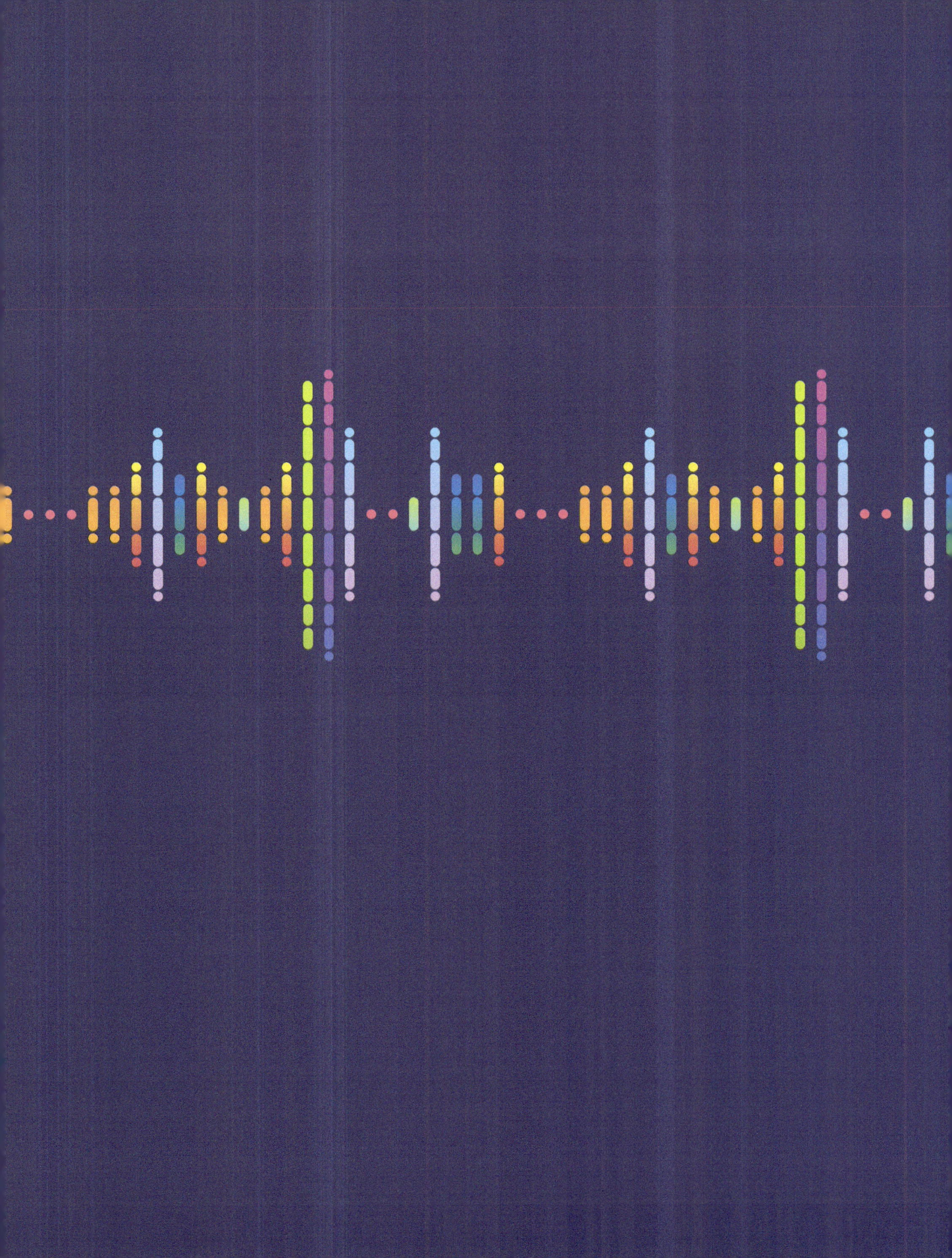

PART IV
APPENDICES

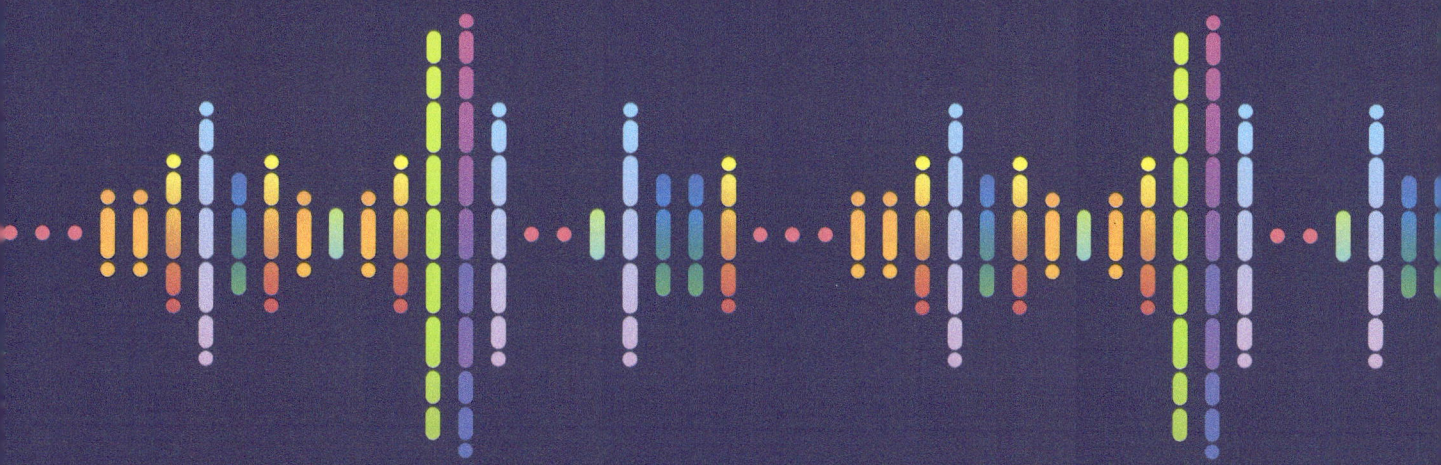

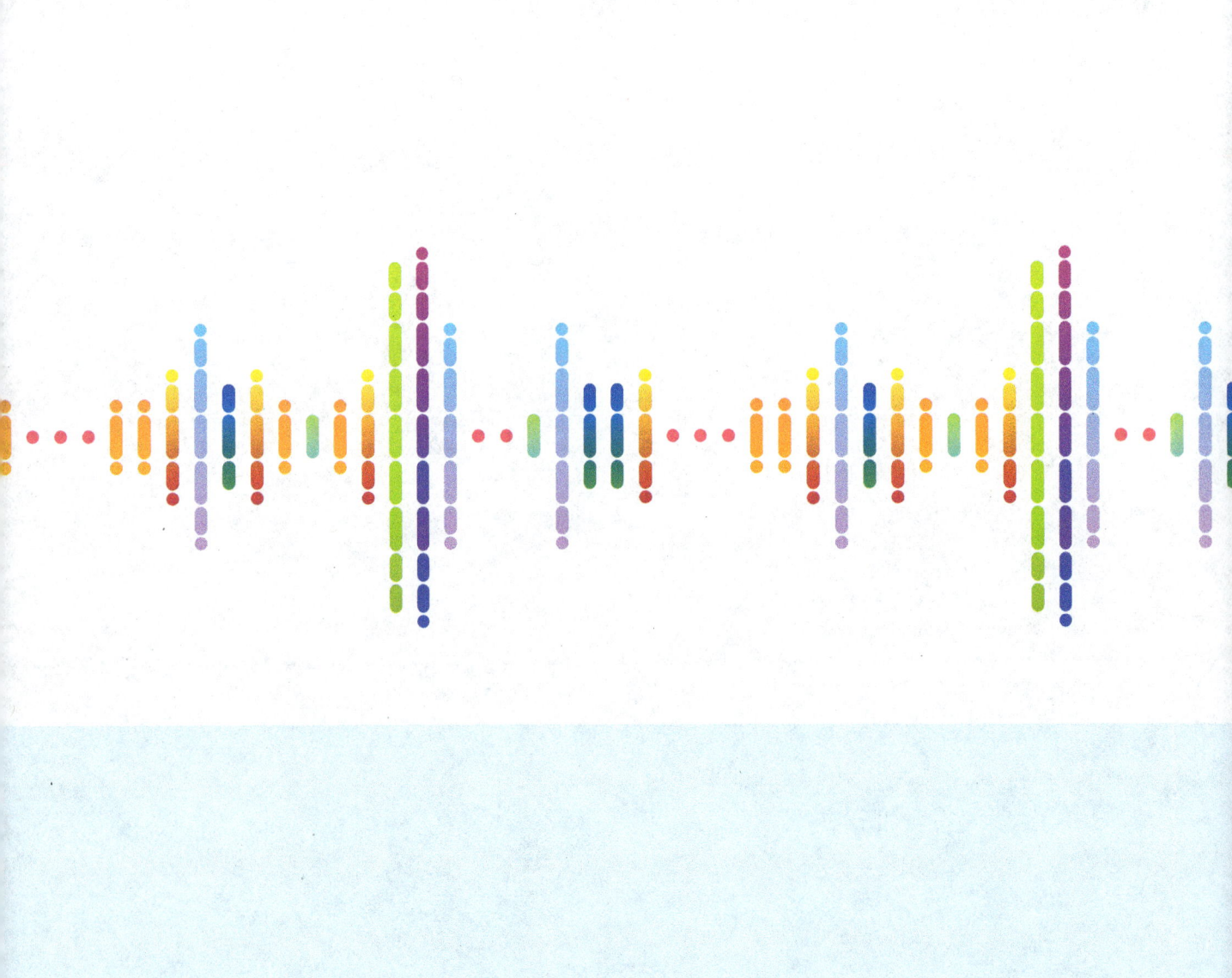

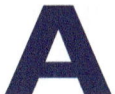

EBP PROJECT STEPS AND OVERVIEW

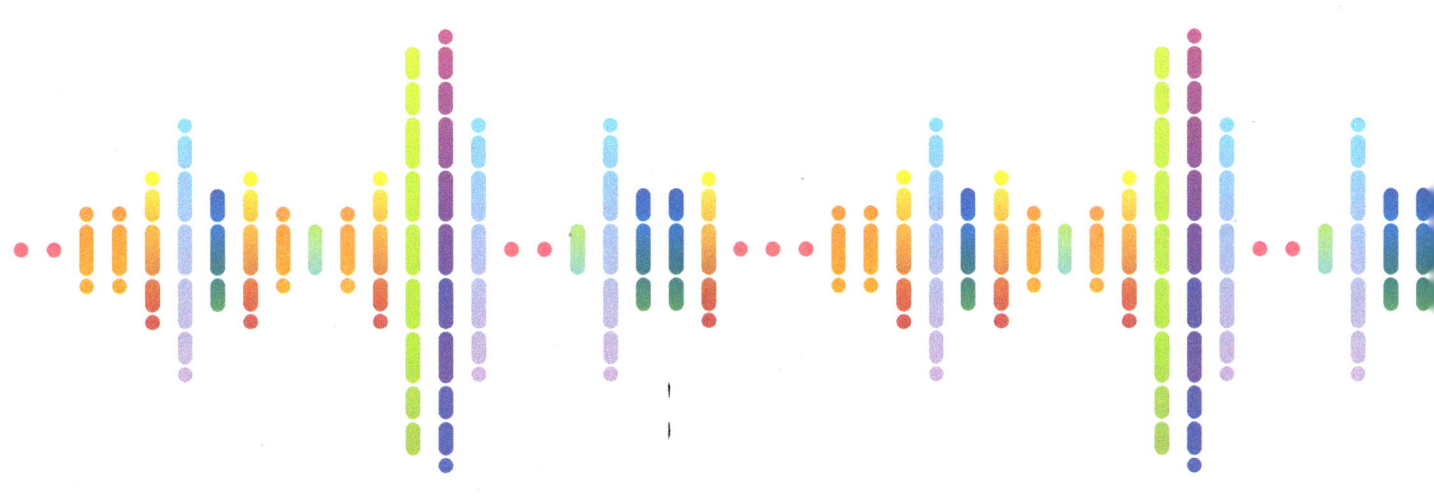

EBP Project Steps and Overview

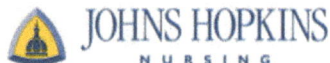

Purpose: This appendix outlines the steps in the PET process and factors the team should consider throughout the project. The tools to facilitate the steps are listed according to the process phase. Additionally, the decision tree guides teams in determining if an EBP project is the correct path and what kind of evidence search is required.

Steps	Phase	Associated Tool (Appendix)
1. Explore & describe the problem 2. Develop the problem statement 3. Write the EBP question	Practice Question	Question Development Tool (B)

Review On-Going Considerations

Steps	Phase	Associated Tool (Appendix)
4. Conduct best-evidence search & appraisal 5. Conduct targeted search OR exhaustive search and screening 6. Appraise the evidence 7. Summarize the evidence 8. Organize the data 9. Synthesize the findings 10. Record best evidence recommendations	Evidence	Searching and Screening Tool (C) Appraisal Tool Selection Algorithm (D) Pre-appraised Evidence Appraisal Tool (E1) Single Study Evidence Appraisal Tool (E2) Anecdotal Evidence Appraisal Tool (E3) Evidence Terminology and Considerations Guide (F) Best-Evidence Summary Tool (G1) Individual Evidence Summary Tool (G2) Summary, Synthesis, & Best-Evidence Recommendation Tool (H)

Review On-Going Considerations

Steps	Phase	Associated Tool (Appendix)
11. Assess the risk, fit, feasibility, & acceptability of best evidence recommendations 12. Identify practice-setting specific recommendations 13. Identify an implementation framework 14. Create an implementation/action plan 15. Implement 16. Monitor sustainability & identify next steps	Translation	Translation Tool (I) Implementation and Action Planning (A3) Tool (J)

On-Going Considerations

> Maintain project plan, including timeline & responsibilities

> Ensure appropriate team & impacted groups are involved

> Monitor project alignment with organizational priorities

> Communicate & disseminate

© 2025 Johns Hopkins Health System

Evidence Phase Decision Tree:

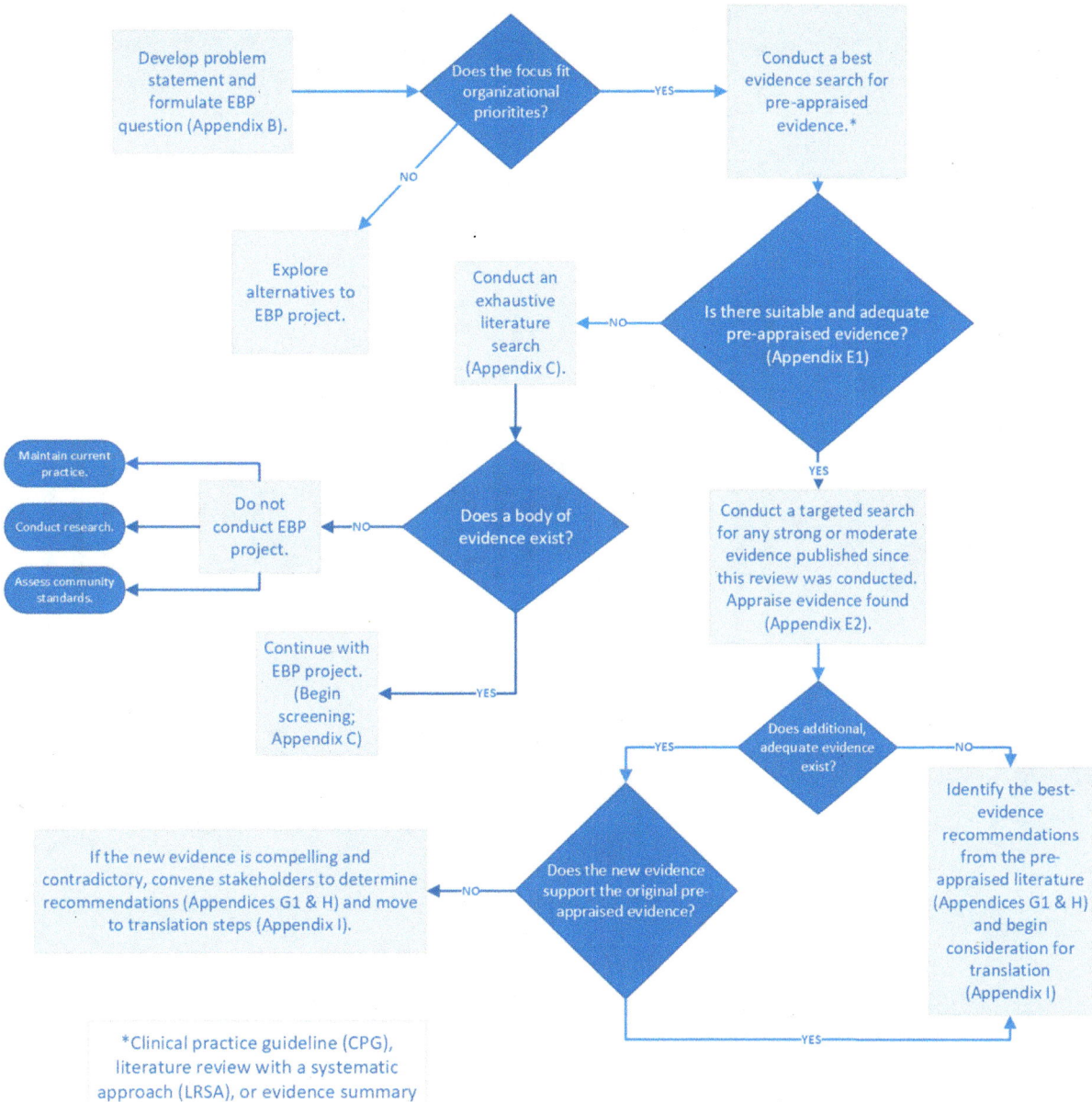

*Clinical practice guideline (CPG), literature review with a systematic approach (LRSA), or evidence summary

© 2025 Johns Hopkins Health System

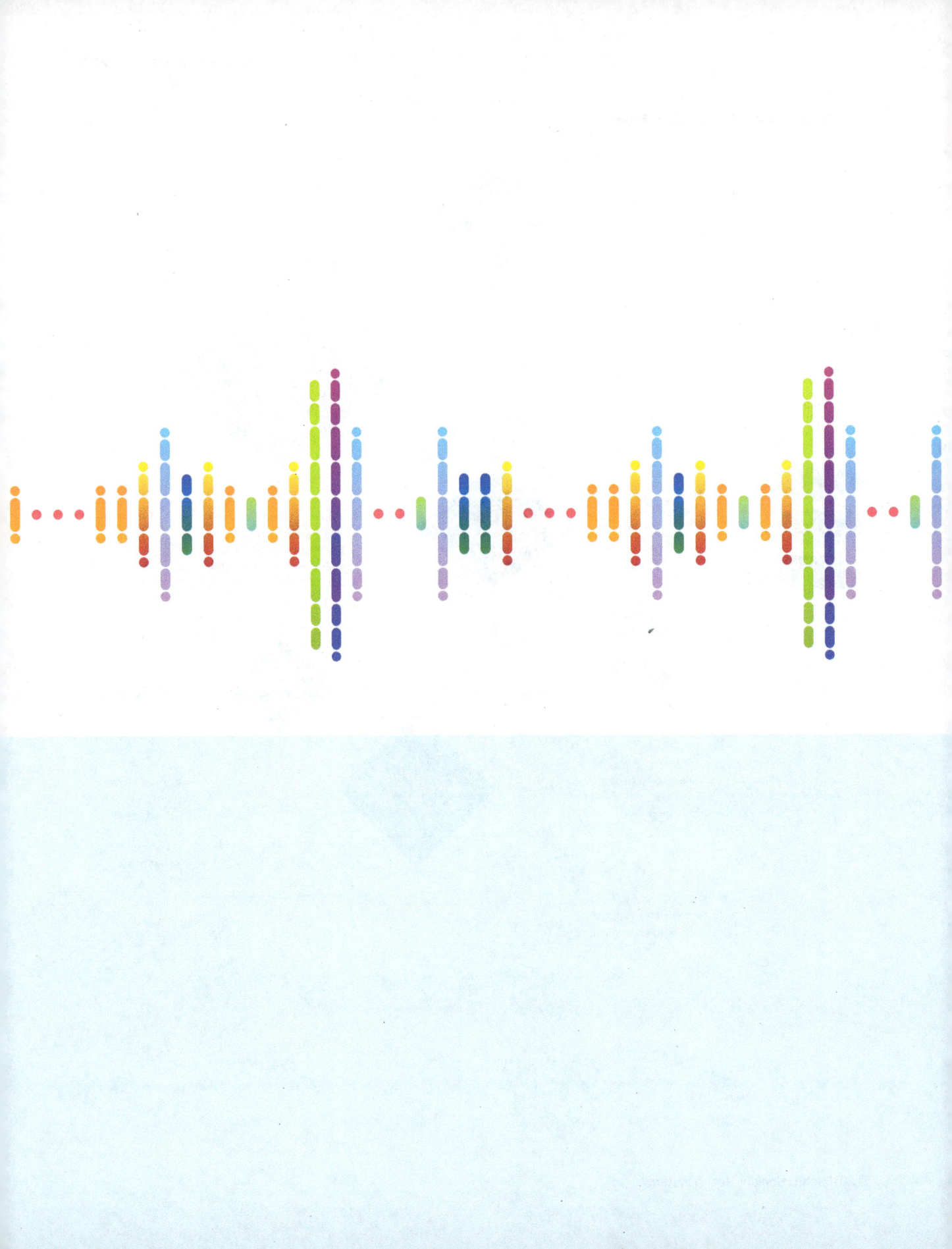

QUESTION DEVELOPMENT TOOL

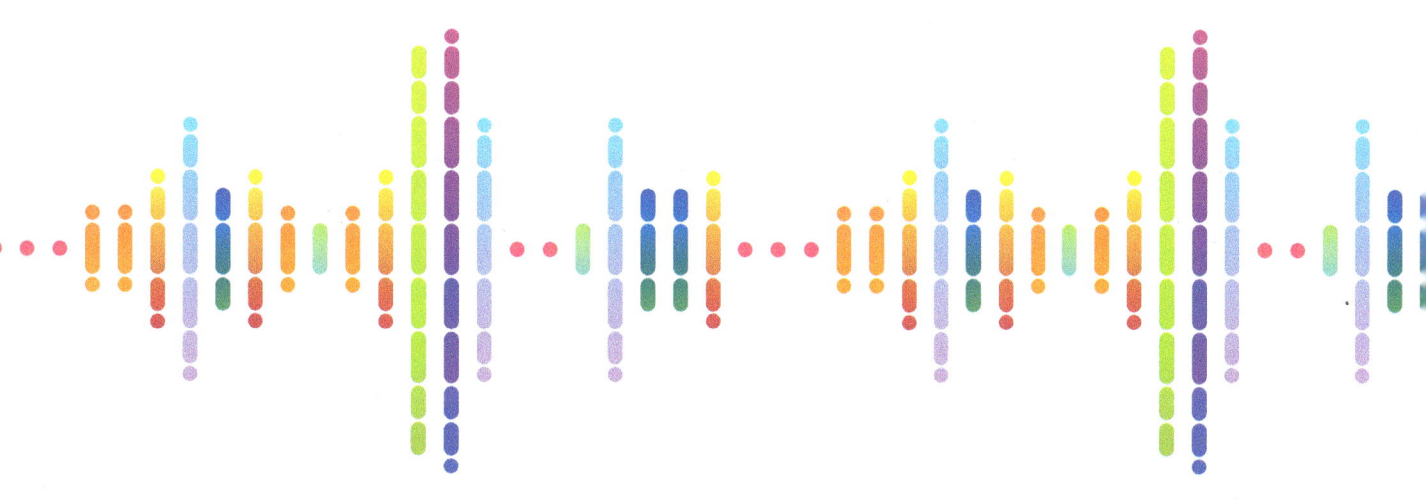

Question Development Tool

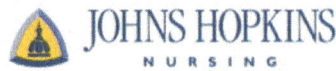

> Purpose: This form guides the EBP team in developing an answerable EBP question. It is meant to be fluid and dynamic as the team engages in the question development process. As the team becomes familiar with the evidence base for the topic of interest, they revisit, revise, and refine the question, search terms, search strategy, and sources of evidence.

If viewing this online, hover over bold text for more information

What is the local problem? *(the response can be a bulleted list or phrases)*

Why is this problem important and relevant? What would happen if it was not addressed?

What is the current practice in the EBP team's setting?

What data from the EBP team's setting indicates there is a problem?

Considering all of the information above, create a concise problem statement below.

Will this be a broad or intervention EBP question?
☐ Broad   ☐ Intervention

© 2025 Johns Hopkins Health System

Identify the relevant elements of the EBP question *(some items may not be used)*	
Population	
Setting	
Topic (for broad questions) or **Intervention**(s) (for intervention questions)	
Outcomes (as needed)	

Use the information above, and the sentence templates below, to construct the EBP question.

For Broad EBP Questions:

In/among _____ , what are best practices/strategies/interventions for/regarding _____ ?
      (*population and/or setting*)   (*topic*)

For Intervention EBP Questions:

According to the evidence, in/among _____ , what is the impact of _____ on _____ ?
                              (*population and/or setting*)   (*intervention**)   (*outcome*)

*If comparing more than one intervention, provide the interventions and separate them with the phrase "as compared to"

Record the completed EBP question below.

If needed after a preliminary evidence search/review, record an updated or revised EBP question here.

© 2025 Johns Hopkins Health System .

Instructions for the Question Development Tool

What is the local problem? *(The response can be a bulleted list or phrases)*
Describe the topic or problem that needs to be addressed in the team's local setting. This can be a quick and informal report of what is happening or the results of the group's brainstorming session.
Why is this problem important and relevant? What would happen if it was not addressed?
Establish a sense of importance and urgency for a practice problem to help build support for the EBP project and on-board other stakeholders. Emphasize why the problem must be addressed and the potential consequences of not doing so. This is the place to establish your "burning platform" for practice change.
What is the current practice in the EBP team's setting?
Define the current practice in the team's local setting, as it relates to the problem by identifying the gap or performance issue. Think about current unit or departmental policies and procedures as well as adherence to these guidelines. What is commonly considered acceptable among the staff related to their daily practice? Do policy and practice align? What do you see?
What data from the EBP team's setting indicates there is a problem?
Confirm the problem with concrete, rather than anecdotal, information from the team's specific setting. Concrete information exists in the form of staff or patient safety concerns, data demonstrating unsatisfactory process or outcome measures on the unit level, financial reports, identification of the lack of evidence for current organizational practice, or unsatisfactory quality indicators. Formal information or observations may demonstrate variations within the practice setting or the community. These elements are not mutually exclusive, and the problem may be evidenced in multiple areas.   Consider the following (provide actual data or examples, if available):   • Safety and risk management concerns   • Quality indicators   • Financial information   • Practice observations   • Lack of evidence for current practice   • Other data
Considering all of the information above, create a concise problem statement below.
Write a short paragraph to capture the problem. It should be succinct (one or two concise sentences) and robust (strongly constructed. Articulating a well-developed problem statement provides a comprehensive understanding of the population of interest (e.g., patients, families, staff, and their characteristics), how they are affected (e.g., morbidity, mortality, satisfaction), and why it matters.
Will this be a broad or intervention EBP question?
☐ Broad   ☐ Intervention
Select if you intend to write a broad or an intervention best practice question. Broad questions are expansive and produce a wide range of evidence to establish best practices when the team has little knowledge, experience, or expertise in the area of interest. Broad questions do not include any interventions or outcomes. Intervention questions are focused and may include a specific comparison of two or more ideas or interventions, as well as an outcome of interest. Intervention questions often flow from an initial broad question and evidence review.
Identify the relevant elements of the EBP question *(some items may not be used)*

Population	*Who is the group of interest? What types of patients, clients, healthcare providers, or people? Consider attributes such as age, gender, symptoms, diagnosis, or roles (e.g., pediatric, adult, nurses, pharmacists, post-operative patients, patients with congestive heart failure).*
Setting	*Where does the problem need to be addressed? What are the characteristics of the environment? Consider factors such as general location (e.g., in-patient, out-patient, home-based) and specific care areas (e.g., oncology, peri-operative, surgical, critical care).*
Topic (for broad questions) or **Intervention**(s) (for intervention questions)	*What is the problem or issue? Provide the general topic or the specific intervention(s) under investigation.*
Outcomes (as needed)	*Why is there a problem? What is the metric the team is hoping to address (e.g., fall rates, infection rates, length of stay)?*

Use the information above, and the sentence templates below, to construct the EBP question.

For Broad EBP Questions:

In/among _____ , what are best practices/strategies/interventions for/regarding _____?
      (population and/or setting)   *(topic)*

For Intervention EBP Questions:

According to the evidence, in/among _____ , what is the impact of _____ on _____?
                                                 (population and/or setting)   *(intervention*)*   *(outcome)*

*If comparing more than one intervention, provide the interventions and separate them with the phrase "as compared to"

Enter the **EBP Question** below.

Write the EBP question. Use the information you identified in the above section to complete the fill-in-the-blank sentence structure. Ensure you are using the correct format, depending on if you are writing a broad or intervention EBP question. You will also need to select if you would like to use the word "in" or among." Additionally, for broad questions, select "practices," "strategies" or "interventions" and "for" or "regarding," depending on that makes the sentence easiest to read.

After a preliminary evidence search/review, a revised EBP question can be developed if necessary.

Often the question that you start with will not be the final EBP question. Needed revisions to the EBP question may not be evident until after the initial evidence review, which may indicate a need to focus or broaden the question, update terminology, and/or consider additional measures of success.

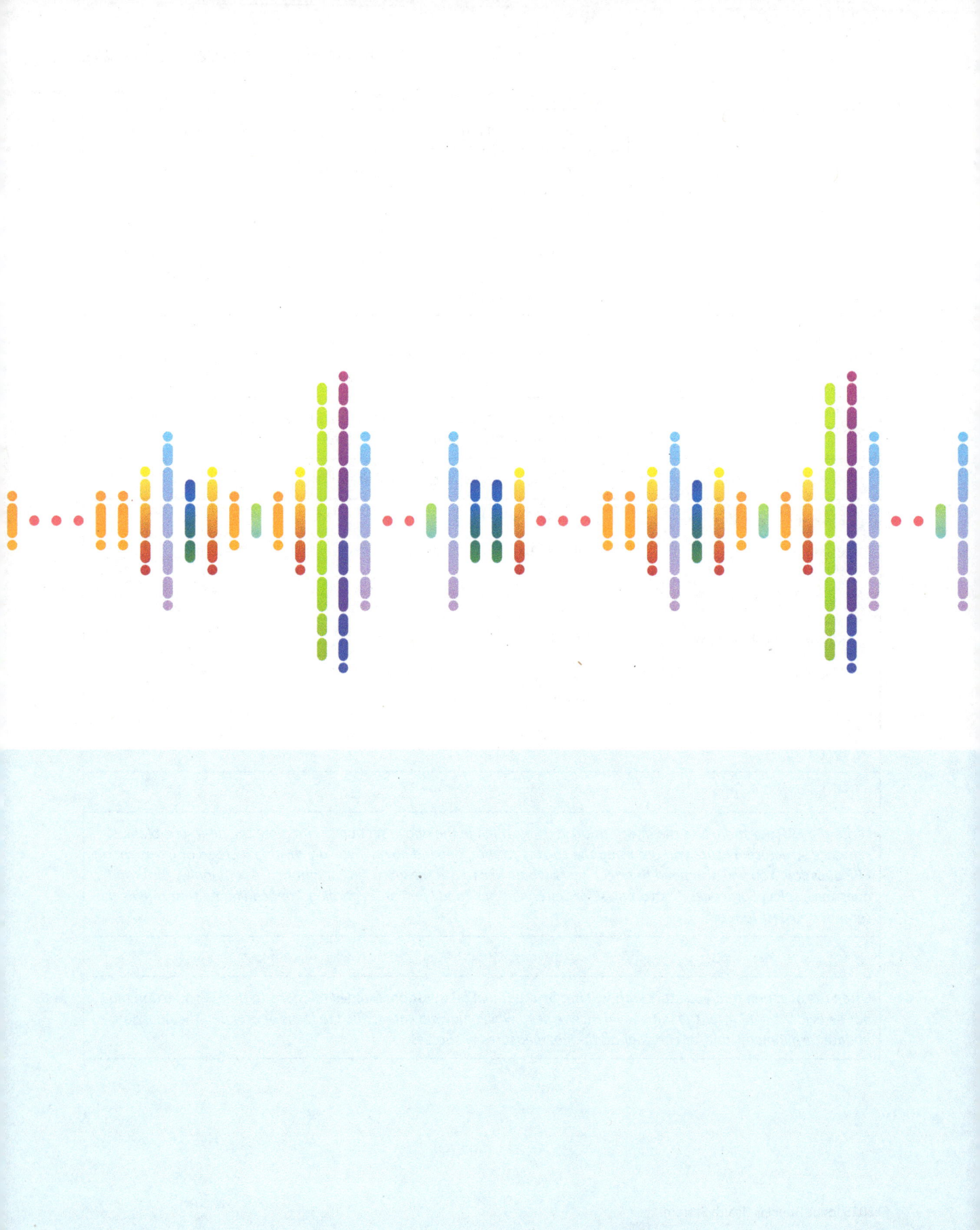

C

SEARCHING AND SCREENING TOOL

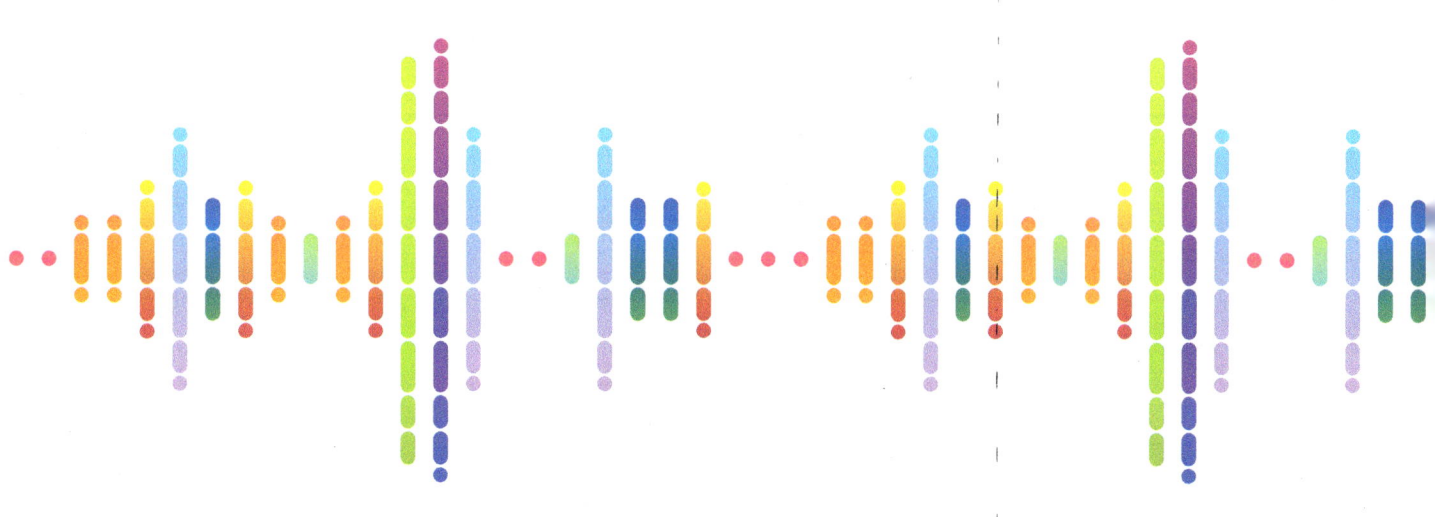

Searching and Screening Tool

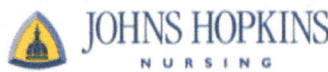

Purpose: This tool guides the team through the steps of searching for evidence that answers their EBP question and tracking the process. The team will first look for pre-appraised evidence in a best-evidence search. The results of that investigation will guide the next steps (a targeted or exhaustive search). Recording the evidence identification process creates confidence in the eventual project recommendations by demonstrating a thorough and unbiased approach.

Section I: Key Elements of the EBP Question

Identify the key elements of the EBP question (*from the Question Development Tool*)

Population	
Setting	
Topic or Intervention(s)	
Outcomes (as needed)	

Section II: Best-Evidence Search

Does pre-appraised evidence exist in the form of clinical practice guidelines (CPGs), literature reviews with a systematic approach (LRSAs), or evidence summaries?

☐ Yes → Appraise using the Pre-appraised Evidence Appraisal Tool (Appendix E1)
   o Is the evidence suitable and of adequate quality?
      ☐ Yes → Complete targeted search for additional evidence based on search date in pre-appraised evidence to determine if relevant evidence has been published in the interim
      ☐ No → Skip to Section III (Exhaustive Search)

☐ No → Skip to Section III (Exhaustive Search)

Section III: Exhaustive Search and Screening

Complete the table below using the population, setting, topic or intervention(s), and outcomes identified in Section I. List the element and associated terms to build a full search concept.

EBP Question Element	Possible Search Terms (*synonyms, alternative spellings, or brand names*)
1)	
2)	

© 2025 Johns Hopkins Health System

3)	
What databases will you search?	
☐ CINAHL ☐ MEDLINE (PubMed) ☐ Embase	☐ PsychINFO ☐ Epistemonikos ☐ Other:

What are the inclusion and exclusion criteria?	
Inclusion:	Exclusion:

What date limit will you use and why?

What is the date the team conducted the search?

What are the search strings and number of results from each database?

Database	Search String	Number of Results

How will the team systematically screen the results to identify evidence that answers the EBP question and meets the inclusion/exclusion criteria (*select all that apply*)?

☐ Use software or web-based program to track (e.g., Google Forms, Excel, Abstrackr)
☐ Have at least two independent reviewers for each record
☐ Inclusion or exclusion disagreements resolved by third reviewer
☐ Other:

Complete the screening flow chart below

© 2025 Johns Hopkins Health System

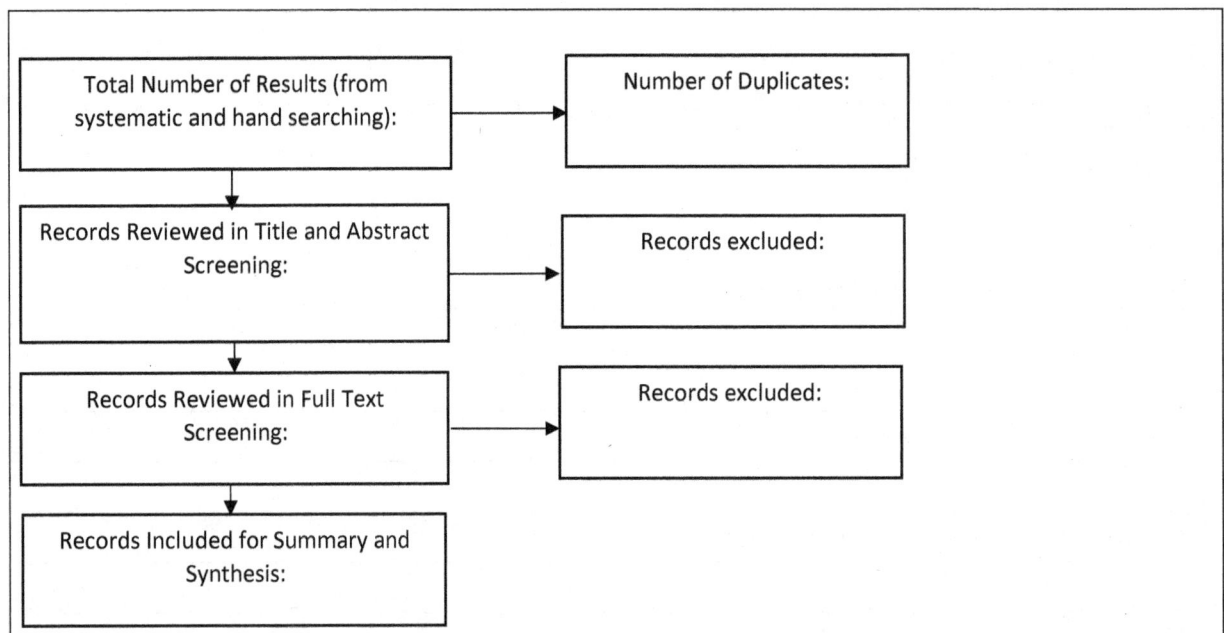

Instructions for the Search and Screening Tool

Section I: Key Elements of the EBP Question

Identify the key elements of the EBP question (from the Question Development Tool)

Population	Record the details of the population outlined in the EBP question.
Setting	If not captured in the population, record any additional details about the setting the EBP question pertains to.
Topic or Intervention(s)	Record the topic or intervention the EBP team is interested in investigating. If comparing two interventions, list them both here.
Outcomes (as needed)	If needed, list any specific outcomes of interest. Only list outcomes if you intend to make them a part of the literature search.

Section II: Best-Evidence Search

Does pre-appraised evidence exist in the form of clinical practice guidelines (CPGs), literature reviews with a systematic approach (LRSAs), or evidence summaries?

Some sources of pre-appraised of evidence include Cochrane Library, Joanna Briggs Institute (JBI), The National Institute for Health and Care Excellence (NICE), US Preventative Services Taskforce (USPSTF), ECRI Guidelines Trust®, and Trip Database. See Chapter 7 for more information on which type of information to prioritize.

☐ Yes → Appraise using the Pre-appraised Evidence Appraisal Tool (Appendix E1)
  ○ Is the evidence suitable and adequate quality? *This is determined by a series of questions on the Pre-appraised Evidence Appraisal Tool. Complete the appraisal and come back here to answer the question.*
    ☐ Yes → Complete targeted search for additional evidence based on search date in pre-appraised evidence to determine if relevant evidence has been published in the interim
    Locate the date the search was completed in the pre-appraised evidence. Complete a targeted search to specifically look for evidence that can provide moderate and strong support for decision-making that has been published since the authors completed their search. For a list of possible databases to query, see Section III.

    ☐ No → Skip to Section III (Exhaustive Search)

☐ No → Skip to Section III (Exhaustive Search)

Section III: Exhaustive Search and Screening

Complete the table below using the population, setting, topic or intervention(s), and outcomes identified in Section I. List the element and associated terms to build a full search concept.

EBP Question Element	Possible Search Terms (*synonyms, alternative spellings, or brand names*)
1) Write the word or phrase that captures one element of the EBP question from the table in Section I.	Brainstorm possible synonyms for the concepts, including alternative spellings, brand names and alternative terms.
2) Repeat steps from element 1.	Repeat steps from element 1.

© 2025 Johns Hopkins Health System

3) *Repeat steps from element 1.*	*Repeat steps from element 1. You may have more or fewer concepts than the boxes provided here. Remember, team should not search on directional words such as "increase," "improve," etc., because it can bias the search.*

What databases will you search? *Highlight or select each of the databases the team plans to search. If a database is not listed, select "other" and record the name*
☐ CINAHL   ☐ PsychINFO   ☐ MEDLINE (PubMed)   ☐ Epistemonikos   ☐ Embase   ☐ Other:

What are the inclusion and exclusion criteria? *While this may be similar to the EBP question, it helps the team think through the details of exactly what they ARE and ARE NOT looking for. These discussions help to ensure the team has a mutual understanding of the focus of the project. The group should revisit the list throughout the process to provide further clarifications and refine evidence search results.*	
Inclusion: *Record characteristics of the evidence the team wants to explicitly INCLUDE beyond the elements of the EBP question. They may relate to the type of evidence, the year it was published, or more granular specifics of the setting, population, or interventions.*	Exclusion: *Record characteristics of the evidence the team wants to explicitly EXCLUDE. Common characteristics include date of publication, type of publication, language, population, type of setting, or specifics of the intervention.*

What date limit will you use and why?
Record the data limit the team will use for the search and the reason for selecting the parameters. Remember, data cut-offs are topic-dependent and require consideration and justification. Do not simply include the outdated five-year cut-off without specific reasoning.

What is the date the team conducted the search?
Record the date the official search was run.

What are the search strings and number of results from each database?		
Database	Search String	Number of Results
Record the database searched	*Copy/paste the exact search string entered into the search field of the database.*	*Record the number of results retrieved*
Record the database searched	*Copy/paste the exact search string entered into the search field of the database.*	*Record the number of results retrieved*
Record the database searched	*Copy/paste the exact search string entered into the search field of the database.*	*Record the number of results retrieved*

How will the team systematically screen the results to identify evidence that answers the EBP question and meets the inclusion/exclusion criteria (*select all that apply*)?
☐ Use software or web-based program to track (e.g., Google Forms, Excel, Abstrackr)   ☐ Have at least two independent reviewers for each record   ☐ Inclusion or exclusion disagreements resolved by third reviewer   ☐ Other: *Select the strategy the team will use to screen the results of their literature search. This should represent a systematic and unbiased approach to ensure the final evidence is representative of the true state of the literature on the topic.*

Complete the screening flow chart below

C SEARCHING AND SCREENING TOOL

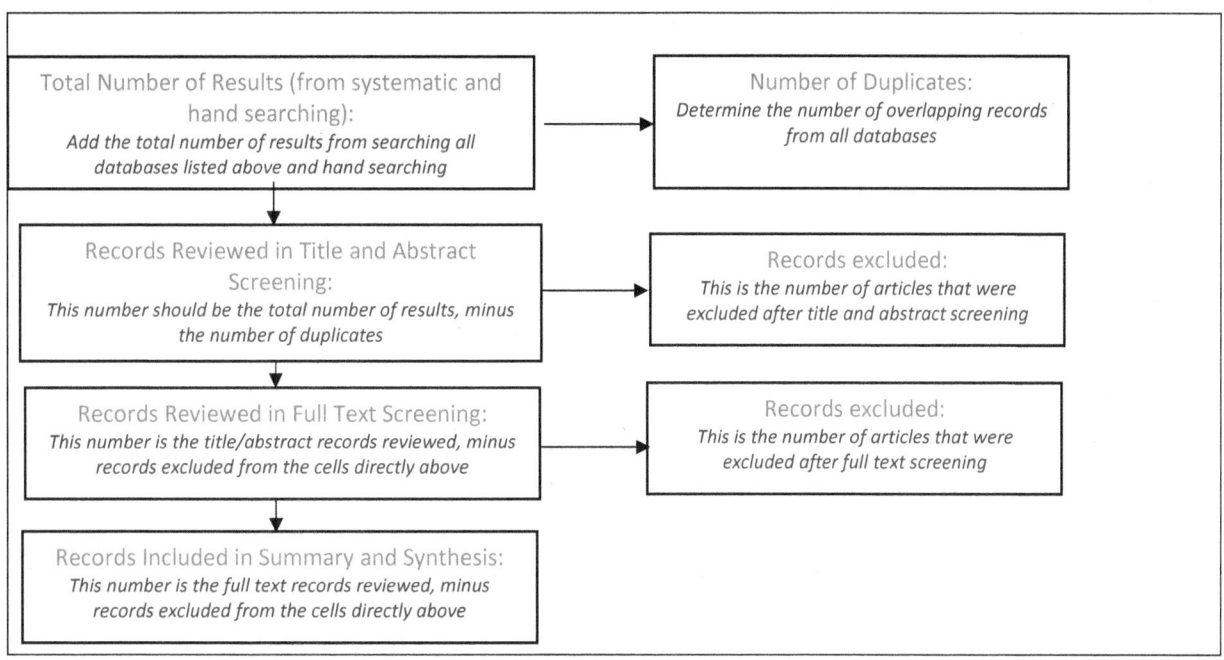

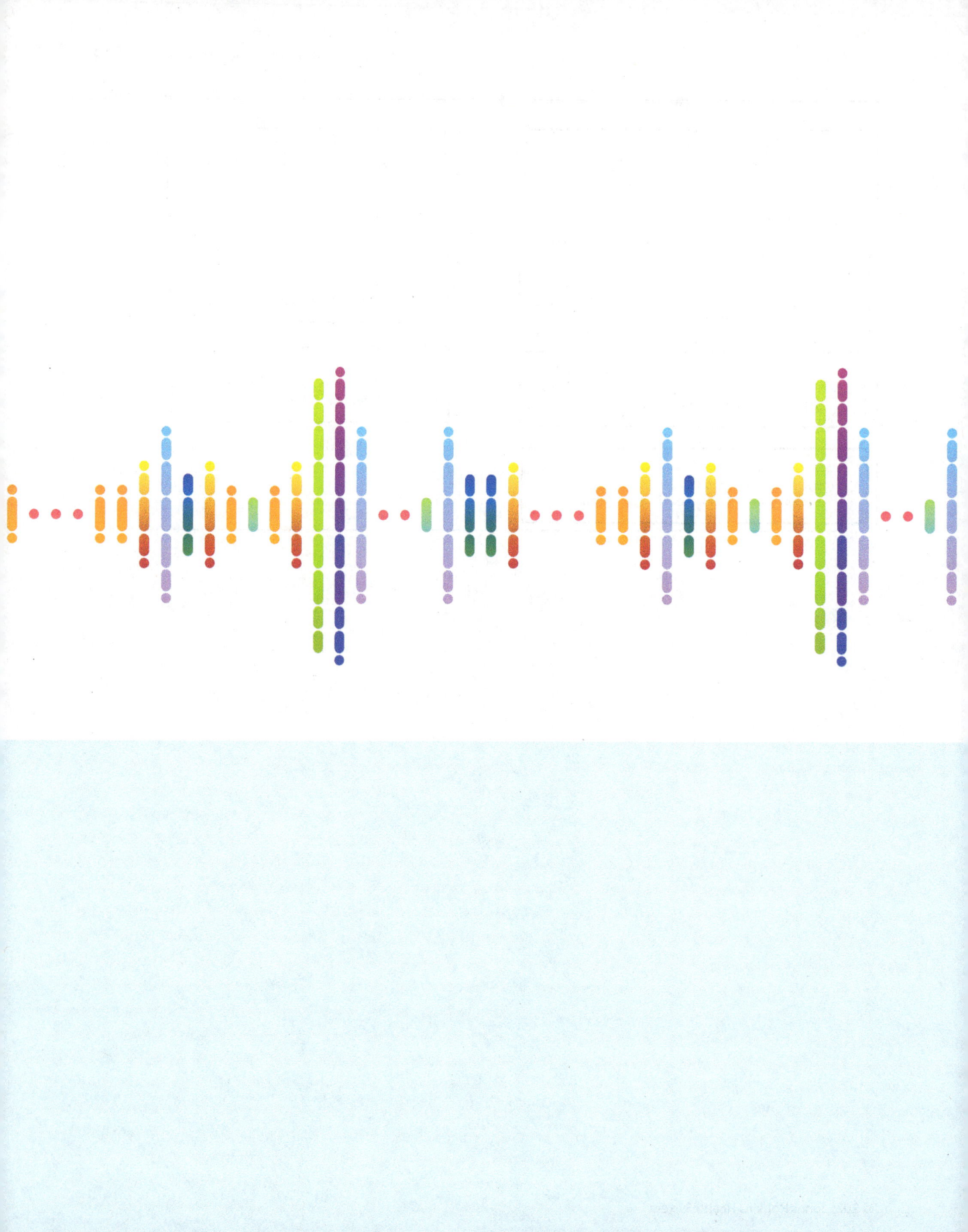

APPRAISAL TOOL SELECTION ALGORITHM

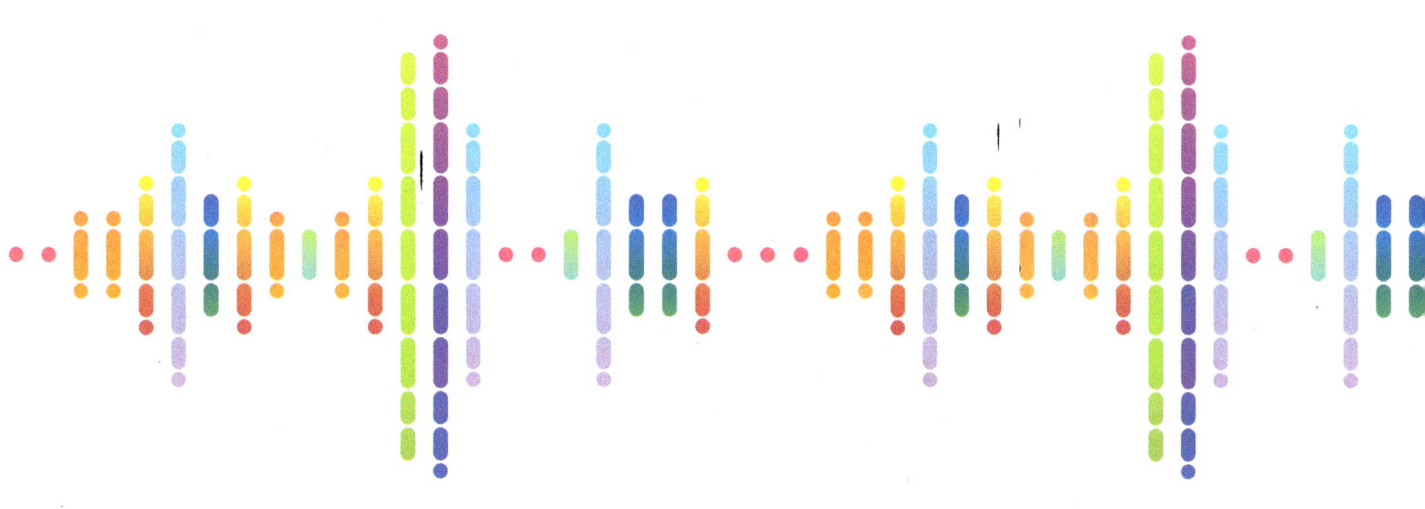

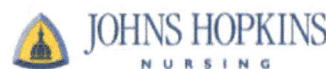

Appraisal Tool Selection Algorithm

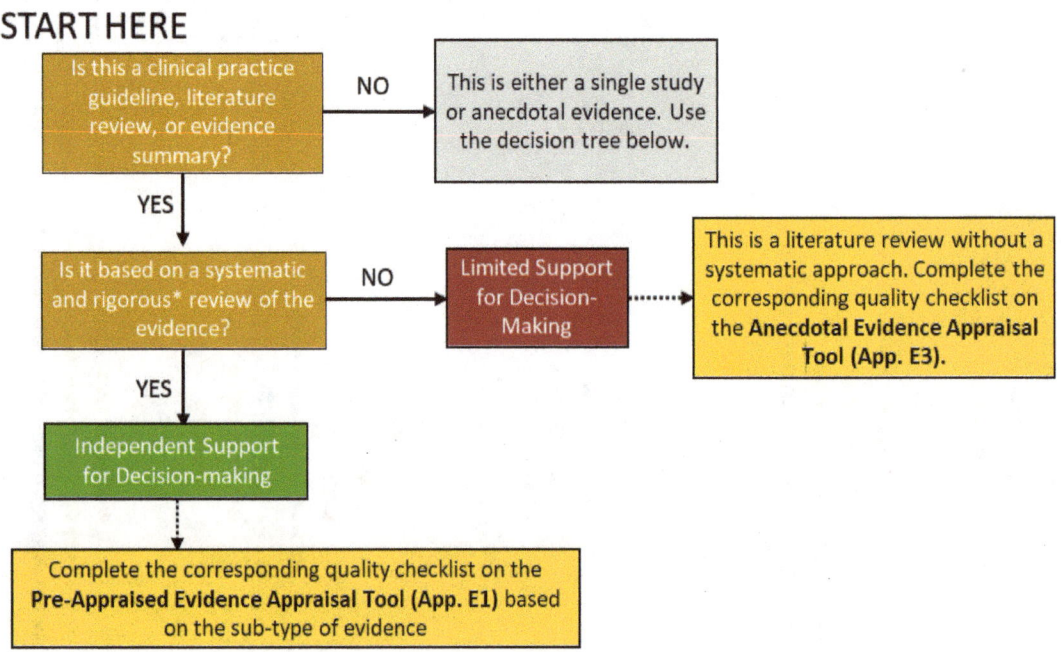

*To be considered systematic and rigorous, a review should include:
- A pre-planned method or protocol
- A question the authors are attempting to answer
- Clear and explicit inclusion and exclusion criteria
- A documented search strategy, including sources and terms
- Use of tables to provide pertinent characteristics of the studies included
- An explicit approach to assess the quality (risk of bias) of included evidence
- Exploration of the data to identify consistencies as well as gaps
- Tables or figures to support the interpretation of data
- Appendices or supplemental files to provide further details

Note: This may not be readily apparent. Teams may need to consult organizational websites and delve deeper into their methods.

Adapted from Booth, 2021

© 2025 Johns Hopkins Health System

SINGLE STUDY OR ANECDOTAL EVIDENCE DECISION TREE

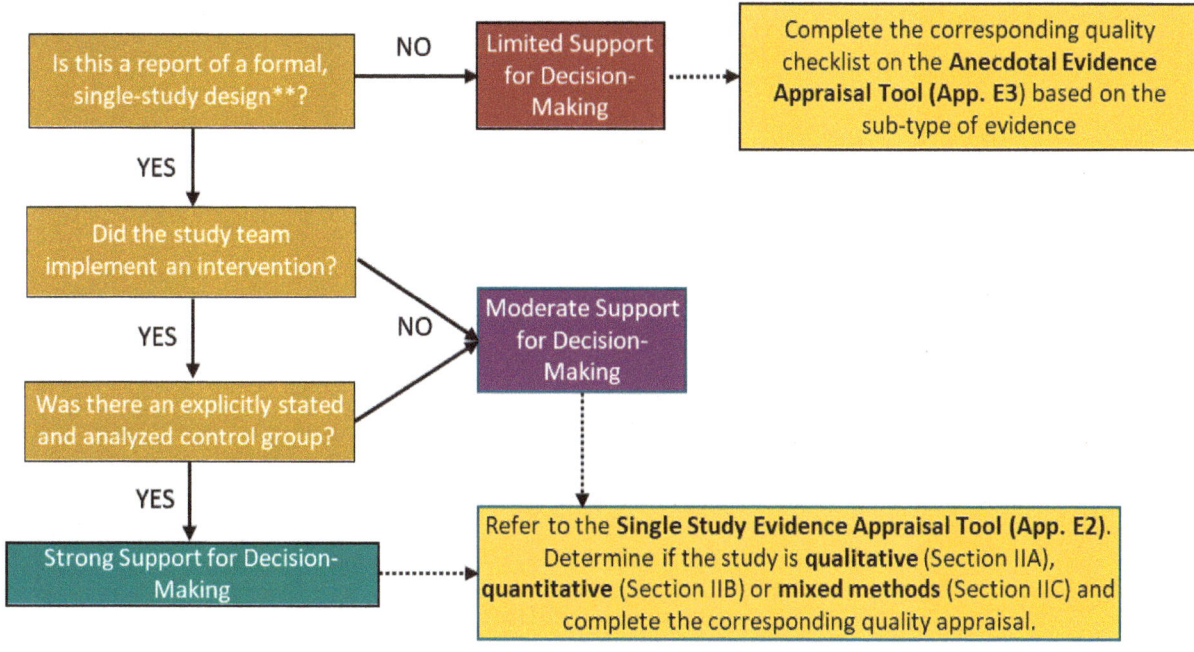

**Study designs should be explicit and formal. A report is considered to have a formal study design if it meets most of the following criteria:
- Was pre-planned (before investigators initiated intervention or data collection)
- Received ethical review (by the institutional review board)
- Has formal and systematic data collection and data analysis
- Uses specific qualitative and/or quantitative information gathered for the investigation
- The study team is not also a subject of the intervention
- Has a clear aim, reproducible methods, results, and discussion
- Do not only recount the authors' personal, organizational, or literature-based experience.

© 2025 Johns Hopkins Health System

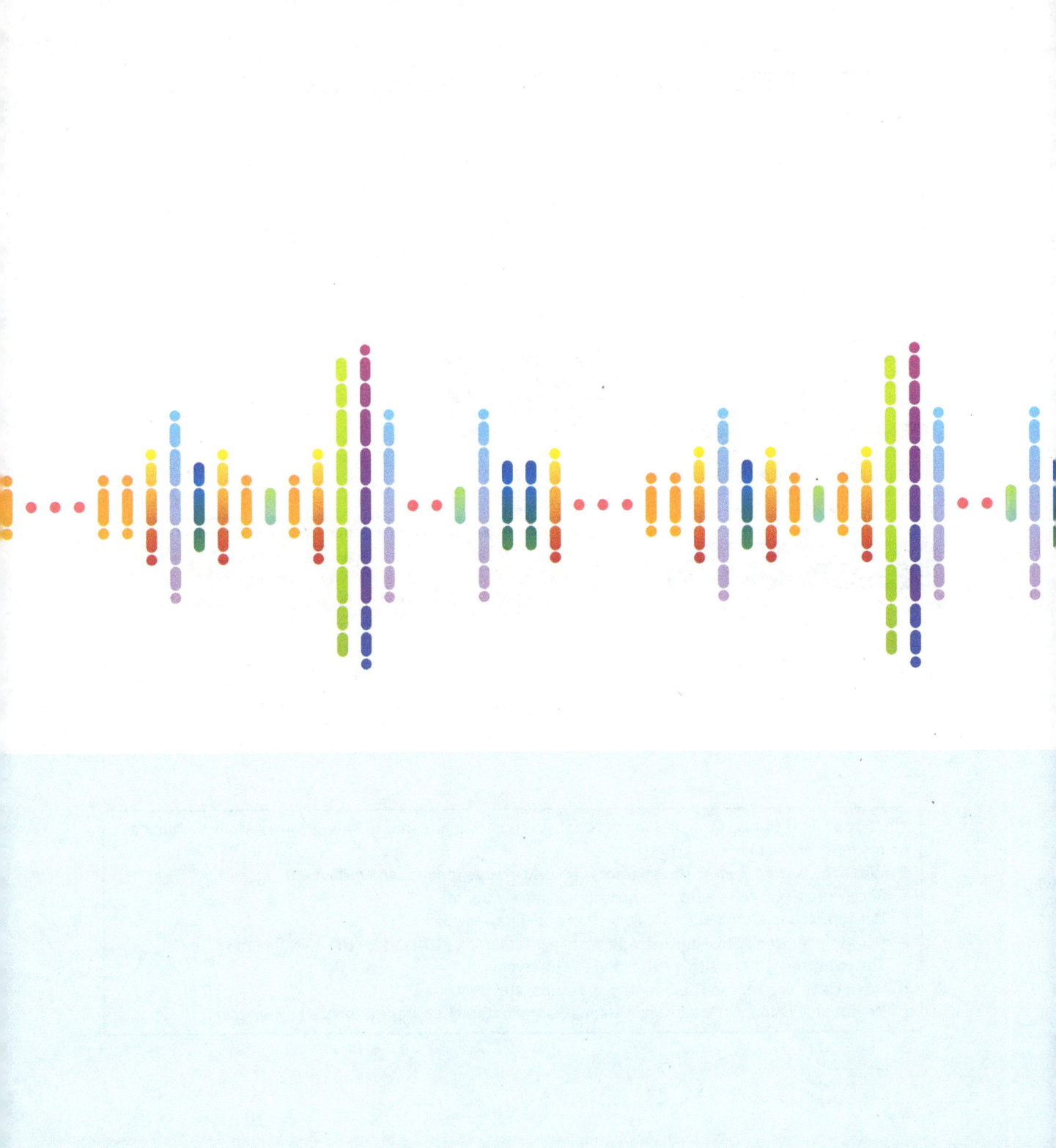

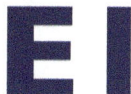

PRE-APPRAISED EVIDENCE APPRAISAL TOOL

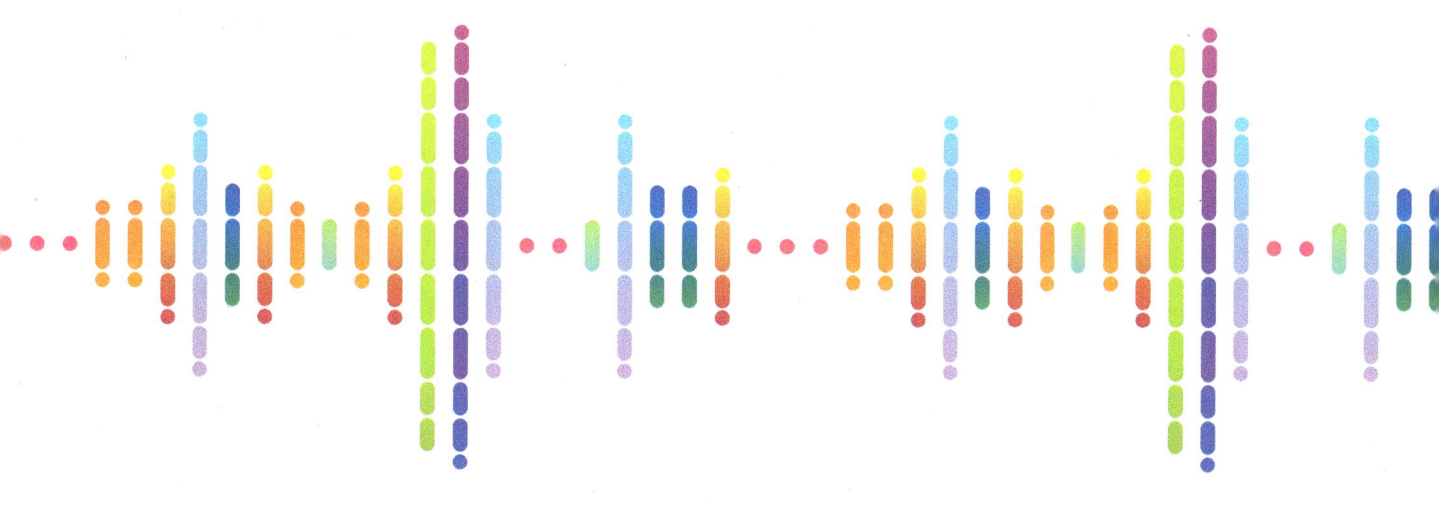

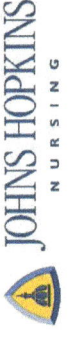

Pre-Appraised Evidence Appraisal

Fill in this data collection table after completing the suitability and quality assessments below.

Article Number	Author, date, title	Type of pre-appraised evidence	Topic or intervention	Population	Setting	Recommendations that answer the EBP question

*For definitions of terms in **bold print** see **Appendix F: Evidence Terminology and Considerations Guide**

Section I: Suitability

Only complete this section if you are using this evidence as potential independent support for decision-making. **If you gathered this evidence in an exhaustive search, skip to Section II: Quality Appraisal.**

	Yes	No	Unclear	N/A
Is the topic or intervention the same or similar to the topic of interest?				
Is the population the same or similar to your population of interest?				
Is the setting the same or similar to your setting of interest?				
If applicable, are the **outcomes** the same or similar to your **outcomes** of interest?				
How recent are the references (*provide date*)?				
Are the references recent enough to be reasonably applied to the practice setting (this will depend on the intervention and changing nature of the topic at hand)				

Notes:

*For independent support for decision-making, all responses must be YES. If the topic, population, setting, or outcome is similar, but not the same, include in the notes section the team's rationale for how the provided information can be reasonably compared to the elements in the team's EBP question. **If suitable, complete the corresponding quality assessment below.**

If the evidence is not fully suitable, but it informs the EBP question, complete the appraisal below. If the quality is adequate, this is strong support for decision-making, record the information on Appendix G2: The Individual Evidence Summary Tool.

© 2025 Johns Hopkins Health System

Section II: Quality Appraisal

Complete the checklist below for the corresponding sub-type of evidence.

Evidence Summary (point-of-care clinical decision support produced by a reputable organization)

	Yes	No	Unclear	N/A
1. Was the summary produced by a reputable organization?				
2. Does the organization use a clear, systematic, and comprehensive method for selecting evidence?**				
3. Does the organization use a clear, well-established process for evaluating evidence (e.g. rapid review protocol, systematic review)?**				
4. Is the **review question** or summary topic clearly stated?				
5. Are the details of the included evidence provided (including types of studies, intervention(s), settings, populations, and **grading**)?				
6. Is there a direct and obvious link between recommendations and the provided evidence?				
7. Are recommendations clear and complete (including a **level of certainty/confidence**)?				
8. Does the **level of certainty/confidence** of each of the recommendations align with the evidence used to support them?				
9. Did the review undergo an independent peer review?				
10. Are funding and **conflicts of interest** addressed?				
** This may be directly provided or available on the organization's website				

Consider all of your responses above. Do you think the quality of this article is adequate to provide independent support for decision-making?

☐ Yes → Include, complete data collection table on page 1
☐ No → Exclude, set aside, and note exclusion for tracking

Clinical Practice Guidelines

	Yes	No	Unclear	N/A
1. Is the review group made up of experts who have proven expertise or skills related to the topic?				
2. Is the target population of the recommendations clear?				
3. Is the process for making the recommendations provided (e.g. evidence review, reaching consensus)?				
4. Are recommendations clear and complete (including a level of certainty/confidence)?				
5. Was there an external, peer-review of the guidelines?				

© 2025 Johns Hopkins Health System

	Yes	No	Unclear	N/A
6. Does the level of certainty/confidence of each of the recommendations align with the evidence used to support them?				
7. Are funding and conflicts of interest addressed?				

Complete the below checklist to determine the quality of the literature review used to generate the guidelines.

Literature Reviews with a Systematic Approach (LRSAs)

	Yes	No	Unclear	N/A
Background/Introduction				
1. Is a logical background and rationale for the review explained regarding current literature?				
2. Is the review question clear?				
Methods				
1. Did the review follow a model or guideline (e.g. PRISMA, AMSTAR II, etc.)?				
2. Do the authors clearly state what they are trying to measure or describe?				
3. Was the literature search thorough and could it be replicated (this includes providing keywords, inclusion/exclusion criteria, and at least 2 formal databases searched)?				
4. Was there an independent double-check system in the review process (this includes an independent assessment for eligibility, critical appraisal, and data extraction by at least 2 reviewers for each article)?				
5. Was the quality of each included study formally assessed and listed?				
6. Was the risk of introducing bias into the literature selection and review process addressed and minimized?				
7. If applicable, were data pooling (meta-analysis or meta-synthesis) methods clear and appropriate?				
8. In addition to the items above, did the authors answer all of your questions about how they conducted their review [include notes about additional concerns]?				
Results				
1. Was there a flow diagram that included the number of studies eliminated at each stage of the review?				
2. Were details of included studies provided (e.g. design, sample, methods, results, outcomes, limitations, the strength of evidence)?				
3. If applicable, are themes identified?				
4. If applicable, are statistics shown clearly?				

© 2025 Johns Hopkins Health System

E1 PRE-APPRAISED EVIDENCE APPRAISAL TOOL

	Yes	No	Unclear	N/A
Discussion				
1. Does the discussion match what is reported in the results section?				
2. Do the authors examine what they found and compare it to other literature on the topic?				
3. Are limitations included with an explanation of how they were handled?				
4. Do the authors provide implications of their study for practice and future investigation?				
General				
1. Is all the information in the paper congruent (consistent throughout the aims, methods, results, and discussion sections)?				
2. Are funding and conflict(s) of interest addressed?				
Consider all of your responses above. Do you think the quality of this article is adequate to provide independent support for decision-making?	☐ Yes → *Include, complete data collection table on page 1* ☐ No → *Exclude, set aside, and note exclusion for tracking*			

© 2025 Johns Hopkins Health System

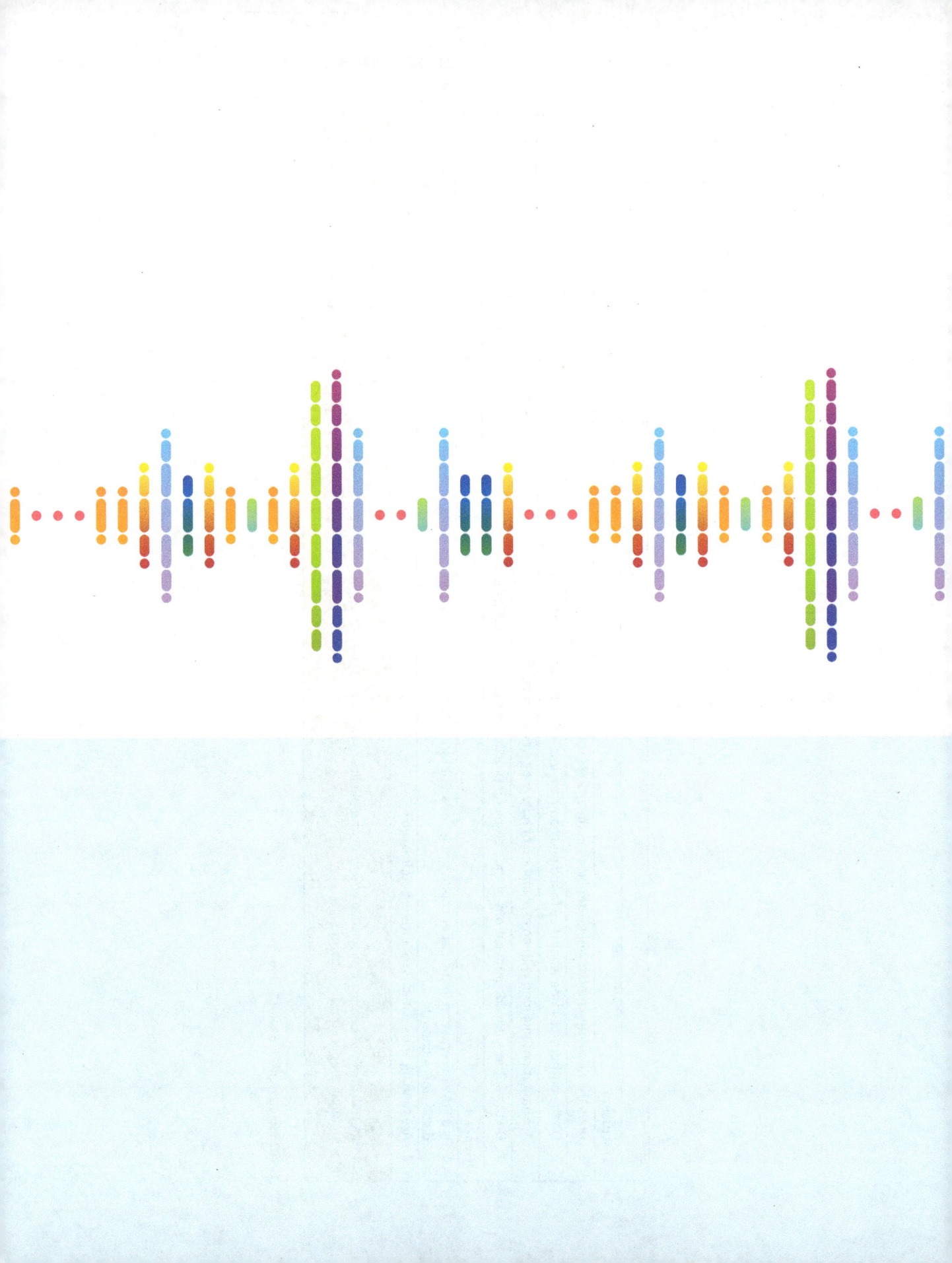

E2

SINGLE STUDY EVIDENCE APPRAISAL TOOL

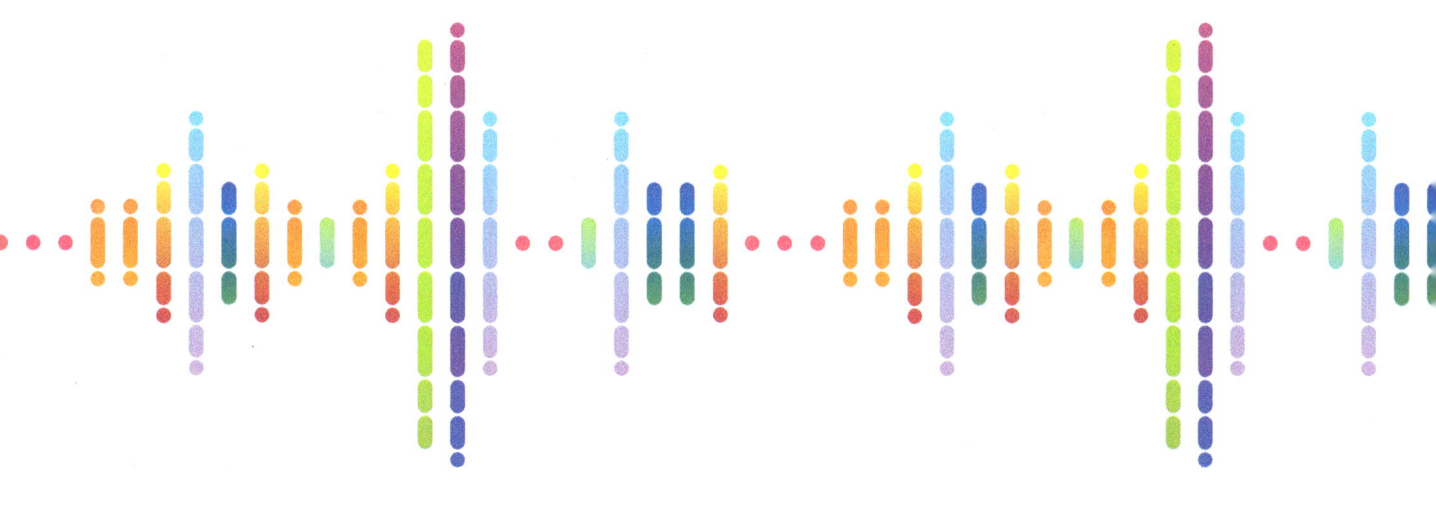

Single Study Evidence Appraisal Tool

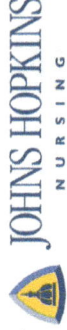

Section I: Level of Support for Practice Change

Complete the decision tree below to determine the level of support for practice change.

- **Is this a report of a single study?** — NO → Do not use this tool, use **Appendix D: Appraisal Tool Selection Algorithm** to determine the correct appraisal tool.
- YES ↓
- **Does the evidence report a formal study design?** — NO → Do not use this tool, use **Appendix D: Appraisal Tool Selection Algorithm** to determine the correct appraisal tool.
- YES ↓
- **Did the study team implement an intervention?** — NO → Moderate support for decision-making
- YES ↓
- **Was there an explicitly stated and analyzed control group?** — NO → Moderate support for decision-making
- YES ↓
- **Strong support for decision-making**

→ Determine if the research is **qualitative** (Section IIA), **quantitative** (Section IIB), or **mixed methods** (Section IIC) and complete the corresponding quality appraisal checklist.

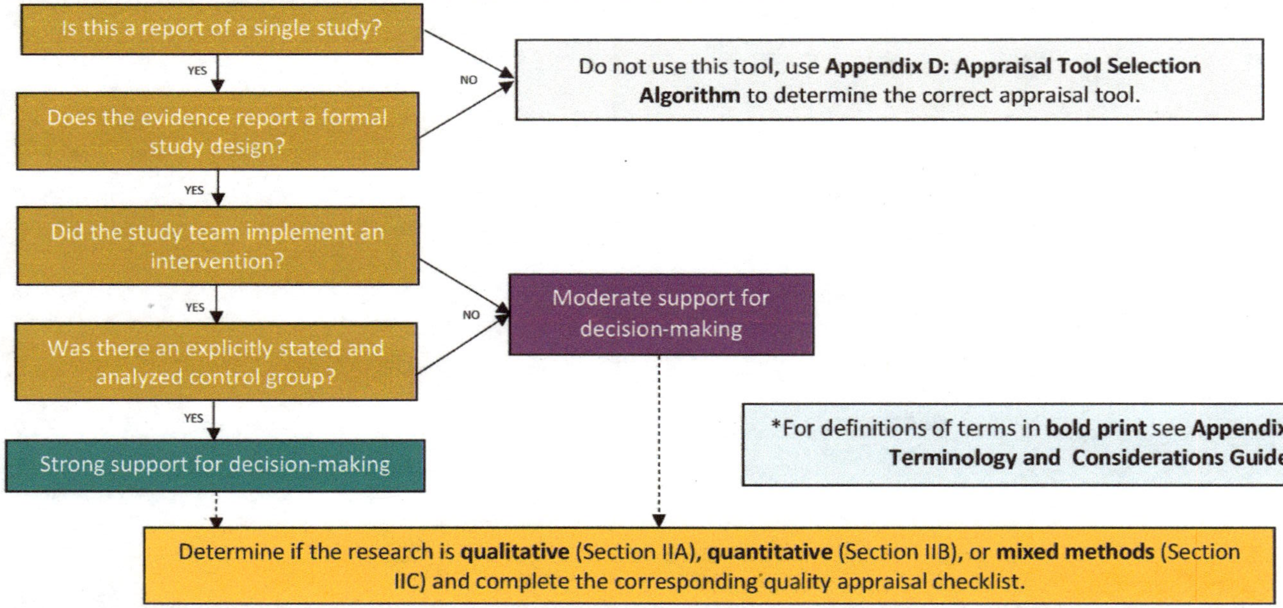

*For definitions of terms in **bold print** see **Appendix F: Evidence Terminology and Considerations Guide**

Fill in this data collection table after completing the quality assessment below (see Instructions in **Appendix G2: Individual Evidence Summary Tool** for more information)

Article Number	Author, date, title	Type of evidence	Population, size, and setting	Intervention	Findings that help answer the EBP question	Measures used	Limitations	Level of support for decision-making

© 2025 Johns Hopkins Health System

E2 SINGLE STUDY EVIDENCE APPRAISAL TOOL

Section II: Quality Appraisal

Complete the checklist below for the corresponding type of evidence.

Section IIA: Qualitative Evidence

	Yes	No	Unclear	N/A
Introduction/Background				
1. Is a logical background and rationale for the study explained using **current** literature?				
2. Is the purpose/objective of the study clear?				
Methods				
1. Is the **study design** and guiding theory or model provided with the reason it was chosen?				
2. Is the **study setting** clearly described (including location, dates, and other important details) to enhance **transferability**?				
3. Is the process for recruiting participants (**sampling**) explained clearly and does it match with the study aim(s)?				
4. Do **eligibility** criteria (rules for who can join the study) make sense and are they easy to understand?				
5. Is the **sample size** adequate, as shown by reaching data **saturation**?				
6. Are important characteristics of the group they studied (**sample**) provided (e.g. how many participants or encounters were involved, demographics, or other details about the participants or things being studied)?				
7. Did the authors address **reflexivity** (how their background or experience might have affected the study)?				
8. Are the **data collection** methods clear and appropriate (this includes how they gathered and recorded the information)?				
9. Are **data processing** methods clear and appropriate (this includes how the data was transcribed and checked) to enhance **credibility**?				
10. Are the methods to **analyze** the data well explained (this includes what computer programs they used and how they coded the data to find patterns or themes) to enhance **confirmability**?				
11. Are the **intervention**(s) clearly described?				
12. Is there information on the **ethical review** provided?				
13. In addition to the items above, did the authors answer all of your questions about how they conducted their study [include notes about additional concerns]?				
Results/Findings				
1. Do the findings make sense and are they easy to understand?				

© 2025 Johns Hopkins Health System

	Yes	No	Unclear	N/A
2. Are **themes or patterns** identified clearly?				
3. Do the authors provide enough quotations, detailed observations, or other proof to support their findings?				
Discussion				
1. Does the discussion match what is reported in the results section?				
2. Do the authors examine what they found and compare it to other literature on the topic?				
3. Are **limitations** included with an explanation of how they were handled?				
4. Do the authors provide implications of their study for practice and future investigation?				
General				
1. Is all the information in the paper **congruent** (consistent throughout the aims, methods, results, and discussion sections)?				
2. Are funding and **conflicts of interest** addressed?				
Consider all of your responses above. Do you think the quality of this article is adequate to provide dependable information to answer your EBP question?	☐ Yes → Include, complete data collection table on page 1 ☐ No → Exclude, set aside, and note exclusion for tracking			

Section IIB: Quantitative Evidence

	Yes	No	Unclear	N/A
Introduction/Background				
1. Is a logical background and rationale for the study explained using **current** literature?				
2. Is the purpose/objective of the study clear?				
Methods				
1. Is the **study design** clearly stated?				
2. Is the **study setting** clearly described (including location, dates, and other important details) to enhance **generalizability**?				
3. Is the process for recruiting participants (**sampling**) explained clearly and does it match with the study aim(s)?				
4. Do **eligibility** criteria (rules for who can join the study) make sense and are they easy to understand?				
5. Is the **sample size powered** adequately (a calculation or other explanation for how the authors decided how many participants or observations to include)?				
6. Did the authors clearly state what they wanted to measure?				

© 2025 Johns Hopkins Health System

	Yes	No	Unclear	N/A
7. Are the **data collection** methods clear and appropriate (this includes how they gathered and recorded the information)?				
a) If applicable, were all the tools **reliable**?				
b) If applicable, were all the tools **valid**?				
8. Are the methods to analyze the data well explained (this includes what computer programs they used, how they made calculations or anything else they did to explore the data)?				
9. If applicable, are the intervention(s) clearly described?				
10. If there was **randomization**,				
a) Was true **randomization** used to put people in the **control** and **intervention** groups?				
b) Other than the intervention being studied, were the **intervention** and **control** groups treated similarly?				
11. Is there information on the **ethical review** provided?				
12. In addition to the items above, did the authors answer all of your questions about how they conducted their study [include notes about additional concerns]?				
Results/Findings				
1. Do the findings make sense and are they easy to understand?				
2. Are characteristics of the participants provided (this may include demographics or other important details about the participants or things being studied)?				
3. If applicable, was the survey **response rate** provided?				
4. If applicable, are **attrition** rates provided (this includes how many people remained with the study at each stage)?				
5. Is data provided for each item the authors stated they wanted to measure?				
6. If applicable, are the baseline characteristics of the **intervention** and **control** groups similar?				
7. Are any statistics shown clearly?				
Discussion				
1. Does the discussion match what is reported in the results section?				
2. Do the authors examine what they found and compare it to other literature on the topic?				
3. Are **limitations** included with an explanation of how they were handled?				
4. Do the authors provide implications of their study for practice and future investigation?				

© 2025 Johns Hopkins Health System

	Yes	No	Unclear	N/A
General				
1. Is all the information in the paper **congruent** (consistent throughout the aims, methods, results, and discussion sections)?				
2. Are funding and **conflicts of interest** addressed?				
Consider all of your responses above. Do you think the quality of this article is adequate to provide dependable information to answer your EBP question?	☐ Yes → *Include, complete data collection table on page 1* ☐ No → *Exclude, set aside, and note exclusion for tracking*			

Section IIC: Mixed Methods Evidence

	Yes	No	Unclear	N/A
Background/Introduction				
1. Is a logical background and rationale for the review explained regarding **current** literature?				
2. Is the purpose/objective of the study clear?				
Methods				
1. Is the **study design** and mixed methods approach clearly stated with an explanation of why it was chosen?				
2. Is the **study setting** clearly described (including location, dates, and other important details) to enhance **generalizability**?				
3. Is the process for recruiting participants (**sampling**) explained clearly and does it match with the study aim(s)?				
4. Do **eligibility** criteria (rules for who can join the study) make sense and are they easy to understand?				
5. Is the **sample size** adequate...				
a) For the qualitative portion (this includes evidence of data saturation)?				
b) For the quantitative portion (this includes adequate **power**, a calculation, or other explanation for how the authors decided how many participants or observations to include)?				
6. Did the authors clearly state what they wanted to measure or describe?				
7. Did the authors address **reflexivity** (how their background or experience might have affected the study)?				
8. If applicable, are the **intervention**(s) clearly described?				
9. Are the **data collection** methods clear and appropriate (this includes how they gathered and recorded the information)?				
a) If applicable, were all the tools **reliable**?				

© 2025 Johns Hopkins Health System

	Yes	No	Unclear	N/A
b) If applicable, were all the tools **valid**?				
10. In the qualitative section, are data processing methods clear and appropriate (this includes how the data was transcribed and checked) to enhance **credibility**?				
11. Are the methods to **analyze** the data well explained…				
a) For the qualitative section (this includes coding and generation of themes)?				
b) For the quantitative section (this includes what computer programs they used, how they made calculations, or anything else they did to explore the data)?				
12. If there was **randomization**,				
a) Was true **randomization** used to put people in the **control** and **intervention** groups?				
b) Other than the intervention being studied, were the **intervention** and **control** groups treated similarly?				
13. Do the authors truly use and integrate both qualitative and quantitative methodologies to collect and analyze data?				
14. Is there information on the **ethical review** provided?				
15. In addition to the items above, did the authors answer all of your questions about how they conducted their study? [include notes about additional concerns]				
Results				
1. Do the **findings** make sense and are they easy to understand?				
2. Are characteristics of the participants provided (this may include demographics or other important details about the participants or things being studied)?				
3. If applicable, was the survey **response rate** provided?				
4. If applicable, are **attrition** rates provided (this includes how many people remained with the study at each stage)?				
5. Is data provided for each item the authors stated they wanted to measure or describe?				
6. In the qualitative section, do the authors provide enough quotations, detailed observations, or other proof to support their findings?				
7. In the quantitative section, are statistics shown clearly?				
8. If applicable, are the baseline characteristics of the **intervention** and **control** groups similar?				
9. Are any statistics shown clearly?				

© 2025 Johns Hopkins Health System

	Yes	No	Unclear	N/A
Discussion				
1. Does the discussion match what is reported in the results section?				
2. Do the authors fully integrate the qualitative and quantitative data to create a deeper understanding?				
3. Do the authors examine what they found and compare it to other literature on the topic?				
4. Are **limitations** included with an explanation of how they were handled?				
5. Do the authors provide implications of their study for practice and future investigation?				
General				
1. Is all the information in the paper **congruent** (consistent throughout the aims, methods, results, and discussion sections)?				
2. Are funding and **conflicts of interest** addressed?				
Consider all of your responses above. Do you think the quality of this article is adequate to provide dependable information to answer your EBP question?	☐ Yes → *Include, complete data collection table on page 1* ☐ No → *Exclude, set aside, and note exclusion for tracking*			

© 2025 Johns Hopkins Health System

E3
ANECDOTAL EVIDENCE APPRAISAL TOOL

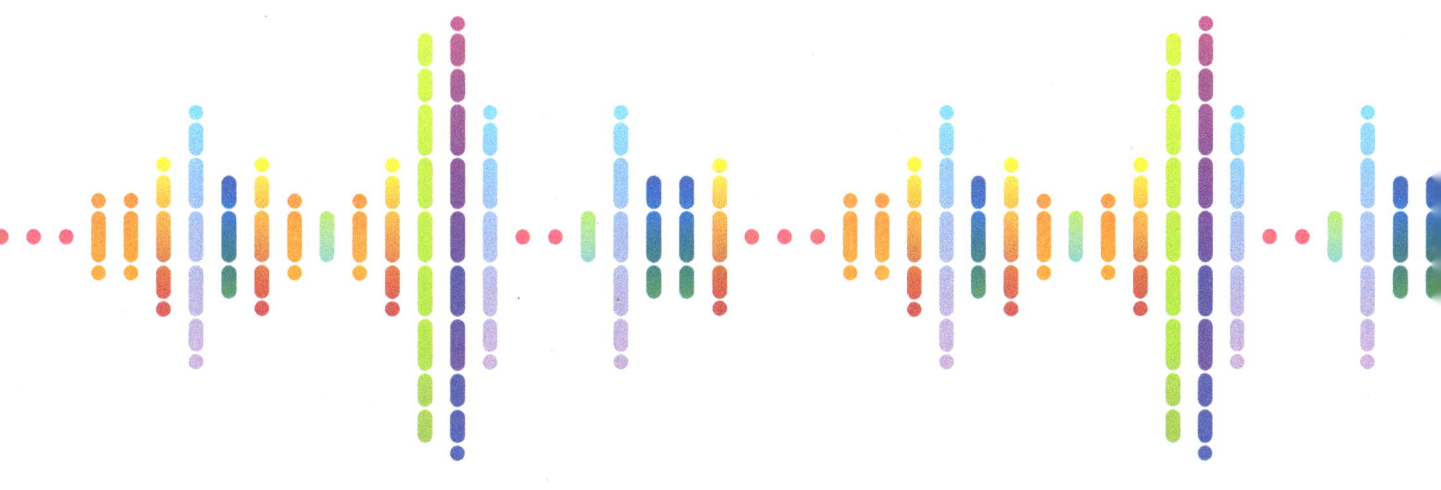

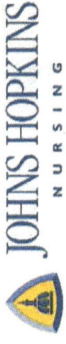

Anecdotal Evidence Appraisal Tool

Fill in this data collection table after completing the quality assessment below (see Instructions in **Appendix G2: Individual Evidence Summary Tool** for more information).

Article Number	Author, date, title	Type of evidence	Population, size, and setting	Intervention	Findings that help answer the EBP question	Measures used	Limitations	Level of support for decision-making?
								Limited

Section I: Quality Appraisal

Complete the checklist below for the corresponding sub-type of evidence. Note, that the headers within each checklist are used for organization and may not match the exact language from the article or report being appraised.

*For definitions of terms in **bold print** see **Appendix F: Evidence Terminology and Considerations Guide**

Expert Opinion, Position Statements, and Book Chapters

	Yes	No	Unclear	N/A
Author(s) expertise				
1. Does the author(s) know about the topic of interest as evidenced by previous publications on the topic, relevant professional or academic **affiliations**, related education/training, or other activities that suggest their **expertise**?				
Purpose/objectives				
1. Is the purpose/objective(s) clearly stated?				
Reference to evidence				
1. Is there a thorough reference to **current** literature on the topic?				
2. Do the author(s) provide meaningful **analysis** (through insights or commentary) of existing evidence on the topic?				
Summary/conclusions				
1. Is it clear and logical how the authors reached their conclusion(s)?				
2. Are recommendations clear?				

© 2025 Johns Hopkins Health System

E3 ANECDOTAL EVIDENCE APPRAISAL TOOL

	Yes	No	Unclear	N/A
General				
1. Are funding and **conflicts of interest** addressed?				
Consider all of your responses above. Do you think the quality of this article is adequate to provide dependable information to answer your EBP question?	☐ Yes → *Include, complete data collection table on page 1* ☐ No → *Exclude, set aside, and note exclusion for tracking*			

Case Report

	Yes	No	Unclear	N/A
Introduction				
1. Is there a short introduction to the case, including why it is relevant or important?				
Patient information				
1. Is patient-level data provided to address the clinical focus of the case study (this can include patient history, clinical findings, diagnosis, or timeline)?				
2. Is there a thorough explanation of diagnostic and/or therapeutic intervention(s)?				
3. Did the patient or caregiver provide informed consent?				
Discussion				
1. Is there meaningful interpretation of the patient information (see above)?				
2. Are "lessons learned" clearly stated and based on the provided patient information?				
3. Is there an insightful discussion of the case presentation regarding relevant medical literature?				
General				
1. Are funding and **conflicts of interest** addressed?				
2. Is the information provided in a logical manner that is easy to follow?				
Consider all of your responses above. Do you think the quality of this article is adequate to provide dependable information to answer your EBP question?	☐ Yes → *Include, complete data collection table on page 1* ☐ No → *Exclude, set aside, and note exclusion for tracking*			

© 2025 Johns Hopkins Health System

Programmatic Experiences	Yes	No	Unclear	N/A
Introduction				
1. Is there a short introduction to the project, including **why** it is relevant or important?				
2. Is the purpose/objective of the project clear?				
Project Information				
1. Is there adequate information regarding the context of the project, including the setting and people involved?				
2. Is what the project team did (interventions) clearly described?				
3. Was a tool, model, or framework used to plan and implement the project?				
4. Are the findings or impact of the project provided?				
Discussion				
1. Does the author(s) provide insights into the project's successes and areas for improvement?				
2. Are "lessons learned" clearly stated?				
3. Is the project discussed in the context of **currently** available information on the intervention or problem it was addressing?				
General				
1. Are funding and **conflicts of interest** addressed?				
2. Are you able to follow what the group did to implement and measure the success of the project?				
Consider all of your responses above. Do you think the quality of this article is adequate to provide dependable information to answer your EBP question?	☐ Yes → *Include, complete data collection table on page 1* ☐ No → *Exclude, set aside, and note exclusion for tracking*			

Reviews with an Unsystematic Approach (e.g. Scoping, Critical, Literature Reviews)	Yes	No	Unclear	N/A
Background/Introduction				
1. Is a logical background and rationale for the review explained regarding current literature?				
2. Is the review question clear?				
Methods				
1. Did the review follow a model or guideline?				

	Yes	No	Unclear	N/A
2. Do the authors clearly state what they are trying to measure or describe?				
3. Do the authors explain how they selected the articles included in their review?				
Results				
1. Are findings from the included articles presented clearly?				
Discussion				
1. Does the discussion match what is reported in the results section?				
2. Is it clear how the authors arrived at their conclusions?				
General				
1. Are funding and **conflicts of interest** addressed?				
Consider all of your responses above. Do you think the quality of this article is adequate to provide dependable information to answer your EBP question? ☐ Yes → *Include, complete data collection table on page 1* ☐ No → *Exclude, set aside, and note exclusion for tracking*				

© 2025 Johns Hopkins Health System

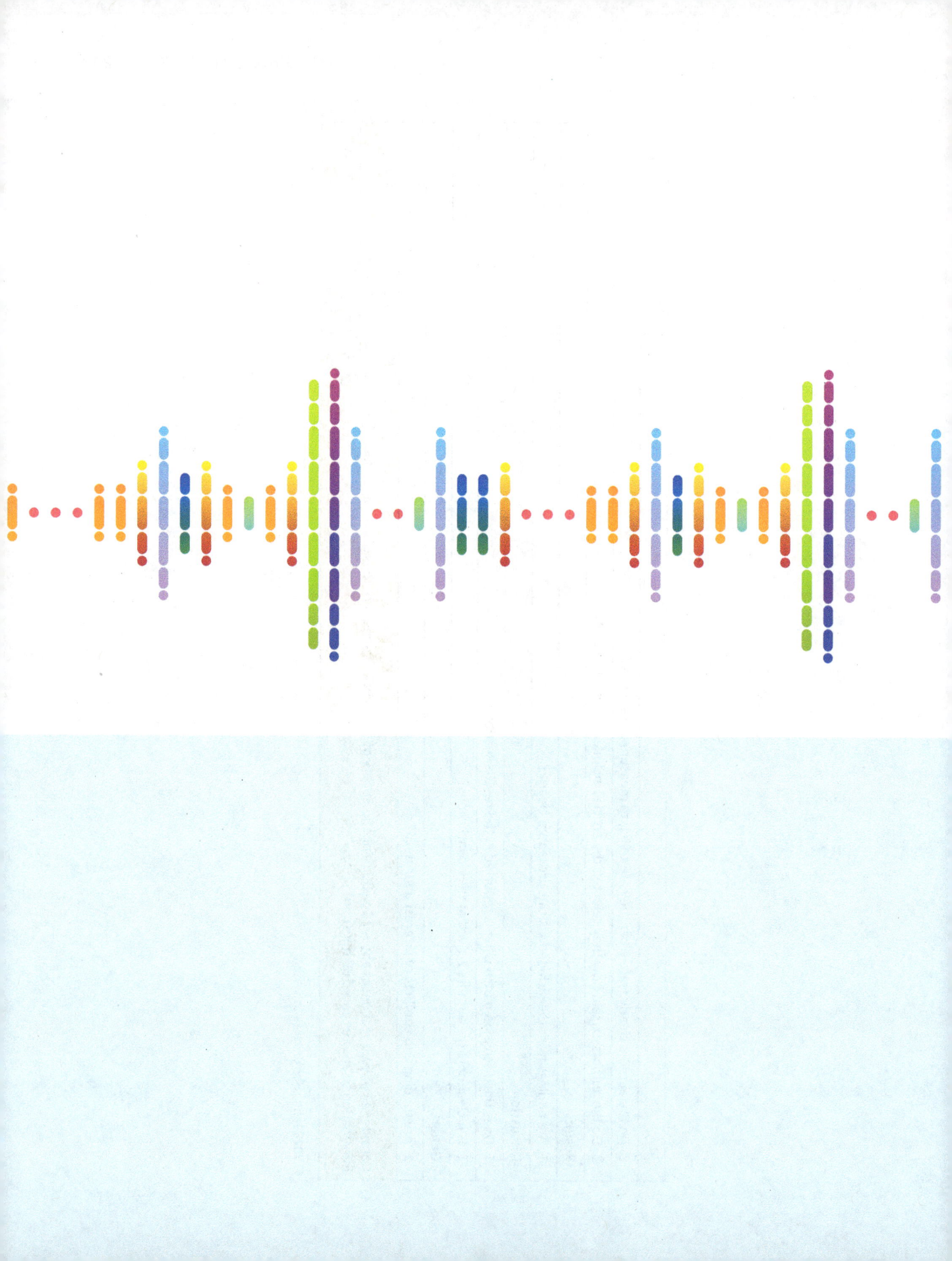

EVIDENCE TERMINOLOGY AND CONSIDERATIONS GUIDE

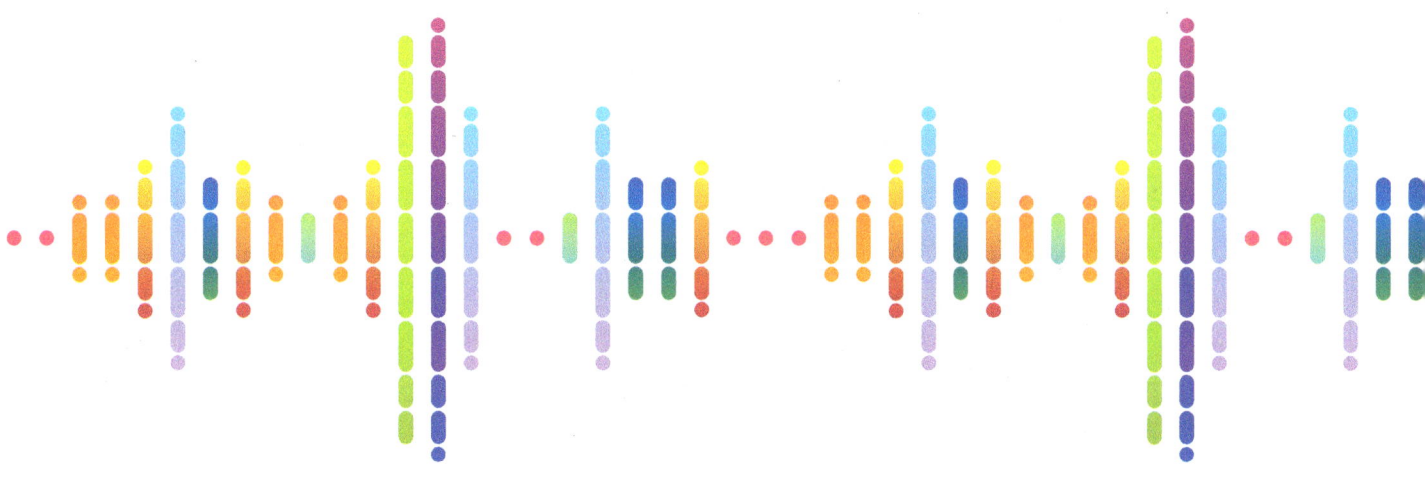

Evidence Terminology and Considerations

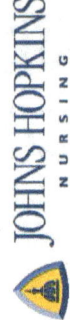

Term	Definition*	Appraisal Considerations
AMSTAR II	A critical appraisal tool for systematic reviews (Shea, 2017)	The use of this instrument by authors is an indication they used a formal, well-established approach to their review
Affiliation	A formal link between an author and one or more organizations or groups that often provide support or recognition.	Affiliations may help the EBP team to determine if an author or team member has relevant training and professional standing. If not explicitly listed in a report, the team can do an internet search of a person's name for more information.
Analysis	The systematic processes to describe, summarize, or evaluate data to create greater meaning through description and evaluation.	Authors should provide very clear and explicit information on the process they used to interpret their data, including what software was used. For quantitative analysis, this should also include statistical calculations. For qualitative analysis, this should include the process to code narrative data and generate themes, including how many people performed each step.
Attrition	The loss of participants during the course of a study, which can affect the validity and reliability of study outcomes.	Some loss to follow-up in a study is normal, but if those dropping out aren't comparable to those remaining in, this can generate results that may not represent the truth of the subject of study. It is important to report attrition, as well as how this may have affected study results.
Bias	An influence that produces a distortion or error and results in the systematic alteration from the truth (McDonagh et al., 2013).	Biases can cause the findings from studies or reviews to not accurately reflect the truth. There are many types of biases, and it is the responsibility of study teams and reviewers to make efforts to mitigate them and include these efforts in their report. Of note, the terms "quality assessment" and "bias assessment" are often used interchangeably but do not mean the same thing. Quality assessment looks at the inclusion of safeguards to minimize bias and bias assessment evaluates the effectiveness of those safeguards (Furuya-Kanamori et al., 2021; Banzi et al., 2018)
Case-control study design	A type of epidemiological study design that compares two groups, people with an outcome of interest (cases) and a similar group without the outcome (controls) and looks back (retrospectively) into their lives to examine if the cases are more likely than the control to have been exposed to a risk factor (Polit & Beck, 2021)	This is a common type of observational study when a disease or condition is rare, or it would be unethical to expose a group to a risk factor (e.g. cigarette smoking). In these studies, it is important that both groups are similar other than the outcome of interest and there are measures taken to minimize recall bias since they are looking into people's historic behaviors and data.
Causation	A relationship where one event is the result of the other's occurrence; more than correlation, causation indicates a direct effect.	EBP teams should ensure statements about causation are fully supported and authors are not implying causation when correlation (two things are related, but one doesn't necessarily cause the other) is more appropriate. Causation is usually established with randomized control trials, and sometimes quasi-experimental studies.

© 2025 Johns Hopkins Health System

F EVIDENCE TERMINOLOGY AND CONSIDERATIONS GUIDE

Term	Definition*	Appraisal Considerations
Certainty/ confidence (level of)	A rating or assessment of how assured reviewers are in the body of evidence or their specific recommendations. This is usually based on data analysis and a quality or bias evaluation.	Different reviews use different approaches to establishing levels of certainty or confidence. The authors should explicitly state which approach they used and the level of certainty or confidence in each recommendation or outcome. They are sometimes expressed as "high to low" or with letters "A, B, or C."
Clinical Practice Guidelines (CPGs)	Reports that generate recommendations on a specific healthcare topic based on rigorous collection of data, analyses, and processes to achieve consensus by a group of experts.	All CPGs are not created equal. EBP teams should look carefully at the methodology of a CPG (either provided in the document itself or on the organization's website) to ensure it meets all necessary standards.
Conflict of interest	A situation in which a person or affiliation might compromise professional judgment or integrity due to a potential for personal gain.	All conflicts of interest should be disclosed by authors and considered when assessing information from a report or study. For example, if an author is employed by a company that produces the product a study is endorsing, the team should keep this in mind when reading and interpreting the findings.
Confounding	A situation in a scientific study where the effect or association between an independent and dependent variable is distorted by another factor.	EBP teams should look for study teams' efforts to reduce confounding. This can include matching among groups, randomization and using statistics to control for different factors.
Congruency	The alignment of each of the parts of a study (aims, methods, results, discussion, and conclusions).	EBP teams should ensure that study teams have used and reported methods that adequately address their aims, all data introduced in the methods is reported in the results, all results have associated methods, and conclusions are based on those results. This helps establish the study was well done and all data is accounted for.
Control	The standard to which comparisons are made in a study. Often refers to a group of subjects that does not receive the intervention or treatment being tested.	Control groups should be similar to the group receiving an intervention. Exact similarities will depend on the nature of the intervention (e.g. sex, age, medical history). Keep in mind, control groups do not necessarily receive no intervention, they may be the standard of care or a placebo intervention. This helps control for things like time spent with a member of the study team (e.g. an orientation to the hospital vs the intervention of disease process education) or the expectation of a positive result (e.g. a sugar pill vs the intervention of an antidepressant).
Correlation	Relationship(s) between variables that indicate an association, but not that one is the result of the other	Studies that investigate correlational relationships observe things that are happening naturally and use statistical calculations to describe negative and positive relationships between two or more variables. They are useful in situations where conducting an experiment is not possible (e.g. the area where a person grows up and their highest education level achieved). Epidemiologic studies such as case-control and cohort studies are examples of correlational studies.

© 2025 Johns Hopkins Health System

Term	Definition*	Appraisal Considerations
Credibility	A component of trustworthiness. The confidence that findings and conclusions of a qualitative study represent the truth.	Study teams can increase credibility in both how they conduct the study and demonstrate it in their report by keeping details records, accounting for personal biases, data triangulation, including rich descriptions, transparency in data processing and interpretation, and respondent validation. This term speaks to the same idea as "internal validity" in quantitative studies (Noble & Smith, 2015).
Cross-sectional study design	A type of observational study that analyzes data from a population at a specific point in time.	Cross-sectional study designs typically collect data with surveys, observations, and sometimes secondary data analysis. It is often used to assess the prevalence of phenomena or current conditions within a particular population. It does not introduce an intervention but rather describes a phenomenon that is occurring naturally.
Current	Recent, occurring, or existing in the present time (Merriam-Webster)	The concept of "current" is subjective and the EBP team should determine what is a reasonable timeline for their topic at hand. Additionally, the inclusion of older literature on a topic should not necessarily be seen as a sign that a literature summary is not current, but rather it may be referring to foundational information on a subject (see seminal literature).
Data collection	The formal process for gathering information for analysis	Data collection should be explicitly and clearly described. This includes details of the tool(s) used, how the data was recorded (e.g. electronically, paper survey), and where that data was collated for future analysis. Data collection tool descriptions should include the number and types of questions and specific metrics gathered (e.g. blood pressure, Likert-scale feedback, open-ended questions).
Data pooling	The process of combining information from multiple studies or sources to allow for new statistical calculations that can increase the power and generalizability of results	This is a common technique when combining information from multiple studies in a systematic review with meta-analysis. To pool data, studies need to have similar populations, designs and analyses, and metrics (i.e. homogeneity).
Descriptive studies	A type of observational study designed primarily to describe the nature or status of the situation as it occurs naturally	Descriptive studies describe characteristics of a population or phenomenon using observational methods such as surveys, prevalence, and incidence data. It does not involve relationships between variables; instead, it aims to create a picture of a variable, condition, or situation of interest.
Delphi technique	A research approach to generate consensus among subject-matter experts on a topic that lacks robust, science-based data, to set priorities, or to create a stance where one has not existed before (McPherson, 2018)	Descriptive studies describe characteristics of a population or phenomenon using observational methods such as surveys, prevalence, and incidence data. It does not involve relationships between variables; instead, it aims to create a picture of a variable, condition, or situation of interest.
Eligibility criteria	The pre-determined list of criteria that outline the characteristics of who will and will not be included in a study.	Eligibility criteria should be clearly listed and should define the exact characteristics of who can and cannot be included in a study. It can be based on what is feasible and ethical, as well as who or what the team is truly trying to study.

© 2025 Johns Hopkins Health System

F EVIDENCE TERMINOLOGY AND CONSIDERATIONS GUIDE

Term	Definition*	Appraisal Considerations
Ethical Review	The process by which an institutional review board (IRB) assesses research proposals to ensure they are ethically acceptable.	In general, all research studies should undergo ethical review (there may be some exceptions based on the country in which a study is conducted and the amount of interaction with participants). Citing the ethical review process is an essential part of the report of a research study. Review boards may deem studies "approved" or "exempt." Other non-research activities, such as quality improvement (QI) can also undergo ethical review. If this occurs, the study team should provide the process and confirm the IRB deemed their project to be acknowledged as QI and outside of the IRB's scope.
Evidence Summary	A peer-reviewed synthesis of scientific literature written by organizations following pre-determined methods to select and evaluate evidence. Information is presented in a succinct and actionable way for a broad audience with the intent to support point-of-care decision-making (Petkovic, 2016; Jordan, 2019).	The EBP team should ensure an evidence summary was completed using robust methods for selecting and appraising evidence. It may be helpful to reference organizations that are well-known for producing high-quality evidence summaries (e.g. UpToDate and JBI). Because of the goal of making the report easy to read, many times the methodology is not included in the document itself, and the team will need to look for further details on an organization's website.
Experiment	In true experiments, a study team manipulates an independent variable and randomly assigns it to an intervention or control group.	Experimental studies use highly structured designs to establish cause-and-effect relationships. See Randomized Control Trials for further information.
Expertise	Special skills or authoritative knowledge of a topic (Merriam-Webster)	Expertise is not always readily apparent from looking at the listed authors in a publication. Further information can be found in their listed affiliations and by performing an internet search. Items to look for are their professional affiliations, publications on the topic at hand (see H-index), and credentials.
Findings	The results of systematic inquiry usually in the form of data or narrative information	Authors should provide both the data they are analyzing and the results of that analysis. Often this is displayed in tables or figures. The findings should be presented without commentary and reflect the information exactly as it was gathered and analyzed. The findings should help inform the study's aim and the process to generate them should be explained in the methods.
Forest plot	A graphical display designed to illustrate the relative strength of the effects of an intervention from multiple quantitative studies addressing the same question	These are a hallmark of systematic reviews with meta-analysis. EBP teams should ensure they are easy to read and match the results and discussion sections.

© 2025 Johns Hopkins Health System

Term	Definition*	Appraisal Considerations
Funding	Money provided to aid in conducting and reporting studies or other reports. It can come from government grants, private foundations, corporations, or academic institutions.	Studies can be commissioned by various organizations with various interests or priorities. Investigations have shown that commercially sponsored studies (e.g. from technology or drug companies) are more likely to have findings that favor a sponsor's product than independently funded studies. Publications should include a statement addressing any funding received, if it poses a conflict of interest, and if so, how it was addressed.
Generalizability	The extent to which the findings from a study can be applied or extended to other settings, populations, or time periods. High generalizability means the conclusions are likely relevant beyond the study's specific conditions. Sometimes also called "external validity."	Study teams should make an effort to ensure their participants truly reflect the larger population, such as random sampling or subgroup analysis, and clearly report these measures. Authors should also provide detailed information about where the study took place and the included participants. They should do this in a way that allows the reader to determine if the findings can be applied not only to the larger population but also to their specific setting and population. Of note, quality improvement projects do not have a main goal to be generalized, and these efforts may be minimal in this type of report.
Grading	A systematic way to assess and assign a rating to the quality or bias of evidence.	Reviewers can use a variety of tools/models to assess or "grade" their evidence. They should explicitly state the model used and list the grade or rating assigned for all the provided evidence or recommendations.
Gray literature	Scholarly output that is not formally published in peer-reviewed journals. This can include theses, dissertations, government reports, conference papers, and internal documents from organizations.	EBP teams should assess the source of their gray literature and ensure it is reputable. The report itself should provide sufficient information to conduct a formal assessment. Occasionally, this literature does not meet the requirements to be included in the evidence synthesis, but it may provide helpful background information.
H-index	A calculation to measure the amount and impact of scientific publications by an individual. The number is related to the number of published papers by the author and how many times each has been cited (Schreiber, 2019).	This can be a helpful metric to determine someone's expertise on, and scientific contributions to, a topic. It can be found using search engines such as Scopus or Google Scholar. There is no required value, but for context, in the medical field, assistant professors tend to have h-indexes between 2 and 5, associate professors between 6 and 10, and full professors between 12 and 24 (Schreiber, 2019).
Incidence	A measure of the occurrence of new cases of a disease or condition in a specified population within a certain timeframe. It provides information about the risk of contracting the disease or condition.	This metric is often used to report on the outcome of interest. It is usually expressed as a rate, meaning a count over a certain time frame. When possible, authors should provide incidence rates in a well-recognized format (e.g. number of falls per 1,000 patient bed days).

F EVIDENCE TERMINOLOGY AND CONSIDERATIONS GUIDE

Term	Definition*	Appraisal Considerations
Inclusion/Exclusion criteria	The set of rules, markers, or guidelines used to determine who or what is eligible to be included in a study or evidence review.	In the context of literature reviews, the inclusion/exclusion criteria are the list of characteristics a study must HAVE or NOT HAVE to be included in the data analysis. In literature reviews with a systematic approach, they should be directly recorded in the report itself or supplemental content. The EBP team should ensure they are present and fit the question the reviewers are trying to answer. The team should also assess the given criteria for biases (e.g. excluding evidence from one region of the world without reasonable justification).
Institutional Review Board (IRB)	A group, usually associated with an academic organization, that reviews study proposals to evaluate their ethical implications. See "ethical review" for more information.	This term is primarily used in the United States. Authors should list their specific IRB and the designation assigned to a study. Other terms include Ethics Review Committee, Ethics Review Board, Research Ethics Board, and Independent Ethics Committee.
Intervention	An action or item purposefully introduced into a study to test its effects on outcomes of interest.	Interventions can be used in any type of experimental or quasi-experimental study and are often used to assess effectiveness of treatments, drugs, or techniques. An intervention should be deliberate and described in enough detail so that the reader could replicate it.
Likert scale	A scale for measuring attitudes or opinions that uses a fixed number range with associated descriptions for each of the values in that range.	Likert scales typically ask people for their level of agreement, likelihood, or other opinions using a number range (usually between 3 and 7 options) with each side of the scale representing the extremes of each option. Although they are assessing subjective information (e.g. attitudes), Likert-scales are a type of quantitative measurement because they assign a numeric value to the measurement.
Limitations	The recognized flaws, constraints, or weaknesses within a study that may affect the results or implications of the findings.	All studies have limitations. If they are not provided, this is a limitation in and of itself. Ideally, authors provide limitations as well as explanations of how they were mitigated.
Literature Reviews with a Systematic Approach (LRSAs)	LRSAs use explicit methods to search the scientific evidence, analyze the information, extract data, and summarize the included studies.	These reviews go by different names (e.g. systematic, integrative, rapid, umbrella). To determine if a review uses a systematic approach the EBP team should look for the following: • An explicit pre-planned method or protocol • A clear question • Clear and explicit inclusion and exclusion criteria • A documented search strategy, including sources and terms • Use of tables to provide pertinent characteristics of the studies included • An explicit approach to assess the quality (risk of bias) of included evidence • Exploration of the data to consistencies and gaps • Use of tables or figures to support interpretation *Some of this information may be provided in appendices or supplemental files (Booth, 2021)

Term	Definition*	Appraisal Considerations
Longitudinal	A study design that involves repeated observations or measurements of the same variables, among the same individuals, over time. This can span years or even decades.	Longitudinal studies involve multiple data collection points and are useful in understanding long-term efforts or changes. It is common in developmental psychology, sociology, and medicine.
Manipulation	The study team's control over the independent variable (intervention) to observe its effect on the dependent variable.	Manipulation of a variable essentially means a study team "did something." They intervened or changed a situation in some way to measure how that change affected other metrics (variables) of interests. This can range anywhere from introducing a program to giving a patient a medication or treatment.
Meta-analysis	A statistical technique that combines the results of multiple scientific studies addressing the same question to integrate findings and measure an overall effect size. This method enhances the overall understanding of the variable of interest by increasing the sample size and statistical power.	Meta-analysis is usually conducted after reviewers have completed a systematic search and selection of literature on their topic and outcome of interest. Essentially, in a rigorous and replicable way, reviewers attempt to gather all studies that answer their review question and meet their inclusion/exclusion criteria (see corresponding section), to pool data that measures the same variable in the same way. They can then combine those numbers to create a larger, more convincing statistical calculation.
Meta-synthesis	A method used in qualitative research to integrate, evaluate, and interpret findings from multiple qualitative studies. The goal of meta-synthesis is to build a greater narrative or comprehensive understanding about a phenomenon.	Meta-synthesis is the qualitative counterpart to meta-analysis. The analysis process begins after reviewers have systematically gathered and selected evidence that addresses their topic of interest. It uses systematic methods to not just pull information together but to create new interpretations and deeper insights that go beyond the findings of individual studies. This approach attempts to make the whole greater than the sum of its parts.
Mixed methods methodology	An approach that combines elements of both qualitative and quantitative methods to provide a more comprehensive analysis of the topic of interest than either method could offer alone.	Authors should provide their reasoning for selecting a mixed methods approach and how they used one type of data to inform the other. Both the quantitative and qualitative portions should be equally explained and analyzed with true integration of data.
Observational Study design	A type of study in which the investigators observe the natural course of events with minimal or no intervention in the study subjects.	Observational design includes both descriptive and analytical studies (e.g. cohort, case-control, or cross-sectional studies). It is used to describe topics or outcomes of interest as they occur naturally and can simply describe a phenomenon or can suggest relationships between different variables.

© 2025 Johns Hopkins Health System

Term	Definition*	Appraisal Considerations
Outcome	The result or effect of an intervention or exposure, which is measured to determine the impact of the independent variable in a study.	EBP teams should ensure all outcomes of interest are clearly listed. Authors should explain how they gathered and analyzed data to assess each one.
Participant	A person taking part in a study.	Authors should include information about how they selected and recruited participants, including the percentage of how many agreed to participate. They should also provide details about the participants that help the reader understand who the findings could be applied to.
Peer review	The process by which scholarly work (such as papers, reports, or proposals) is checked by a group of experts in the same field to ensure it meets the necessary standards before it is published or funded.	The purpose of peer review is to ensure that scientific and scholarly work is based on sound methods and that the findings are trustworthy. Peer review adds an additional level of scrutiny to published work and is an important part of the generation of clinical practice guidelines (CPGs) and evidence summaries, as well as work published in scholarly journals. While it is assumed for most journal work, the peer-review process should be explicitly explained in the methods for evidence summaries and CPGs
Phenomenon	A fact, situation, or concept	In qualitative studies, this is the concept the study team is exploring. Authors should explicitly state the phenomena of interest, and their methods should clearly match what they are attempting to explore. This can be considered the counterpart to "variable" in quantitative studies.
Prevalence	The proportion of a population who have a specific characteristic in a given time period. In epidemiology, it often refers to the proportion of people with a particular disease or condition.	This metric is often used to report the number of people who have a disease or condition among those at risk. It is usually expressed as a percentage or the number of cases per set number of people (e.g. 2.5 cases per 1,000 people).
The Preferred Reporting Items for Systematic Reviews and Meta-Analyses (PRISMA) diagram	A flow chart that depicts the different phases of a literature review with a systematic approach (LRSA) and illustrates the flow of studies screened, included, and excluded from the search and appraisal.	PRISMA diagrams, or similar flow charts, should be included with all LRSAs. They help the reader understand the scope of the literature search and ensure the process was systematic and comprehensive. Keep in mind, sometimes these diagrams are included as supplementary material and are not available in the article or report itself. The diagram is a portion of a larger reporting checklist (see https://www.prisma-statement.org/).
Prospective	A design that gathers data from the beginning of the study period and forwards in time. Data collection can occur once or several times.	Prospective studies do not look back at any historical or previously collected data. They only collect and analyze data for the study period. This allows the study team to ensure they are gathering complete information and adjust their design as needed.

© 2025 Johns Hopkins Health System

Term	Definition*	Appraisal Considerations
Qualitative methodology	Qualitative studies collect and analyze narrative data to gain an in-depth understanding of a phenomenon or experience, including opinions, meanings, and motivations. They provide insights into the problem or help to develop ideas or hypotheses for potential quantitative inquiry.	Considerations for qualitative designs are outlined in the Qualitative Appraisal Checklist in Appendix E2. See Chapter 6 for more details. Some words to look for that are associated with qualitative designs and may help the EBP team determine if they are looking at this type of study are: narrative, thematic, coding, phenomenology, ethnography, grounded theory, critical theory, or data saturation.
Quantitative methodology	Quantitative studies involve the collection and analysis of number-based data to quantify a problem by generating numerical information that can be transformed into usable statistics.	Considerations for quantitative designs are outlined in the Quantitative Appraisal Checklist in Appendix E2. See Chapter 6 for more details. Some words to look for that are associated with quantitative designs and may help the EBP team determine if they are looking at this type of study are: randomized control trial, experimental, quasi-experimental, statistics, calculations, power, significance, Likert, incidence, prevalence, case-control, or cohort.
Quasi-Experimental Studies	Quasi-experimental studies have an intervention but lack randomization and sometimes lack a control group. They can help to establish causal relationships, but because they are limited in their ability to control for confounding factors, are not as compelling as true experiments (Randomized Control Trials; RCTs).	Quasi-experimental designs are used when it is not ethical or feasible to randomly assign people to an intervention. Words commonly associated with this approach are pre/post, nonrandomized, nonequivalent, natural experiment, or opt-in.
Randomization	The process of assigning participants into different groups in a study to ensure each participant has an equal chance of being assigned to any group.	Randomization reduces bias by increasing the likelihood that groups are comparable at the beginning of a study. EBP teams should ensure participant assignments are truly random (e.g. random number generator, coin flip) and not haphazard (e.g. dividing a list in half) or introduce bias in another way (e.g. grouping patients by time of day they present to a clinic).
Randomized Control Trial (RCT)	RCTs are considered "true experiments" and are considered the gold standard for establishing causal relationships. They have three core components, randomization, control, and manipulation of a variable.	EBP teams should assess if RCTs truly used random methods that ensured each participant had the same likelihood of being in the intervention or control group, the control group was otherwise similar to the intervention group and the intervention is clear and well-described. RCTs typically follow very robust methods and use advanced statistical calculations that are approved by an institutional review board. To increase confidence in the study findings, the EBP team can look to see if the trial protocol was registered or published.

© 2025 Johns Hopkins Health System

F EVIDENCE TERMINOLOGY AND CONSIDERATIONS GUIDE

Term	Definition*	Appraisal Considerations
Reflexivity	The study team members' awareness of their own influence on the study process and outcomes.	Study team members should reflect and provide information on their own biases, values, and decisions and how this might have affected the conduct of their study. This helps ensure transparency and objectivity.
Reliability	Reliability refers to the consistency of a measure or instrument. A reliable tool will yield the same results under consistent conditions across different times and settings.	Authors should provide specific information about the reliability of their data collection tools. This can sometimes be expressed with a statistic called Cronbach's alpha (>.7 is usually considered adequate) or intra-class correlation coefficients (ICC). Other types of reliability relate to having consistent measurements regardless of who is collecting/analyzing the data (inter-rater reliability), and consistent measurements from multiple tests describing unchanged conditions (test-retest reliability).
Research	Research is a systematic investigation into, and study of, materials and sources to establish facts and reach new conclusions. It is an organized way to learn and understand more about a specific question or problem.	Research should be rigorous and replicable with the intention of creating new knowledge.
Response rate	The proportion of individuals who respond to or participate in a survey or study out of all those invited or selected to participate.	Response rates should be provided because they are an important indicator of the representativeness of the data collected. Low response rate may introduce bias, especially if those who did respond are fundamentally different than those who did not. Authors should provide the exact number of people they attempted to recruit for all data collection points and the number of those people who responded (usually expressed as a percentage). There is not one "gold standard" for acceptable response rates. For context, one systematic review found the average response rate in patients is 70% and 53% for doctors (across all modalities; Meyer et al., 2022).
Retrospective	A retrospective study design involves looking back at events that have already occurred.	Retrospective studies do not collect data generated during the study period but rather look back at previously recorded information (e.g. retrospective chart review) or through recollections of participants. This can make the conduct of a study more feasible or ethical, but also can lead to incomplete data because study teams cannot fill in missing information or participants' memories might be limited. It is often contrasted with prospective studies, which follow participants into the future.
Review or research question	A clear and focused question that outlines the topic the study or review seeks to answer.	In the context of a review, the question should be explicitly listed in order for a reader to understand who, what, and where the review applies to. It defines the scope of the investigation, often expressed as a PICO question (Population, Interventions, Comparisons, and Outcomes of interest). It guides the literature search and inclusion/exclusion criteria for studies.

© 2025 Johns Hopkins Health System

Term	Definition*	Appraisal Considerations
Sample	The subset of individuals, cases, or data points selected from a larger population for the purpose of conducting a study. The goal of using a sample is to obtain conclusions that can be generalized to the entire population while being cost-effective and more manageable in terms of size and practicality.	A sample should ideally represent the characteristics of the larger population from which it is drawn. This allows for the generalization of results back to the population. Authors should provide relevant details about their sample (e.g. demographics, past medical history, diagnoses) clearly and explicitly to help the reader understand the groups the findings apply to.
Sample size	The number of participants or data points included in a study.	Study teams should provide the number of people they intended to recruit, and how they arrived at that number (this can be based on a statistical calculation, power, or other methods such as comparison to similar studies that have been previously published). Authors should also provide the number of participants they successfully recruited at each data collection point in their report in a way that is easy to find and interpret. Larger samples generally provide more reliable estimates but are costlier and more time-consuming to manage.
Sampling	The process of selecting the participants for a study.	Authors should explicitly provide their methods for selecting potential participants for their study. This helps the reader determine if the eventual participants truly represent the larger group they were pulled from. Various methods include random sampling, stratified sampling (breaking the larger population into sub-groups that share similar characteristics and recruiting from each), convenience sampling (selecting participants who are easily and readily available), systematic sampling (selecting individuals at a pre-determined interval, e.g. every 5th person), cluster sampling (selecting entire groups) and snowball sampling (using participants to identify other participants). Snowball sampling can be used when populations are difficult to access, or a disease or condition is rare.
Saturation	In qualitative studies, the point at which data collection is not revealing any new information and themes or patterns are redundant. Saturation indicates that the data collection process can be concluded.	In qualitative studies, saturation is an indication the study team has collected enough data, and the sample size was adequate. They should explicitly explain how they determined saturation had been reached.
Search Strategy	A formal process used to retrieve evidence by identifying databases and creating search strings that include key concepts and synonyms with database-specific syntax (Booth, 2021; Bramer, 2018).	For literature reviews with a systematic approach (LRSAs), search strategies should be provided. This might not appear in the report itself but in online supplemental materials or technical development reports.

Term	Definition*	Appraisal Considerations
Seminal paper	Works of central importance to a topic or area of study. They often report a major breakthrough, insight, or a new theory. This kind of paper may describe a study that changes our understanding of a topic or describes and illustrates a new and highly useful scientific method. Also called pivotal, classic, or landmark studies.	When EBP teams are assessing the reference list of an article or report to ensure citations are recent, they may come across much older entries. This does not necessarily mean it is out-of-date, but they include foundational information in the form of a seminal paper (e.g. Benner's Novice to Expert paper). There is no specific label to identify these works, rather the team may need to do further investigation to determine their status—citation analysis is one method.
Study Design	An approach or set of methods and procedures used to collect and analyze information (Ranganathan, 2018).	Study designs should be explicit and formal. A report is considered to have a formal study design if it meets most of the following criteria: • Was pre-planned (prior to investigators initiating intervention or data collection) • Received ethical review (by the institutional review board) • Has formal and systematic data collection and data analysis • Uses specific qualitative and/or quantitative information gathered for the purposes of the investigation • The study team are not subjects of the intervention • Has a clear aim, reproducible methods, results, and discussion • Do not only recount the authors' personal, organizational, or literature-based experience.
Study setting	The physical location where data collection for a study takes place	Authors should include details about the environment in which a study takes place. This can include the type of facility (e.g. hospital inpatient, nursing home, school), the geographic location (e.g. region and country), and other information about the location that will help a team determine if it applies to their setting (e.g. academic hospital, rural hospital). It is common for authors to not use the name of the organization but general descriptors.
Triangulation	The use of multiple methods, data sources, investigators, or theoretical perspectives to cross-validate and corroborate findings.	Authors should explicitly address their efforts to enhance credibility and confirm their findings through triangulation techniques such as having multiple researchers analyze data, collecting data through different approaches or from more than one source, or approaching analysis with different interpretive frameworks.

© 2025 Johns Hopkins Health System

Term	Definition*	Appraisal Considerations
Validity	Validity refers to the extent to which a research instrument or study measures what it is intended to measure.	Authors should describe if the tools they are using are valid, meaning they have undergone a process to ensure they are measuring what they intend to measure. This can be done through a variety of processes (from consultation with subject matter experts to statistical analyses) which establish different types of validity. Types of validity include: • Content Validity: The extent to which a measure represents all facets of a given construct. • Criterion Validity: The extent to which a measure is related to an outcome. • Construct Validity: The appropriateness of inferences made based on observations or measurements (often using a test) of a particular construct. • Face validity: The general perceiving appropriateness of a tool.
Variable	A variable is any characteristic, number, or quantity that can be measured or quantified. Variables can be considered dependent, independent, or confounding.	Authors should list all variables they intend to measure and how they will measure them. The variables they are collecting should link directly to the aim(s) of the study.

*Unless otherwise cited, definitions are attributed to Polit & Beck (2021)

© 2025 Johns Hopkins Health System

Statistics Terms and Definitions

Term	Definition*
Central tendency	A type of descriptive statistic to describe a "typical" value in a set of numbers that uses different calculations to quantify the center of the range of values. It includes mean (average), median (the middle value when data are put in order), and mode (the most frequently occurring value).
Confidence interval (CI)	Expressed as two numbers with an accompanying percentage, CIs are a range of values within which a metric is estimated to fall, at a specified probability (e.g. 95%). The specified probability tells you how confident the person performing the calculation is that the metric does in fact fall within the range. For example, an average of 10 with a 95% CI of 8-12 tells the reader they can be 95% sure the true average is between 8 and 12.
Effect size	The strength of the relationship between variables. Unlike significance tests that provide a yes-or-no answer to whether an effect exists, the effect size tells how substantial the effect is. Common measures include Cohen's d (standardized difference between two means), correlation coefficient (strength of association between two variables), and odds ratio (ratio of the odds of an event occurring in one group to the odds of it occurring in another group).
Odds ratio (OR)	Expressed as percentage or integer, OR is a measure of the likelihood (odds) of an event occurring to a member of a group compared to another (a ratio of event to non-events). A negative OR means the odds of an event occurring in a member of an exposed group is lower than that of a non-exposed group. ORs of 1 indicate there is no difference between group members. Positive ORs mean there are higher odds of an event occurring in a member of the exposed group compared to the non-exposed group. For example, an OR of -.5 comparing the odds of increased body mass index for a member of a group who attended exercise sessions vs the odds of increased BMI for a member of a group person who did not attend the session means a person who went to the exercise sessions were 50% less likely to have an increase in their BMI. ORs explain the odds of something occurring to an individual whereas relative risk explains the probability of something occurring at the population level.
Power analysis	It is a statistical method used to determine the number of participants or observations (sample size) required to detect an effect of a given size with a certain degree of certainty.
Statistical significance	Is a determination made based on the probability that the observed results of a study could have occurred by chance alone. This probability is expressed as a p-value; a p-value less than a chosen significance level (commonly 0.05) indicates that there is a 95% likelihood the observed effects are true and not based on change alone. In some cases, lack of statistical significance is a good indication (e.g. when comparing baseline characteristics between an intervention and control group).
Relative risk (RR)	Expressed as percentage or integer, RR, also known as the risk ratio, is a measure of the probability of an event occurring in the exposed group versus a non-exposed group. For instance, if the relative risk of developing a disease for smokers compared to non-smokers is 2.0, it means that smokers are twice as likely to develop the disease as non-smokers. Relative risk helps in understanding the strength of the association between an exposure and an outcome at the population level.

*Unless otherwise cited, definitions are attributed to Polit & Beck (2021)

For references, refer to Chapter 8.

© 2025 Johns Hopkins Health System

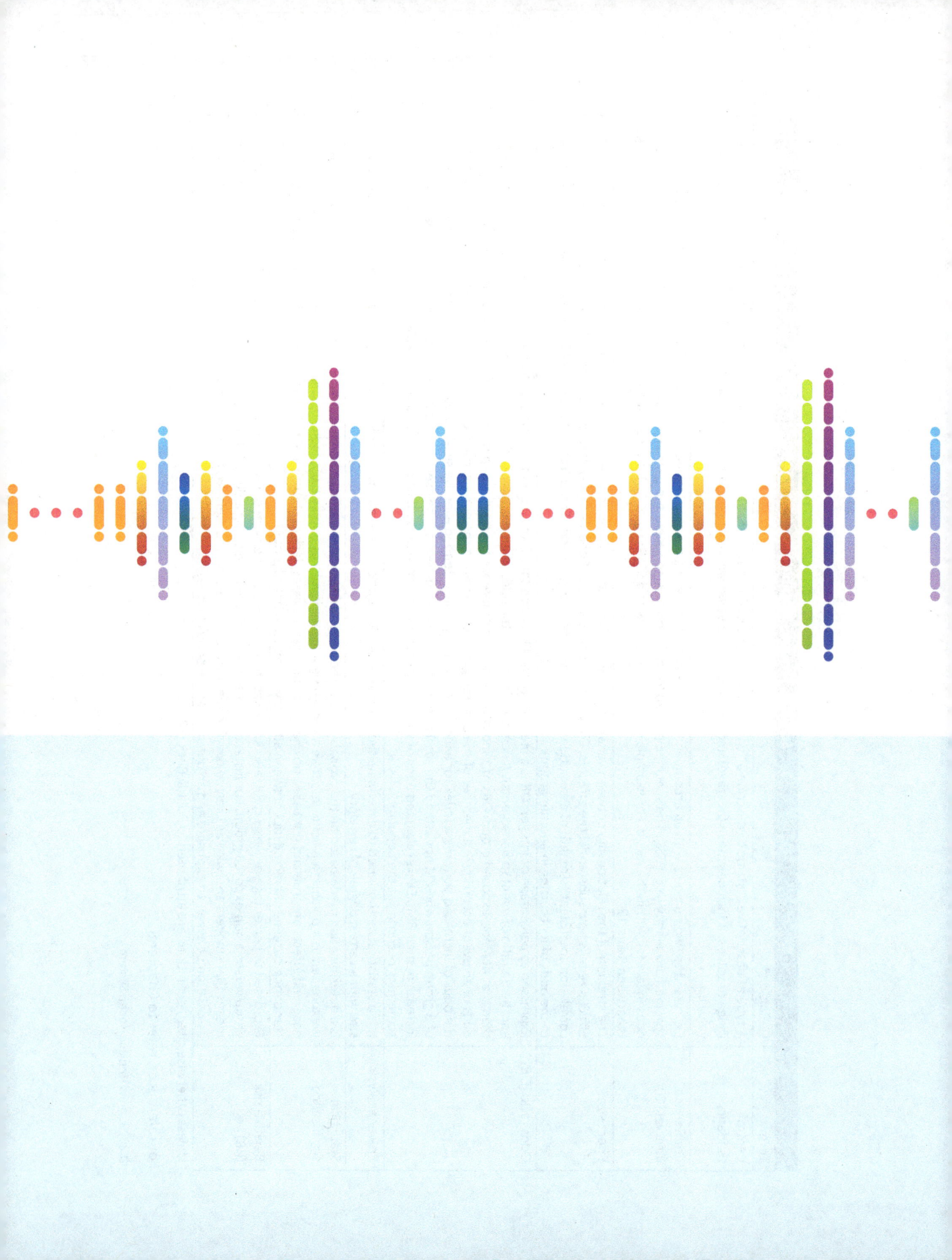

GI

BEST-EVIDENCE SUMMARY TOOL

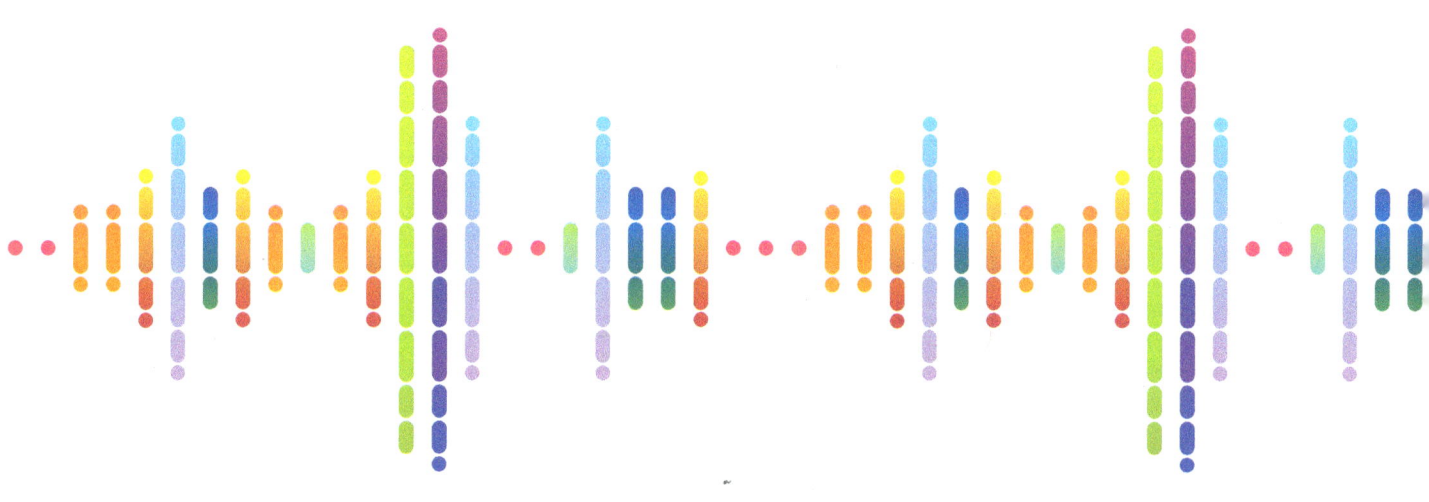

Best-Evidence Summary Tool

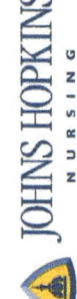

Purpose: This tool collates information from pre-appraised evidence identified in the best-evidence search and other data obtained from a targeted search. It brings all the data into a central document to help the EBP team with the next step of the EBP process, synthesis.

Section I: Pre-Appraised Evidence

Complete the data collection tool below for all included pre-appraised evidence.

Article Number	Author (organization), date, title	Type of pre-appraised evidence	Topic or Intervention	Population	Setting	Recommendations that answer the EBP question

© 2025 Johns Hopkins Health System

G1 BEST-EVIDENCE SUMMARY TOOL

Article number	Reviewer names	Author, date, and title	Type of evidence	Population, size, and setting	Intervention	Findings that help answer the EBP question	Measures used	Limitations	Moderate, or strong support for decision-making?

Complete Section II of Appendix H

© 2025 Johns Hopkins Health System

Instructions for the Best-Evidence Summary Tool

Section I: Pre-Appraised Evidence

Record information from the pre-appraised evidence.

Article Number	Author (organization), date, title	Type of pre-appraised evidence	Topic or Intervention	Population	Setting	Recommendations that answer the EBP question
Assign a unique number to each resource included in the table. This will help with tracking in subsequent steps	Record the name of the organization or authors who produced the evidence. Also include the title and date.	Record the type of pre-appraised evidence. This should be a Clinical Practice Guideline (CPG), literature review with a systematic approach (LRSA), or evidence summary	Record the specific topic or intervention addressed in the pre-appraised evidence. This may be exactly the same as the topic or intervention the team identified in their EBP question or may be more broad and encompass an answer to the EBP team's question.	Record the population(s) the pre-appraised evidence addresses	Record the setting(s) the pre-appraised evidence applies to	List recommendations from the evidence that directly answer the EBP question. These should be considered the "take-away" points from the evidence that help the team better understand solutions to their given problem. When the pre-appraised evidence is broader than the team's scope, only record recommendations that apply to the question at hand.

© 2025 Johns Hopkins Health System

G1 BEST-EVIDENCE SUMMARY TOOL   269

Section II: Reports of Single Studies from the Targeted Evidence Search

Record information from the targeted search evidence.

Article number	Reviewer names	Author, date, and title	Type of evidence	Population, size, and setting	Intervention	Findings that help answer the EBP question	Measures used	Limitations	Moderate, or strong support for decision-making?
Assign a unique number to each resource included in the table. This will help with tracking in subsequent steps.	Record the names of the team members who read the article. This is needed for any follow-up questions and to ensure everyone has completed their assigned readings.	Record the last name of the first author of the article, the publication/ communication date, and the title. This will help track articles throughout the literature search, screening, and review process. It is also helpful when someone has authored more than one publication included in the review.	Indicate the type of evidence provided in this source. This should be descriptive of the study or project design. Consider using descriptors from the word bank below.	Provide a quick review of the population, number of participants, and study location. Location can include the state or country and additional descriptors such as urban, rural, community-based, etc. Consider how the population, size, and setting relate to your EBP question. This may inform the level of detail you choose to record here.	Record the intervention(s) implemented or discussed in the article. This should relate to the intervention or comparison elements of your EBP question. Some studies, such as observational studies, may not have an intervention. However, you can record the focus of the study team's query. Restating the intervention from your EBP question, as the "Intervention" in the summary table, is not useful. Additional details are required.	List findings, or results, from the article that directly answer the EBP question. These should be succinct statements that provide enough information that the reader does not need to return to the original article. Avoid directly copying and pasting from the article. These should be considered the "take-away" points from the evidence that help the team better understand solutions to their given problem.	These are the measures and/or instruments (e.g., satisfaction surveys, patient interviews, focus groups, validated tools, subscales, biometric data, clinical data) the authors used to determine the answer to the research question or the effectiveness of their intervention. These are not the results of what was measured but rather the tool or approach to quantify or qualify the metric(s) of interest.	Provide the limitations of the evidence—both as listed by the authors as well as your assessment of any flaws or drawbacks. Consider not only how well the study or project was implemented, but also how well it was reported. Limitations should be apparent from the team's appraisal checklists. Keep in mind, some limitations are inherent to the type of evidence and don't necessarily negate its findings (e.g. lack of control in an observational study).	Record the type of support for decision-making.

© 2025 Johns Hopkins Health System

Word bank for type of evidence:

No individual study will use a term from each column. Within each grouping, only select one term.

Methodology	Design	Timing
Quantitative Qualitative Mixed-Methods	Randomized Controlled Trial (RCT) Quasi-experimental Interventional Observational (non-experimental) Descriptive Correlational	Prospective Retrospective Cross-Sectional Longitudinal

© 2025 Johns Hopkins Health System

G2

INDIVIDUAL EVIDENCE SUMMARY TOOL

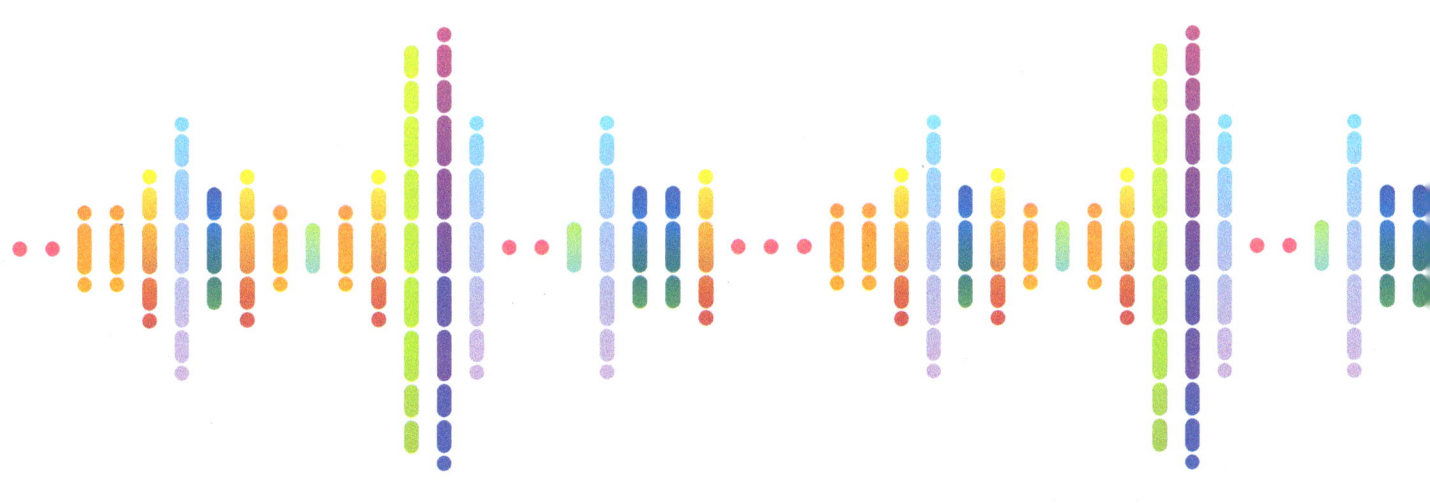

Individual Evidence Summary Tool

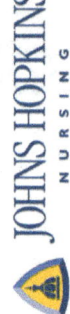

Purpose: This tool collates information from the literature gathered during the exhaustive evidence search. It brings all of the data into a central document to help the EBP team with the next step of the EBP process, synthesis.

Complete the data collection tool below for all included evidence from the exhaustive evidence search.

Article number	Reviewer names	Author, date, and title	Type of evidence	Population, size, and setting	Intervention	Findings that help answer the EBP question	Measures used	Limitations	Level of support for decision-making	Notes to the team

© 2025 Johns Hopkins Health System

Instructions for the Individual Evidence Summary Tool

Record information from the exhaustive evidence search									
Article number	Reviewer names	Author, date, and title	Type of evidence	Population, size, and setting	Intervention	Findings that help answer the EBP question	Measures used	Limitations	Level of support for decision-making	Notes to the team
Assign a unique number to each resource included in the table. This will help with tracking in subsequent steps.	*Record the names of the team members who read the article. This is needed for any follow-up questions and to ensure everyone has completed their assigned readings.*	*Record the last name of the first author of the article, the publication/ communication date, and of the title. This project, will help track articles throughout the literature search, screening, and review process. It is also helpful when someone has authored more than one publication included in the review.*	*Indicate the type of evidence provided by this source. This should be descriptive of the study, project, opinion, or report. Consider using descriptors from the word bank below.*	*Provide a quick review of the population, number of participants, and study location. Location can include the state and country and additional descriptors such as urban, rural, community-based, etc. Consider how the population, size, and setting relate to your EBP question. This may inform the level of detail you choose to record here.*	*Record the intervention(s) implemented or discussed in the article. This should relate to the intervention or comparison elements of your EBP question. Some evidence, such as observational studies or anecdotal evidence, may not have an intervention. However, you can record the focus of the report of the study team's query. Restating the intervention from your EBP question, as the "intervention" in the summary table, is not useful. Additional details are required.*	*List findings, or results, from the article that directly answer the EBP question. These should be succinct statements that provide enough information that the reader does not need to return to the original article. Avoid directly copying and pasting from the article. These should be considered the "take-away" points from the evidence that help the team better understand solutions to their given problem.*	*These are the measures and/or instruments (e.g., satisfaction surveys, patient interviews, focus groups, validated tools, subscales, biometric data, clinical data) the authors used to determine the answer to the study question or the effectiveness of their intervention. These are not the results of what was measured but rather the tool or approach to quantify or qualify the metric(s) of interest.*	*Provide the limitations of the evidence—both as listed by the authors as well as your assessment of any flaws or drawbacks. Consider not only how well the study, project, or review was done, but also how well it was reported. Limitations should be apparent from the team's appraisal checklists. Keep in mind, some limitations are inherent to the type of evidence and don't necessarily negate its findings (e.g. lack of control in an observational study).*	*Record the level of support for decision-making.*	*Use this section to keep track of items important to the EBP process not captured elsewhere on this tool. Consider items that will be helpful to have easy reference to when conducting the evidence synthesis.*

G2 INDIVIDUAL EVIDENCE SUMMARY TOOL 273

© 2025 Johns Hopkins Health System

Word bank for type of evidence:

No individual report will use a term from each column. Within each grouping, only select one term.

Reviews	Methodology	Design/Approach	Timing	Other
-Systematic with or without meta-analysis -Integrative -Rapid -Umbrella -Scoping -Critical -Literature	Quantitative Qualitative Mixed-Methods	Randomized Controlled Trial (RCT) Quasi-experimental Interventional Observational (non-experimental) Descriptive Correlational	Prospective Retrospective Cross-Sectional Longitudinal	-Expert opinion -Book chapter -Position statement -Case report -Programmatic experience

© 2025 Johns Hopkins Health System

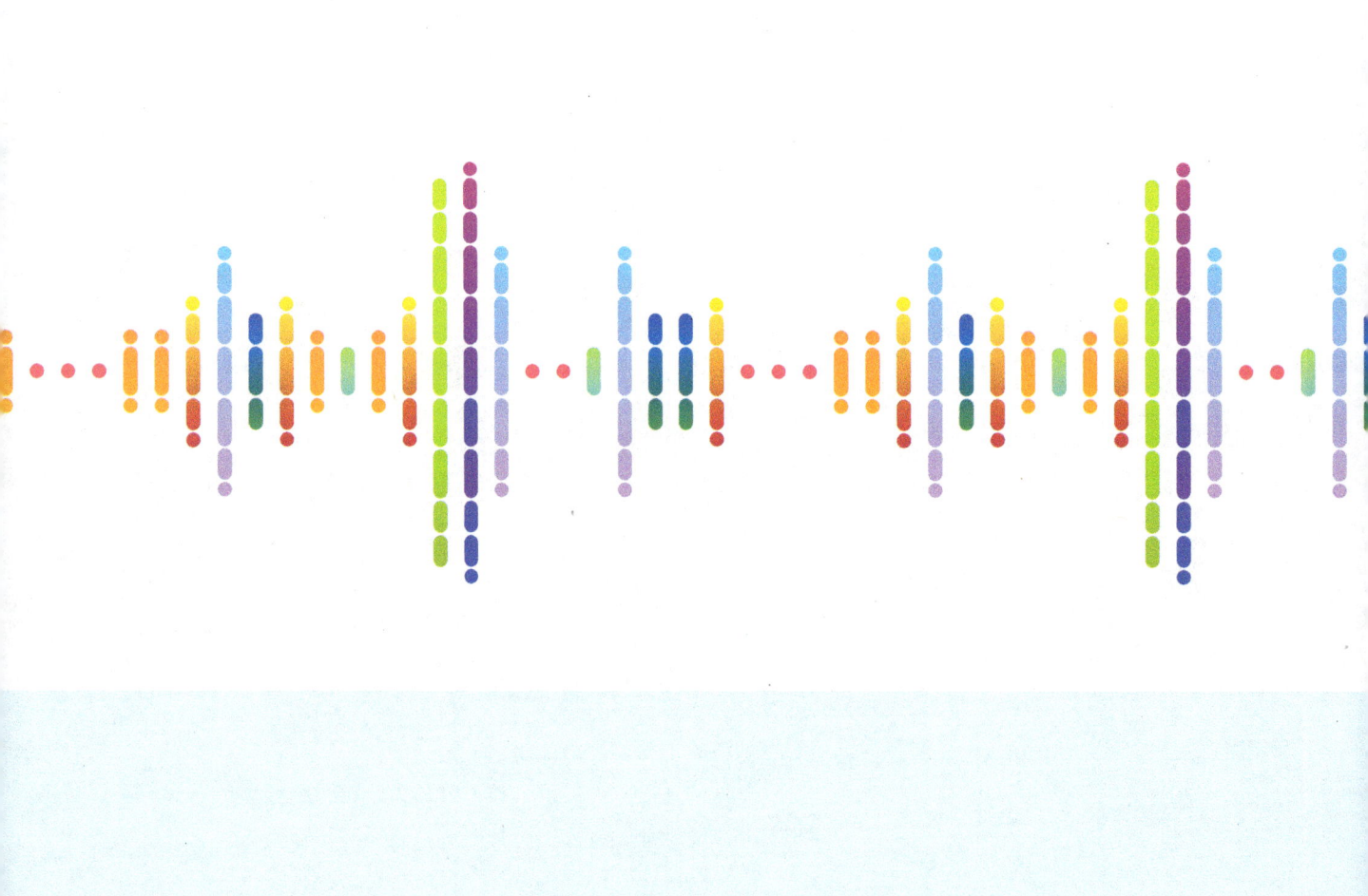

SUMMARY, SYNTHESIS, & BEST-EVIDENCE RECOMMENDATIONS TOOL

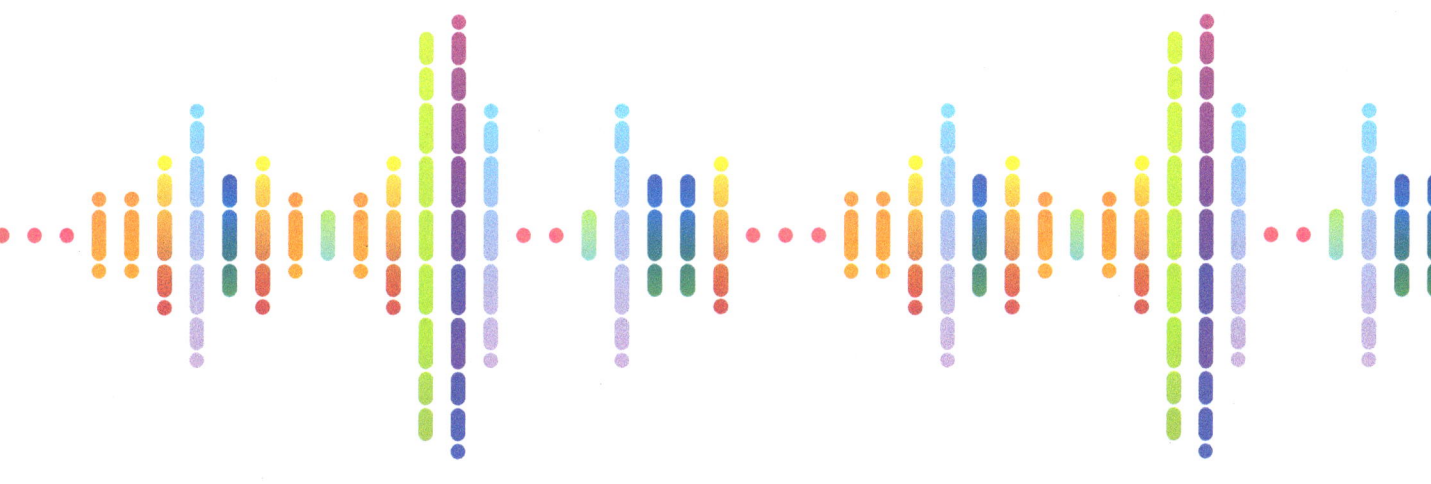

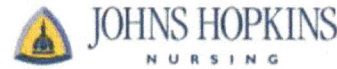

Summary, Synthesis, & Best-Evidence Recommendations Tool

> Purpose: This tool guides the EBP team through the process of synthesizing the pertinent findings from the Best Evidence or Individual Evidence Summary (Appendix G1 or G2) to create an overall picture of the body of the evidence related to the EBP question. The team analyzes the data in each category of support for decision-making, as well as any additional organizational approaches that bring further insights.

Section I: Findings from the Individual Evidence Summary	
Support for Decision-Making	**Synthesized Findings with Article Number(s)** *(This is not a simple restating of information from each individual evidence summary—see instructions)*
Strong Number of sources = _____	
Moderate Number of sources = _____	
Limited Number of sources = _____	

Further Synthesis Based on Additional Organization and Analysis (OPTIONAL)

© 2025 Johns Hopkins Health System

H SUMMARY, SYNTHESIS, & BEST-EVIDENCE RECOMMENDATIONS TOOL

Section II: Best-Evidence Recommendations

The recommendations below are based on:

☐ Pre-appraised evidence identified in a best evidence search → Record each recommendation in the corresponding evidence category in the table below based on the confidence/certainty listed in the clinical practice guidelines, evidence summary, or literature review with a systematic approach

☐ Evidence appraised by the EBP team from a targeted search to supplement the pre-appraised evidence (single studies with a formal study design) → Record any additional or altered recommendations to the pre-appraised evidence in the corresponding evidence category in table below. See instructions for more details.

☐ Evidence appraised by the EBP team from an exhaustive search (single studies, anecdotal evidence, and pre-appraised evidence that does not fully address the EBP question) → Record each recommendation in the table below based on the team's analysis and synthesis of information in Section I

Characteristics of the Recommendation(s)	Best-Evidence Recommendation(s)
High certainty recommendations (Robust, well-documented, consistent & persuasive, based mostly on evidence that provides strong support for decision-making)	
Reasonable certainty recommendations (Good, mostly compelling, consistent evidence, based mostly on evidence that provides moderate to strong support for decision-making)	
Characteristics of the Recommendation(s)	Recommendation(s) Lacking Adequate Evidence
Reasonable to low certainty recommendations (Good but conflicting evidence. Inconsistent results, based mostly on evidence that provides moderate support for decision making)	
Low certainty recommendations (Little to no evidence. Information is minimal, inconsistent and/or based mostly on evidence that provides limited support for decision-making)	

© 2025 Johns Hopkins Health System

Instructions for the Summary, Synthesis, & Best-Evidence Recommendations Tool

Section I: Findings from the Individual Evidence Summary *Only complete Section I if the team completed an exhaustive evidence search and the Individual Evidence Summary Tool (Appendix G2).*	
Support for Decision-Making	**Synthesized Findings With Article Number(s)** *(This is not a simple restating of information from each individual evidence summary—see instructions)*
Strong Number of sources = _____	This table captures key findings that answer the EBP question from an exhaustive evidence search. As a team, review the evidence that provides **strong** support for decision-making in the Individual Evidence Summary Tool (Appendix G2). Look for salient themes, patterns, important takeaways, consistencies, and inconsistencies. After discussing the **strong** evidence and coming to a consensus as a team, record succinct statements in this box that synthesize the information, enhance the team's knowledge, and generate new insight, perspective, and understanding to answer the EBP question. Avoid repeating content and/or copying and pasting directly from the Individual Evidence Summary Tool. Record the article number(s) used to generate each synthesis statement to make the source of findings easy to identify.
Moderate Number of sources = _____	Repeat the process above for evidence that provides **moderate** support for decision-making.
Limited Number of sources = _____	Repeat the process above for evidence that provides **limited** support for decision-making.

Further Synthesis Based on Additional Organization and Analysis (OPTIONAL)
This is an optional section to reflect any additional insights the team has from further organization and analysis of the data. It may include patterns, themes, subgroups, or additional sorting. To determine if this step is necessary, the team should ask themselves, "How can the evidence be organized to explore subtleties or details in order to produce a more comprehensive understanding of the big picture?" See Chapter 9 for more information.

© 2025 Johns Hopkins Health System

H SUMMARY, SYNTHESIS, & BEST-EVIDENCE RECOMMENDATIONS TOOL

Section II: Best-Evidence Recommendations

The recommendations below are based on: *Select boxes below that reflect the type(s) of evidence used to generate the best-evidence recommendations.*

☐ Pre-appraised evidence identified in a best evidence search → Record each recommendation in the corresponding evidence category in the table below based on the confidence/certainty listed in the clinical practice guidelines, evidence summary, or literature review with a systematic approach *Using the certainty or confidence schema used by the authors of the pre-appraised evidence, put each recommendation into the corresponding box.*

☐ Evidence appraised by the EBP team from a targeted search to supplement the pre-appraised evidence (single studies with a formal study design) → Record any additional or altered recommendations to the pre-appraised evidence in the corresponding evidence category in table below. See instructions for more details. *Record any changes to the recommendations from the pre-appraised evidence in the corresponding box. When determining if a recommendation should be updated consider the following:*
- o Does the new evidence provide results that are based on robust methods that the team considers compelling?
- o How does the certainty of any new or altered recommendations compare to the certainty of the recommendation from the pre-appraised evidence?

☐ Evidence appraised by the EBP team from an exhaustive search (single studies, anecdotal evidence, and pre-appraised evidence that does not fully address the EBP question) → Record each recommendation in the table below based on the team's analysis and synthesis of information in Section I *Review the information from Section I. Consider the quantity and quality of information for each recommendation. Based on the descriptions below, record the best-evidence recommendation in the box that corresponds to the characteristics of the evidence used to support it. Recommendations should be succinct statements that distill the synthesized evidence into an answer to the EBP question. The team bases these recommendations on the evidence and does not yet consider their specific setting. Translating the recommendations into action steps within the team's organization occurs in the next step (Translation and Implementation Tools, Appendices I and J).*

Characteristics of the Recommendation(s)	Best-Evidence Recommendation(s)
High certainty recommendations (Robust, well-documented, consistent & persuasive, based mostly on evidence that provides strong support for decision-making)	*Record recommendations the team feels confident in endorsing here. Keep in mind, these can be recommendations FOR or AGAINST an intervention. Sentences can start with phrases such as:* • "The evidence endorses…" • "The evidence recommends…" Or end with • "…is recommended" • "…is indicated" • "…is beneficial" • "…is useful"
Reasonable certainty recommendations (Good, mostly compelling, consistent evidence, based mostly on evidence that provides moderate to strong support for decision-making)	*Record recommendations the team is fairly confident in endorsing here. Sentences can start with phrases such as:* • "the evidence suggests…" Or end with • "…is reasonable" • "…can be useful" • "…can be effective" • "…can be beneficial"

© 2025 Johns Hopkins Health System

Characteristics of the Recommendation(s)	Recommendation(s) Lacking Adequate Evidence
Reasonable to low certainty recommendations (Good but conflicting evidence. Inconsistent results, based mostly on evidence that provides moderate support for decision making)	*Record recommendations the team the team has little confidence in endorsing here. Sentences can start with phrases such as:* • *"Evidence is mixed regarding…"* • *"Evidence is conflicting regarding…"* • *"There is little evidence to support…"* *Or end with:* • *"… may or may not be useful"*
Low certainty recommendations (Little to no evidence. Information is minimal, inconsistent and/or based mostly on evidence that provides limited support for decision-making)	*Record recommendations that team has no confidence in endorses here. Sentences can start with:* • *"There is no evidence to support…"* • *"Evidence is very limited on…"* • *"Recommendations cannot be made on…"* *Or end with:* • *"….is not supported by evidence"*

© 2025 Johns Hopkins Health System

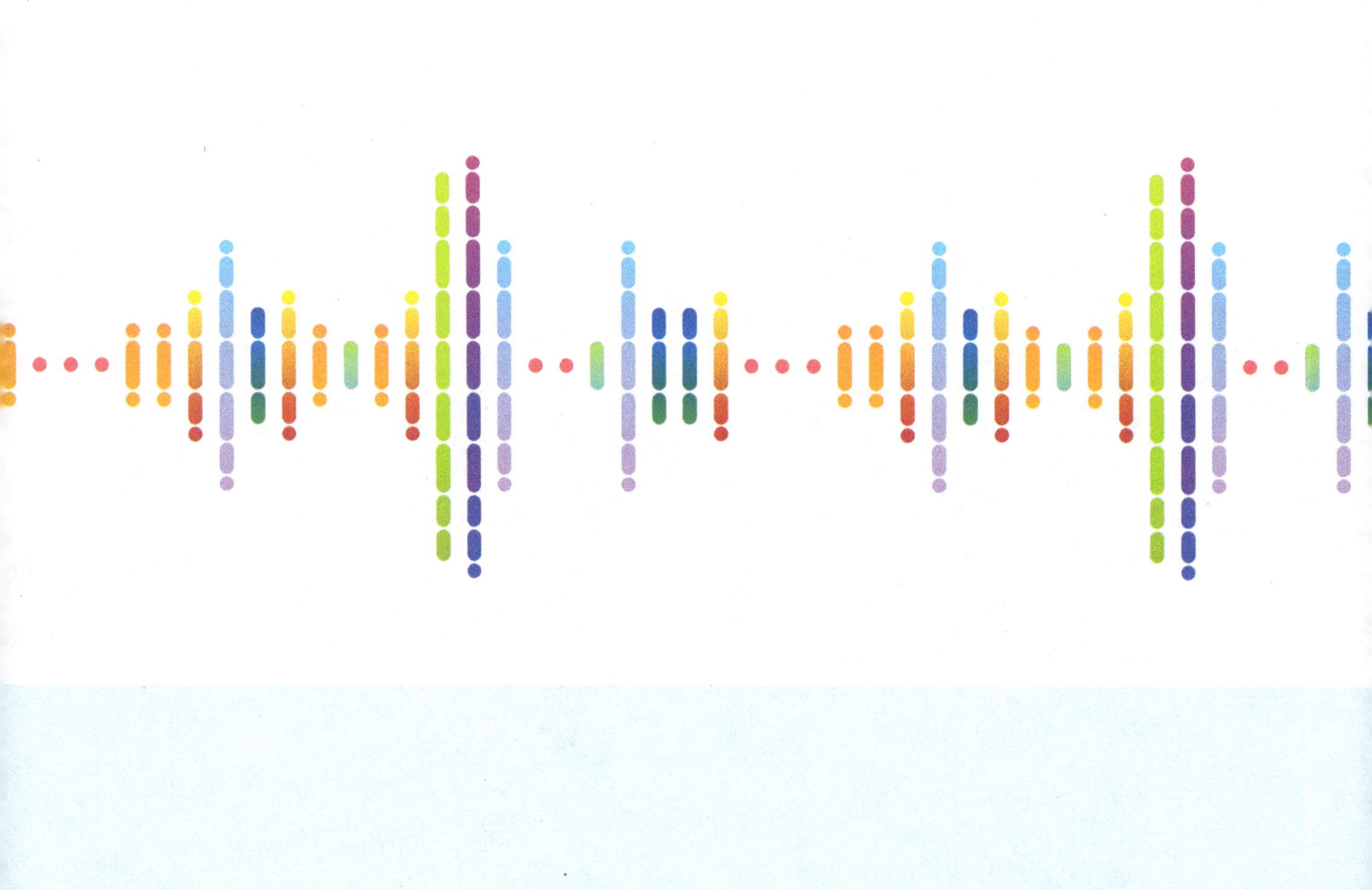

TRANSLATION TOOL

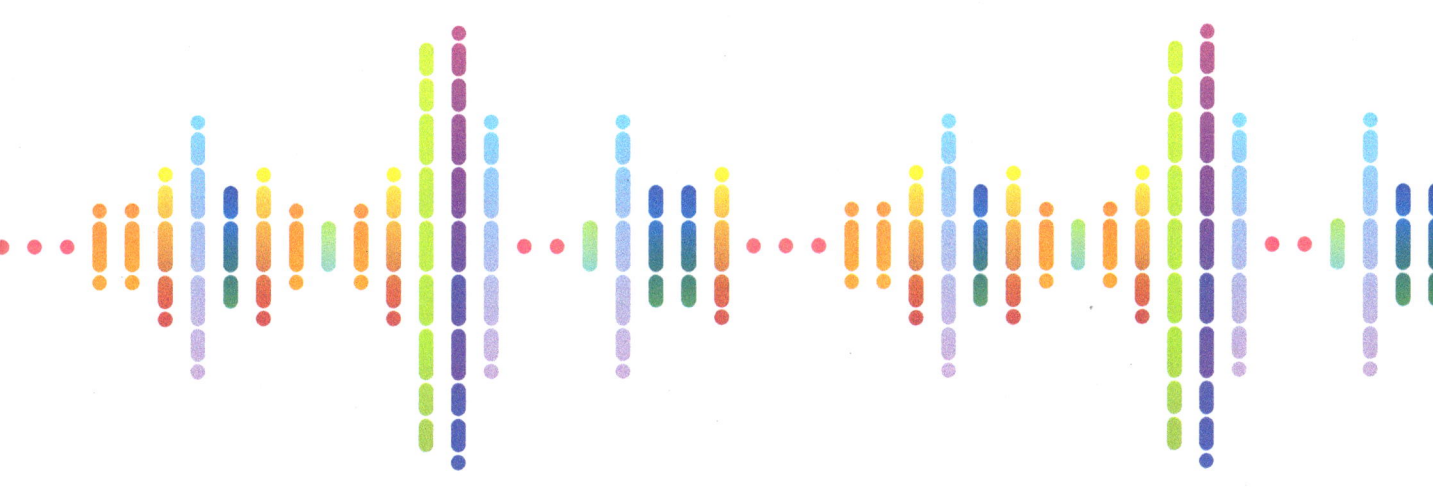

Translation Tool

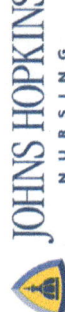

Purpose: This tool guides the EBP team through analyzing the best-evidence recommendations for translation into the team's specific setting. The translation process considers the certainty, risk, feasibility, fit, and acceptability of the best-evidence recommendations. The team uses both critical thinking and clinical reasoning to generate site-specific recommendations.

Refer to the recommendations developed on Appendix H. Consider the certainty of *each* best-evidence recommendation, as well as the fit, feasibility, acceptability, and risk to develop organization-specific recommendations.

Certainty	Risk	Fit	Feasibility	Acceptability
• Do the recommendations have high or reasonable certainty? (Recommendations with reasonable to low and low certainty do not provide adequate support to change current practice, *see instructions below*)	• What is the potential negative impact on patient or staff safety? (Interventions with higher risk require higher certainty evidence to put into practice.)	• How well does the change align with existing practices? • Values? • Norms? • Goals? • Skills?	• Is the change doable and are barriers realistic to overcome? • Is the practice environment ready for change? • Are necessary materials or human resources available? • Can the change be successfully implemented?	• Do impacted groups find the change agreeable? • Does leadership support the change and trust it is reasonable? • Does the change align with organizational priorities?

In concise statements, record the organization-specific recommendations below that address the EBP question.

© 2025 Johns Hopkins Health System

Instructions for the Translation Tool

Referring to the recommendations developed on Appendix H and considering the certainty of *each* best-evidence recommendation, and the fit, feasibility, acceptability, and risk, develop organization-specific recommendations.

Certainty	Risk	Fit	Feasibility	Acceptability
• Do the recommendations have high or reasonable certainty? (Recommendations with reasonable to low and low certainty do not provide adequate support to change current practice.)	• What is the potential negative impact on patient or staff safety? (Interventions with higher risk require higher certainty evidence to put into practice.)	• How well does the change align with existing practices? • Values? • Norms? • Goals? • Skills?	• Is the change doable and are barriers realistic to overcome? • Is the practice environment ready for change? • Are necessary materials or human resources available? • Can the change be successfully implemented?	• Do impacted groups find the change agreeable? • Does leadership support the change and trust it is reasonable? • Does the change align with organizational priorities?

In concise statements, record the organization-specific recommendations below that address the EBP question.

After evaluating the certainty, risk, fit, feasibility, and acceptability of each of the best evidence recommendations, the team should record their organization-specific recommendations here.

There are various scenarios in which an EBP team will determine insufficient evidence to make a change, the risk is too high, or the best-evidence recommendations do not adequately meet the fit, feasibility, and acceptability requirements for implementation at the organization. If this is the case, the EBP team can record a recommendation to wait for more information to become available, consider beginning a research project to fill the knowledge gap or discontinue the project.

Additionally, teams may decide there is insufficient evidence to support a current practice or strong evidence against a current practice. In this case, the team should consider recommending de-implementation.

© 2025 Johns Hopkins Health System

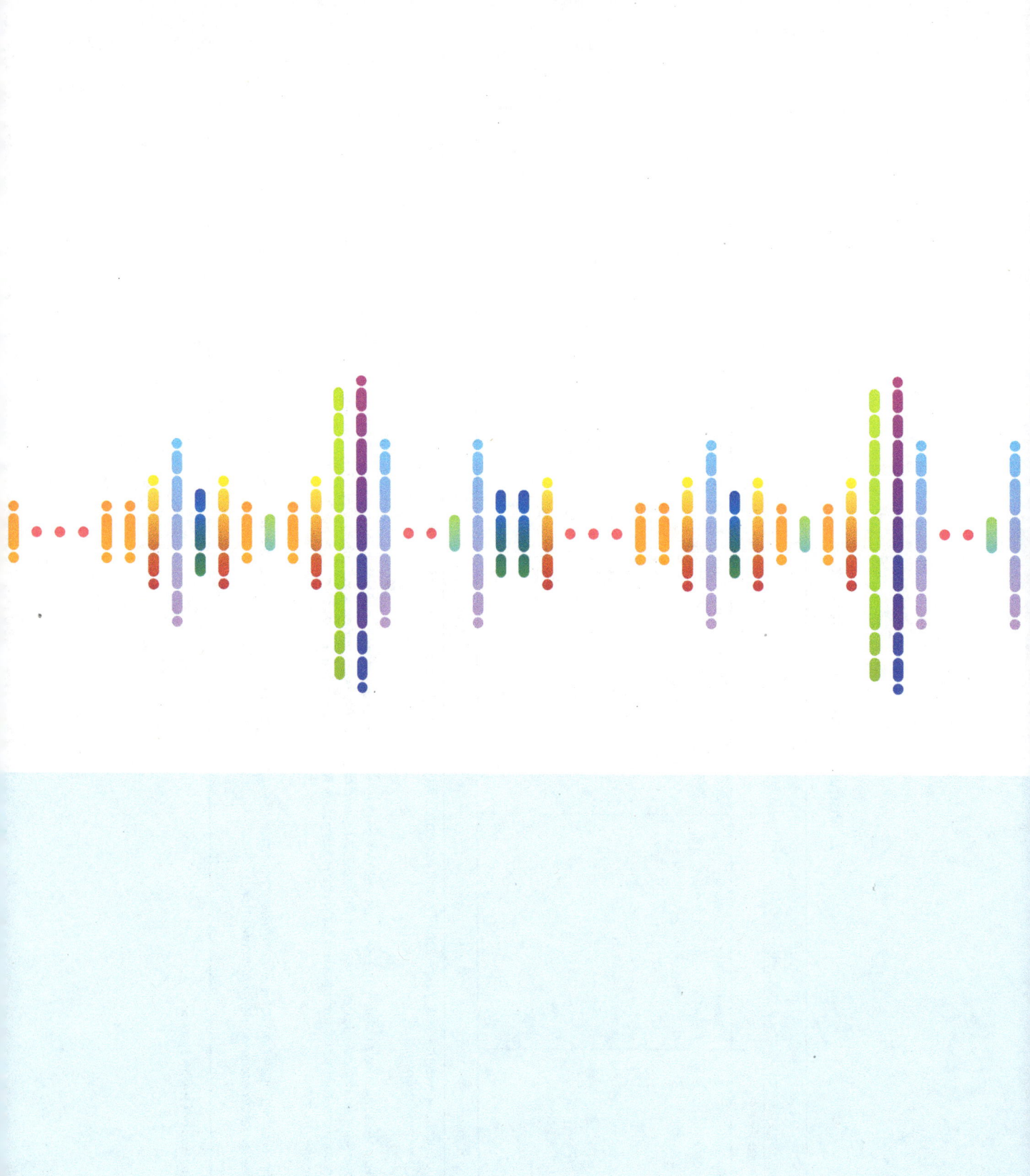

J
IMPLEMENTATION AND ACTION PLANNING (A3) TOOL

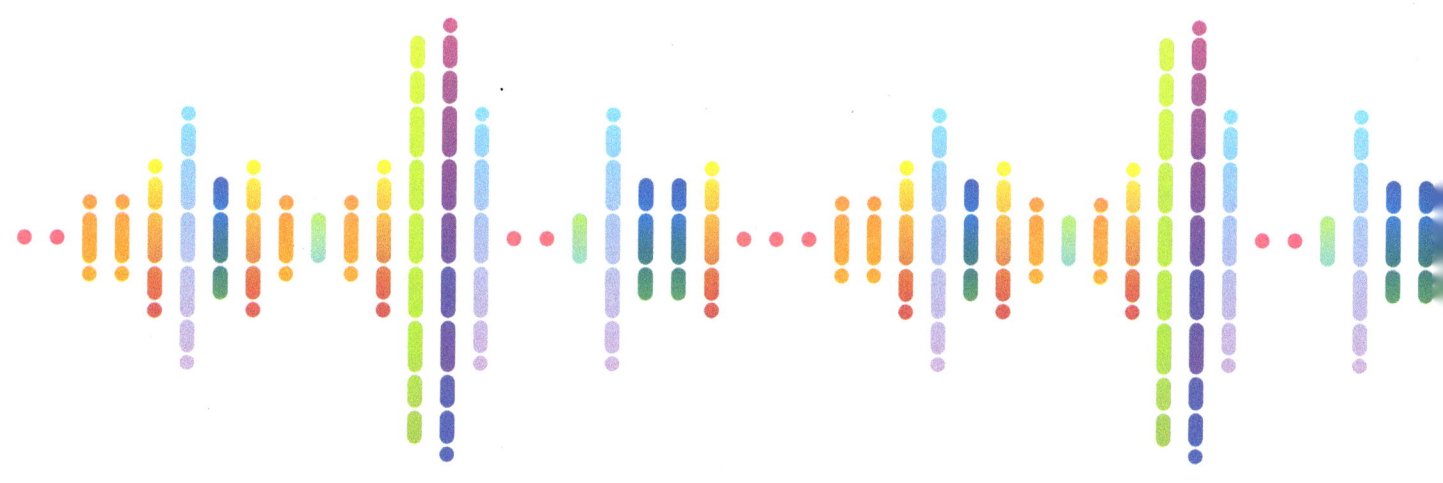

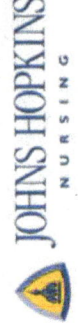

Implementation and Action Planning Tool (A3)

Problem/Evidence (summary of problem, synthesis of evidence)

Goal
SMART Goal aligned with Strategic Priority:

Key Accomplishments using Translation Framework:

Timeline/Milestones (Gantt)

People (Engage)
Project Leader:
Working Group:
Collaborating Groups:
Impacted Groups:
Sponsor:

Implementation (Educate, Execute)

Metrics Progress (Evaluate)

Risk and Risk Mitigation Strategy

Risk	Risk Mitigation Strategy	Status

© 2025 Johns Hopkins Health System

J IMPLEMENTATION AND ACTION PLANNING (A3) TOOL

Work Breakdown Structure (refer to the Timeline/Milestones section of A3 and provide details for each phase of the implementation framework)

Due Date	Task	Dependencies	Accountable Person(s)	Status	Planned Completion	Actual Completion	Resource

Sustainability Plan (Endure)

What are the potential barriers to project sustainability?	What are some mitigation strategies for the potential obstacles?	What additional resources may be needed to support the project?	What additional training may be required?	What responsibilities need to be assigned?	To whom will these responsibilities be assigned?	Are there any additional metrics/outcomes that need to be collected/measured?	How frequently will you monitor and review your outcomes?

© 2025 Johns Hopkins Health System

Instructions for the Implementation and Action Planning Tool (A3)

Problem/Evidence (summary of problem, synthesis of evidence)	Implementation (Educate, Execute)
Establish the problem being solved using national, organizational, and local data. Provide citations. Establish the process measures and patient outcomes that require improvement. Synthesize the evidence around the intervention that will be implemented and how the intervention will address the process measures and patient outcomes identified as problems. Provide citations. **Goal** SMART Goal aligned with Strategic Priority: *The goal should reflect an improvement in the problem identified. Establish how the project can address the process measures and patient outcomes identified as problems. Record what the team hopes to accomplish by implementing the change(s). These can be high-level statements used to inform the measurement plan and implementation. When available, the goal should address the organization's broad strategic priority.* Key Accomplishments using Translation Framework: *Identify each component of the translation framework and the significant accomplishments in each component; identify the stakeholders accountable for each component (the identified stakeholders should be reflected in the People section of the A3). The WBS should go into more detail on how key accomplishments will be completed. The A3 and WBS should go hand in hand and be reflective of each other.*	Note the implementation framework chosen for project translation • May list phases of the framework here • Also, may list tools used, such as PDSA

Timeline/Milestones (Gantt)	People (Engage)
Identify each component of the translation framework and provide a high-level timeline based on the critical accomplishment section of the A3.	**Project Leader:** *The student or the accountable person/group responsible for the project implementation* **Working Group:** *The stakeholders doing the work* **Collaborating Groups:** *The stakeholders who are working with the working group to complete the project* **Stakeholders:** *The stakeholders affected by the implementation, e.g., multi-disciplinary team, organizational/departmental leadership, external community including patients and families, and front-line interprofessional staff (Refer to Stakeholder Analysis Resource). Complete key accomplishments to determine stakeholders.* **Sponsor:** *Identify the accountable leader/group responsible for the improvement.*

© 2025 Johns Hopkins Health System

Metrics Progress (Evaluate) (refer to Chapter 11)

Practice change has different aspects; other measures are frequently used to monitor uptake, attitudes, and outcomes. Select as many as the team feels necessary to gain an accurate picture of ongoing impact. Record the specific metric(s) the team will measure within the outcome categories, how the metrics will be obtained, and how often. Outcomes can be added or changed as the literature review is completed and the translation planning begins. Metrics let you know whether the change was successful. They have a numerator and denominator, typically expressed as rates or percentages. For example, a metric for measuring falls-with-injury would be the number of falls with injury (numerator) divided by 1,000 patient days (denominator). Other examples of metrics include the number of direct care RNs (numerator) on a unit divided by the total number of direct care staff (denominator) or the number of medication errors divided by 1,000 orders.

- *Identify measures of success. This should be related to the goals and the problem identified.*
- *Use process measures, such as compliance to evidence-based practice, attendance to education, etc. (80% compliance to infection prevention bundle)*
- *Use patient/population outcomes, such as improvement in infection rates, length of stay, etc. Be specific- demonstrate improvement comparison from pre-implementation to post-implementation (Reduction of infection by 25% or Reduction of infection rate from 10.0 to 7.5)*
- *Use timelines on when the metrics will be achieved (ex, a month from implementation)*

Example: Implemented a Pressure Injury Prevention Bundle in Unit 5
Process measures:
- 80% of the nurses attended PIP bundle education sessions offered from July 1 2025-August 1, 2025
- 95% of nurses compliant with documentation of the PIP bundle from August 2, 2025, through November 31, 2025

Patient Outcome:
- The acquired Pressure Injury Incidence Rate for Unit 5 improved from 3.0 % of patients admitted from January 1, 2025, to June 31, 2025, to 1.5% of patients admitted from December 1, 2025, through April 1, 2026

Risk and Risk Mitigation Strategy

This analysis allows teams to identify barriers to implementation and potentially mitigate them using inherent strengths and resources. You may find specific challenges that will likely impact the ability to deliver on the action plan. Though these obstacles can get in the way, knowing about them up front is helpful so that you can engage support and create a plan to move forward.

Risk	Risk Mitigation Strategy	Status

Work Breakdown Structure (refer to the Timeline/Milestones section of A3 and provide details for each phase of the implementation framework)

A Work Breakdown Structure (WBS) is a deliverable-oriented prioritized list of the steps needed to accomplish the project objectives and create the required deliverables.

Consider all the categories of work (high-level deliverables) necessary to implement this change. What tasks must be accomplished first for each deliverable to move forward? When must they be completed to stay on track? For example, if a high-level deliverable is needed to implement a protocol, list all the tasks that need to be accomplished. Record when the team must begin and complete the task and which member(s) are responsible. If possible, list a specific person or role to create ownership of work.

© 2025 Johns Hopkins Health System

Due Date	Task	Dependencies	Accountable Person(s)	Status	Planned Completion	Actual Completion	Resource
Month/Day/Year Connect to timeline.	Detailed component of each task within the implementation framework.	What is needed before task completion.	Stakeholder/person responsible for the task.	Planned/ In Progress/ Completed/ Stalled/ Cancelled	Month/Day/Year	Month/Day/Year	Stakeholders, policies, applications, equipment
Sustainability Plan (Endure)							
What are the potential barriers to project sustainability?	What are some mitigation strategies for the potential obstacles?	What additional resources may be needed to support the project?	What additional training may be required?	What responsibilities need to be assigned?	To whom will these responsibilities be assigned?	Are there any additional metrics/outcomes that need to be collected/measured?	How frequently will you monitor and review your outcomes?
Consider resource limitations (e.g. funding, personnel, equipment, supplies), stakeholder engagement, changes in policy or regulations, training needs, and the ability to monitor the program long-term.	Strategies should directly address the barriers identified in the previous column. For example, if there is a concern for long-term funding, other sources of financing can be identified (e.g. grants, donations).	Identify any additional financial, personnel, or equipment resources that will need to be secured. Consider the type of support needed to mitigate obstacles. For example, if pursuing a grant, a grant writer would be a helpful resource.	List the education the end-users and other people supporting the project will need to receive. This may include the who, what, when, where, and/or why of the change.	Beyond the tasks needed to implement the intervention, what will need to be done to support the project in the long term? Considering project monitoring as well as new workflows or responsibilities that will need to be permanently in place.	Assign a person or role to the responsibilities listed in the previous column.	With a new process or practice, consider what additional metrics may need to be collected. For example, a new piece of equipment might require someone to assess the frequency and accuracy of its use.	Record how frequently you will measure the metrics in the previous column. Keep in mind, that as projects continue and results improve or stabilize, it may make sense to decrease monitoring frequency to lessen the burden on staff performing the data collection. This may need to be adjusted if metrics show signs of worsening.

© 2025 Johns Hopkins Health System

INDEX

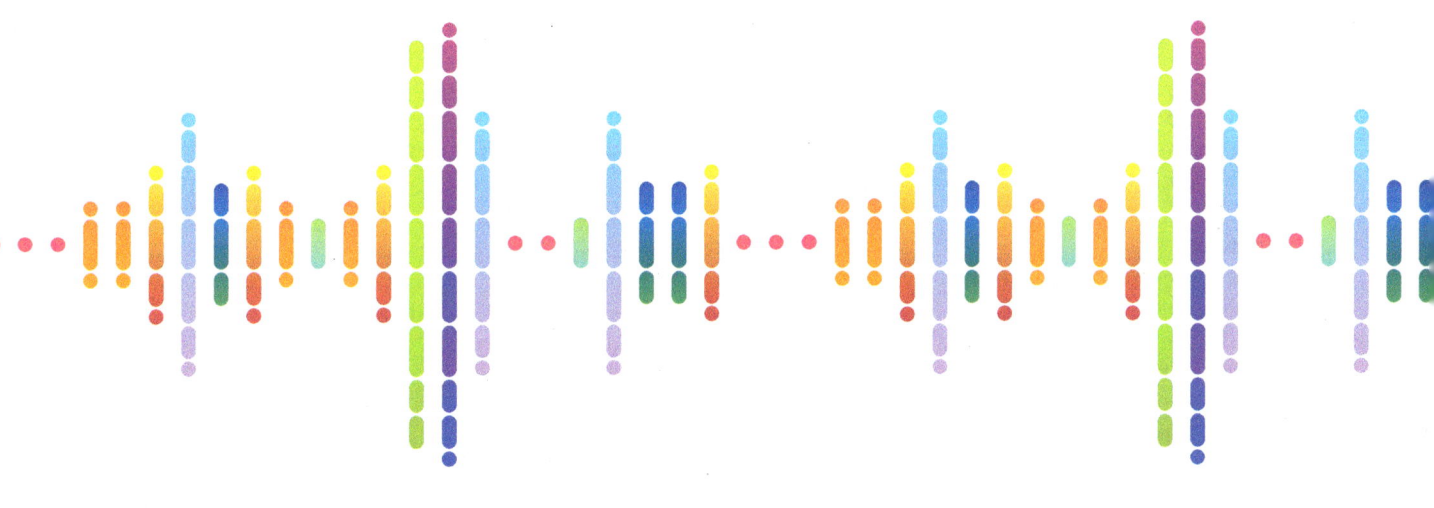

Note: Page references noted with an *f* are figures; page references noted with a *t* are tables.

A

A3 (Implementation and Action Planning) tool, 165, 289–291
abbreviated evidence summaries, 136
abstracts, 112, 122
acceptability, 151, 152
accessibility to information, 6
accountability strategies, 73*t*
accuracy, 134
action, determining best course of, 77*f*
action/implementation plans (PET process #14), 33
action items
 best-evidence searches, 140
 exhaustive searches, 142
 translation, 149–152
 by type of evidence, 121*f*
action plans
 implementation, 165–168
 Implementation and Action Planning (A3) tool, 289–291
adapting problem statements, 52
adopter curves, 68*f*
adoption, 148
affinity diagram, 49*t*
Agency for Healthcare Research and Quality (AHRQ), 95, 172
 Knowledge Transfer model, 159*t*
age of evidence, 123
AHRQ Evidence-based Practice Center (EPC) reports, 96*t*
algorithms, Appraisal Tool Selection Algorithm, 225–227
American Academy of Pediatrics, 95
American Association for Respiratory Care (AARC), 9
American College of Clinical Pharmacy's Standards of Practice for Clinical Pharmacists, 21
American Heart Association, 95
American Nurses Association (ANA), 9
American Nurses Credentialing Center (ANCC), 22, 26
American Occupational Therapy Association (AOTA), 9
American Psychological Association PsychINFO database, 100*t*
analogies, building, 142
analyses
 descriptive analysis, 127
 observational analysis, 127
 root cause, 49*t*
AND operator, 104–106
anecdotal evidence, 87–88, 129
 exhaustive searches, 142
Anecdotal Evidence Appraisal Tool, 243–246
Appraisal Tool Selection Algorithm, 225–227
appraising evidence (PET process #6), 30, 119, 120, 129
 overview of, 120–122
 pre-appraised evidence, 122–126
 quality of, 126
 reviews, 135
articles
 peer-reviewed journal, 181–184
 submitting, 182*f*
artificial intelligence (AI), 10–11
assessing risk (PET process #11), 32, 150
assessment
 bias, 120
 quality, 120, 129
associated designs, support, 30*t*
associated design support, 121*t*
attribute substitution, 114
audiences
 adapting problem statements, 52
 dissemination, 172
authors, citing, 179
authorship roles, 178*t*
availability of literature, 153

B

backgrounds, 57
behavior traits, team members, 67–68
best-evidence recommendations, 139–142, 143
best-evidence searches, 94, 95–98, 135. *see also* searching
 action items, 140
 pre-appraised evidence, 141

Best-Evidence Summary Tool, 135, 265–268
biases
    assessment, 120
    evidence, 113–115
    types of, 113
Boolean operators, 104
brainstorming, 49t
British National Health Service, 7
broad EBP questions, 58, 98
buckets of keywords, 101
building EBP questions, 58

C

care (team engagement strategy), 72t
causation, 127
Centers for Disease Control and Prevention, 9
change champions, 67
character traits, team members, 67
charts, Gantt, 167, 167f
ChatGPT, 10, 11. *See also* artificial intelligence (AI)
CINAHL, 102t
citations
    age of, 123
    management tools, 108
citing authors, 179
clarity, 68
clinical expertise, 7
clinical practice guidelines (CPGs), 76, 97, 122, 218, 221, 257
clinical reasoning, 25–26
clusters of keywords, 101
coach (team engagement strategy), 72t
Cochrane, Archibald L., 7
Cochrane Collaboration, 7
Cochrane Library, 95, 96t
collaboration, 26, 165
communication, 36, 165
    external dissemination, 178f
    plans, 174f, 175f, 178f
    strategies, 173–177
comparison intervention EBP questions, 61
conclusions, 122
conducting search and appraisal (PET process #4), 29
conferences, 179
confirmation bias, 114
confounding factors, 127
congratulate (team engagement strategy), 72t
connect (team engagement strategy), 72t
connectivism, 24
considerations guides, evidence, 249–263
consistency of evidence, 150f
content experts, 134
contribute (team engagement strategy), 72t
control groups, 127, 129
controlled trials, 126–127
controlled vocabularies, databases, 102t
core competencies, 6, 18
    Institute of Medicine (IOM), 66
    overlaps, 22f
correlations, 127
Council of Cardiovascular Prevention and Rehabilitation, 95
COVID-19, 9–10, 12, 61, 123
Covidence, 135
CPGs (clinical practice guidelines), 81
critical evaluation, 122
critical thinking, 25–26
Crossing the Quality Chasm (IOM, 2001), 8
cross-sectional data collection, 127
Cumulative Index to Nursing and Allied Health Literature (CINAHL) indexes, 6
current literature, 123

D

databases
    CINAHL, 102t
    controlled vocabularies, 102t
    Embase, 102t
    healthcare, 100t
    Physiotherapy Evidence Database (PEDro), 97t
    PubMed, 102t
    searching, 94, 95, 98–101 (*see also* searching)
    Trip, 97t
data collection, 86
    cross-sectional, 127
    longitudinal, 127
    organization/preparation, 137–138
data management, 165
decision-making, 30t
    determining level of support, 126
    support, 85–89, 121, 121t, 122–126, 137, 139

dependent variables, 126
descriptive studies, 127, 128
designs
    determining, 126
    observational analysis, 128
    studies, 128*t*
    of studies, 123, 126
developing problem statements (PET process #2), 28
discontinuing projects, 153
discussions, 122
dissemination, 36, 171, 172
    audience, 172
    external, 177–184
    internal, 173–177
    messages, 172
    methods, 172
    plans, 172–173
    purpose of, 172
    timing, 172
    types of, 184
diversity, equity, and inclusion (DEI), 12
DMAIC (Define, Measure, Analyze, Improve, Control), 159
documenting
    screening, 112–113
    searching, 108–109

E

EBP Project Steps and Overview, 207–209
EBP questions, 55, 56. *See also* evidence-based practice (EBP)
    broad EBP questions, 98
    identifying elements to search, 95
    interventions, 59–62
    previous approaches to, 56–57
    teams, 60*f*
    types of, 56–57
    updated EBP questions, 57–62
ECRI (Emergency Care Research Institute) Guidelines Trust, 95, 96*t*
educate (implementing 4 Es), 164
education, 23
effectiveness, 7
effective teamwork
    first meetings, 70–71
        maintaining accountability/engagement, 71–73

efficacy, 7
efficiency, 7, 165
    strategies, 73*t*
Embase database, 100*t*, 102*t*
engage (implementing 4 Es), 164
Enhancing the QUAlity and Transparency Of health Research (EQUATOR) network, 122
Epistemonikos database, 100*t*
errors, random, 113
evaluate (implementing 4 Es), 165
evaluating
    critical evaluation, 122
    evidence, 80 (*see also* evidence)
    literature, 134
    searching, 97, 107–108
evidence, 29–32. *See also* evidence-based practice (EBP)
    abbreviated evidence summaries, 136
    action items by type of, 121*f*
    age of, 123
    anecdotal, 87–88, 129, 142
    appraising evidence, 119, 120 (*see also* appraising evidence)
    best-evidence recommendations, 139–142
    best-evidence searches, 94, 95–98 (*see also* searching)
    bias, 113–115
    considerations guide, 249–263
    defining, 80–81
    introduction to, 79, 80
    matrix example of included populations, 137*t*
    organization/preparation, 137–138
    overview of phase, 76–77
    pre-appraised, 81, 122–126 (*see also* appraising evidence; pre-appraised evidence)
    quality of, 126
    reviews, 153
    screening, 109–113
    searching, 93, 94–109
    strength and consistency of, 150*f*
    suitability of, 123, 124*t*, 125*t*
    summaries, 81, 85, 122, 134–136, 161
    synthesis, 138–139
    terminology, 249–263
    types of, 81–89
    types of literature searches, 95*t*
evidence-based CPGs (clinical practice guidelines), 81
evidence-based medicine, 7, 80

evidence-based practice (EBP)
    artificial intelligence (AI), 10–11
    COVID-19, 9–10
    current state of, 8–9
    defining problems, 45t–46t
    definition of, 6–7
    differentiating between research, quality improvement and, 18–19
    enacting, 26
    health equity, 11–12
    history of, 7–8
    leadership, 9
    narrative approaches to, 138
    PET (Practice Question, Evidence and Translation) process (*see* PET [Practice Question, Evidence and Translation] process)
    project steps and overview, 207–209
    sources of problems, 45t
    teams, 66–70 (*see also* interprofessional teams)
    translation (context in project), 149 (*see also* translation)
Evidence Summary tools, 134, 135
    best-evidence searches, 135
    Evidence Terminology and Considerations Guide, 249–263
examples
    best-evidence recommendations, 143
    included populations, 137t
    information synthesis, 138t
exclusion criteria, screening, 110–111
execute (implementing 4 Es), 164
executing searches, 97, 106
exemplars, 191, 192–203
    certification among perianesthesia nurses, 192–193
    changing practice management, 196–197
    nurse retention, 194–195
    promoting early ambulation, 198–199
    reducing nurse burdens, 200–201
    rehabilitation provider empowerment, 202–203
exhaustive searches (PET process #5), 29–30, 98–109
    action items, 142
expertise
    content experts, 134
    selecting team members, 67
expert opinions, 7

exploring and describing problems (PET process #1), 27–28
external dissemination, 177–184
    communication, 178f

F

feasibility, 151, 152
    tools, 152
feedback, 10
filtered literature, 81, 95, 122
filtering searching, 107
fit, assessing, 151
the Five Whys, 49t, 50f
flexibility, 139
foregrounds, 57
format study designs, 85–87
frameworks
    implementation, 158–165 (*see also* implementation)
    Promoting Action on Research Implementation in Health Services (PARIHS), 160t
full-text screening, 112
The Future of Nursing 2020–2030: Charting a Path to Achieve Health Equity (NASEM, 2021), 8, 11
The Future of Nursing: Leading Change, Advancing Health (IOM, 2011), 8

G

Gantt charts, 167, 167f
gender, health equity of, 12
goals, SMART, 163t
Google Forms, 135
Google Scholar search engine, 100t, 101
groups, control, 129
Guideline Central, 95, 96t
guidelines
    clinical practice guidelines (CPGs), 97
    World Health Organization (WHO), 96t

H

hashtags (#), searching, 102
healthcare
    databases, 100t
    measurements in, 164t
healthcare professionals (HCPs), 18, 29f. *See also* Johns Hopkins Evidence-Based Practice (JHEBP) Model for Nursing and Healthcare Professionals
Health Consumer Assessment of Healthcare Providers and Systems (HCAHPS), 25, 26
health equity, 11–12
health informationists, 97
Health Professions Education: A Bridge to Quality (IOM, 2003), 8, 21
health science librarians, 97

I

identifying recommendations (PET process #12), 32
impact, 68
impacted groups, 35, 69–70, 69t
Impacted Groups Analysis and Communication Resource, 36, 37, 69, 70
implementation
    action plans, 165–168
    barriers to, 161
    definitions, 158t
    identifying frameworks/models, 158–165
    science, 148
    tools, 165
    translation, 157, 158 (*see also* translation)
Implementation and Action Planning (A3) tool, 165, 289–291
implementation frameworks (PET process #13), 33. *See also* implementation
implementation plans (PET process #15), 33–34. *See also* implementation
incidence, 128
included populations examples, 137t
inclusion criteria, screening, 110–111
independent variables, 126, 127
indexes (CINAHL), 6
Individual Evidence Summary Tool, 135, 137, 138, 139, 271–274
informal leaders, characteristics of, 67f

information explosions, 6
information synthesis examples, 138t
inquiry
    definition of, 21
    forms of, 20f
Institute of Medicine (IOM), 6, 8
    core competencies, 66
    goals, 18
internal dissemination, 173–177
internal factors, 26
International Council of Nurses (ICN), 9
internet, accessibility to information, 6
interprofessional teams, 64, 65, 66
    designating leaders, 69
    effective teamwork, 70–73 (*see also* effective teamwork)
    evidence-based practice (EBP) teams, 66–70
    identifying impacted groups, 69–70
    selecting team members, 66–69
interventions, 126
    EBP questions, 59–62
    outcomes, 6
    studies, 127
introductions, 122
Ishikawa Fishbone diagram, 49t

J

JBI (Joanna Briggs Institute), 8, 85, 95, 96t
Johns Hopkins Evidence-Based Practice (JHEBP) Model for Nursing and Healthcare Professionals, 6, 17, 18, 29f
    appraising evidence (*see* appraising evidence)
    components of, 19–24
    description, 24–27
    evidence appraisal updates, 81
    factors influencing, 26–27
    ongoing considerations, 34–37
    PET (Practice Question, Evidence and Translation) process, 24, 25, 27–34, 27f
    types of EBP questions, 56–57
Johns Hopkins Quality and Safety Research Group Translating Evidence Into Practice (TRIP) Model, 159, 161–165, 162f, 166f
journals
    peer-reviewed journal articles, 181–184
    repository websites, 182t
    Worldviews on Evidence-Based Nursing, 8

K

key concepts, searching, 101–104
keywords, 101. *See also* searching
knowledge
    gaps, 44
    translation, 148
knowledge-focused triggers, 44, 45*t*
Knowledge-to-Action model, 160*t*

L

large language models (LLMs), 10
leadership
    communication strategies, 174–177
    designating team leaders, 69
    evidence-based practice (EBP), 9
learning
    cultures, 23
    definition of, 23–24
    education (*see* education)
    transformational, 23
level of influence, team members, 67
lifelong learning, 23
limiting searching, 107
literature
    availability of, 153
    current, 123
    evaluating, 134
    plans, 111
    screening, 109–113
    searching, 93, 94–109
    types of literature searches, 95*t*
longitudinal data collection, 127
LRSAs (Literature Reviews with a Systematic Approach), 81, 82, 84, 97, 122

M

Magnet Recognition Program, 26
maintaining plans, 35
management, 69. *See also* leadership
    data management, 165
    transitions, 173
manipulation of variables, 127
manuscripts, submitting, 183*t*
McMaster University Medical School (Canada), 7
meaning, 68
measurements
    in healthcare, 164*t*
    performance, 163, 164
MEDLINE, 6
message dissemination, 172
methodologies, research, 126
methods, 122
    dissemination, 172
    mixed-methods, 86, 86*t*, 127, 128, 129
    qualitative, 85, 86, 86*t*, 127, 128, 129
    quantitative, 85, 86, 86*t*, 127, 129
Microsoft Teams, 135
mind mapping, 49*t*
mixed-methods, 86, 86*t*, 127, 128, 129
models. *See also* frameworks
    Agency for Healthcare Research and Quality (AHRQ) Knowledge Transfer, 159*t*
    artificial intelligence (AI) (*see* artificial intelligence [AI])
    DMAIC (Define, Measure, Analyze, Improve, Control), 159
    implementation, 158–165 (*see also* implementation)
    Johns Hopkins Evidence-Based Practice (JHEBP) Model for Nursing and Healthcare Professionals, 6, 19–24 (*see also* Johns Hopkins Evidence-Based Practice [JHEBP] Model for Nursing and Healthcare Professionals)
    Johns Hopkins Quality and Safety Research Group Translating Evidence Into Practice (TRIP) Model, 159, 161–165, 162*f*, 166*f*
    Knowledge-to-Action, 160*t*
    large language models (LLMs), 10
    Plan-Do-Study-Act (PDSA) cycle, 159*t*
    Quality Enhancement Research Initiative (QUERI), 160*t*
    RE-AIM, 161*t*
monitoring
    alignment with organizational priorities, 36
    sustainability (PET process #16), 34
mutual trust, 68

N

narrative approaches (EBP), 138
National Academies of Sciences, Engineering, and Medicine (NASEM), 8
National Academy of Medicine (NAM), 6, 8
National Institute for Health and Care Excellence (NICE), 95, 96t
National League for Nursing (NLN), 21
networks, EQUATOR network, 122
Nightingale, Florence, 7
non-experimental studies, 127
non-interventional studies, 127
Notes on Nursing: What It Is, and What It Is Not (Nightingale), 7
"not invented here" bias, 114
NOT operator, 104–106
nursing inquiry, forms of, 18t

O

observational analysis, 127, 128
observational studies, 127–129
ongoing learning, 23
operators, Boolean, 104
opinion leaders, 67
Organisation for Economic Co-operation and Development, 10
organization, 137–138, 165
organizational readiness, 148
organization-specific recommendations, 152–153
organizing data (PET process #8), 31
origins of evidence-based healthcare, 80
OR operator, 104–106
outcomes, 6, 123–126

P

pandemics, 10. *See also* COVID-19
Patient Health Questionnaire (PHQ)-2, 125
Pearson, Alan, 7
peer-reviewed journal articles, 181–184
performance, measuring, 163, 164
PET (Practice Question, Evidence and Translation) process, 24, 25, 27–34, 27f
  evidence (*see* evidence)
  implementation (*see* implementation)
  practice question (*see* practice questions)
  translation (*see* translation)
phenomenon, 128
Physiotherapy Evidence Database (PEDro), 97t
PICO (Patient/Population/Problem, Intervention, Comparison, and Outcome), 57, 101
  PICO questions, 56
Plan-Do-Study-Act (PDSA) cycle, 159t
plans. *See also* action plans
  communication, 174f, 175f, 178f
  dissemination, 172–173
  literature screening, 111
  maintaining, 35
podium presentations, 180–181
populations, 123–126
poster presentations, 179–180
practice
  definition of, 21–22
  forms of, 20f
  questions (*see* practice questions)
practice questions, 27–29
  describing the problem, 44–51
  developing problem statements, 51–52
  EBP questions (*see* EBP questions)
  exploring the problem, 44
  steps of phase, 43, 44
pre-appraised evidence, 81, 122–126. *See also* appraising evidence
  best-evidence searches, 141
  identifying resources for, 95–97, 96t–97t
Pre-Appraised Evidence Appraisal Tool, 229–232
pre-appraised resources, 125
premature closure, 114
preparation, evidence, 137–138
presentations
  podium, 180–181
  posters, 179–180
prevalence, 128
problem-focused triggers, 44, 45t
problems. *See also* practice questions
  accepting first problem identified, 48–51
  defining, 45t–46t
  definition of, 44
  describing the, 44–51
  developing problem statements, 51–52
  exploring the, 44
  focusing on symptoms of, 47
  solution strategies, 47

sources of, 45t
symptoms disguised as, 47t
projects
    discontinuing, 153
    evidence-based practice (EBP), 207–209
    timelines, 167
Promoting Action on Research Implementation in Health Services (PARIHS) framework, 160t
psychological safety, 68
publishing, submitting articles, 182f
PubMed, 102t
purpose of dissemination, 172

Q

qualitative methods, 85, 86, 86t, 127, 128, 129
quality
    appraisal, 121–122
    assessment, 120, 129
    of evidence, 126
Quality Enhancement Research Initiative (QUERI), 160t
Quality Function Deployment (QFD), 152
quality improvement, 6
    differentiating between research, EBP and, 18–19
    research and, 85
quantitative methods, 85, 86, 86t, 127, 129
quasi-experimental studies, 127
Question Development Tool, 95, 211–215
questionnaires, Patient Health Questionnaire (PHQ)-2, 125
questions
    EBP (*see* EBP questions)
    PICO questions (*see* PICO [Patient/Population/Problem, Intervention, Comparison, and Outcome])
    practice, 27–29
    terminology, 58f

R

random errors, 113
randomization, controlled trials with/without, 126–127
randomized control trials (RCTs), 81, 127
randomly assigned participants, 127
RE-AIM, 161t
recommendations
    best-evidence, 139–142
    organization-specific, 152–153
    practice setting-specific, 151
    Summary, Synthesis, & Best-Evidence Recommendations Tool, 277–282
recording recommendations (PET process #10), 31–32
refining searching, 107–108
reflection, 24
Registered Nurses' Association of Ontario (RNAO), 9
relation diagram, 49t
reports
    AHRQ Evidence-based Practice Center (EPC), 96t
    Crossing the Quality Chasm (IOM, 2001), 8
    The Future of Nursing 2020–2030: Charting a Path to Achieve Health Equity (NASEM, 2021), 8, 11
    The Future of Nursing: Leading Change, Advancing Health (IOM, 2011), 8
    Health Professions Education: A Bridge to Quality (IOM, 2003), 8, 21
    Roundtable on Evidence-Based Medicine (IOM, 2007), 8
research, 6
    differentiating between EBP, quality improvement and, 18–19
    introduction to, 120
    methodologies, 126
    Nightingale, Florence, 7
    quality improvement and, 85
resources
    identifying for pre-appraised evidence, 95–97, 96t–97t
    pre-appraised, 125
responsibilities, 35
results, 97, 122. *See also* searching
reviews
    appraising evidence, 135
    evidence, 153
    LRSAs (Literature Reviews with a Systematic Approach), 84
    peer-reviewed journal articles, 181–184
    with systematic approaches, 83t–84t
    with unsystematic approaches, 89t
revising searches, 107–108

risk, assessing. *See* assessing risk (PET process #11)
Robert Wood Johnson Foundation
    best practices for interprofessional teams, 66
Rogers' Theory of Diffusion of Innovation, 67
roles, authorship, 178*t*
root cause analyses, 49*t*
Roundtable on Evidence-Based Medicine (IOM, 2007), 8

S

Sackett, David, 56, 80
screening (PET process #5), 29–30
    abstracts, 112
    bias, 113–115
    documenting, 112–113
    exclusion criteria, 110–111
    full-text, 112
    inclusion criteria, 110–111
    plans, 111
    systematic literature, 109–113
    titles, 112
searching
    best-evidence searches, 135, 140, 141, 143
    bias, 113–115
    conducting search and appraisal (PET process #4), 29
    creating strings, 104–106
    databases, 95, 98–101
    documenting, 108–109
    evaluating, 97, 107–108
    evidence, 80, 93, 94–109 (*see also* evidence)
    executing, 97, 106
    exhaustive searches, 98–109, 142
    filtering, 107
    journals, 181
    key concepts, 101–104
    limiting, 107
    refining, 107–108
    revising, 107–108
    social media, 102
    targeted searches (PET process #5), 29–30
    types of literature searches, 95*t*
Searching and Screening Tool, 217–223
search satisficing, 113
secondary literature, 81, 95, 122
selecting team members, 66–69
settings, 123–126
single intervention EBP questions, 61
single studies, exhaustive searches, 142
Single Study Evidence Appraisal Tool, 235–241
SMART goals, 163*t*
social media, searching, 102
Society for Healthcare Epidemiology of America (SHEA), 97
solution strategies to problems, 47
    approaching with an open mind, 48
    asking why to get more answers, 49–51
    focusing on actual problems, 48–49
specificity, 134
spectrum bias, 113
spirit of inquiry, definition of, 21. *See also* inquiry
staff, adopter curves, 68*f*
statements, developing problem, 51–52
strategies
    accountability, 73*t*
    communication, 173–177
    for defining EBP problems, 45*t*–46*t*
    efficiency, 73*t*
    team engagement, 72*t*
strength of evidence, 150*f*
strings, searching, 104–106
structure, 68
studies
    descriptive, 127, 128
    designs of, 123, 126, 128*t*
    interventions, 127
    observational, 127–129
    quasi-experimental, 127
submitting
    articles, 182*f*
    manuscripts, 183*t*
suitability of evidence, 123, 124*t*, 125*t*
summaries
    abbreviated evidence, 136
    Best-Evidence Summary Tool, 265–268
    evidence, 81, 85, 122, 134–136, 161
    Individual Evidence Summary Tool, 271–274
    SUPPORT, 85
    tools, 135 (*see also* tools)
summarizing evidence (PET process #7), 31
Summary, Synthesis, & Best-Evidence Recommendations Tool, 277–282
support
    associated designs, 30*t*, 121*t*
    decision-making, 30*t*, 85–89, 121, 121*t*, 122–126, 137, 139
    evidence-based practice (EBP), 9
SUPPORT summaries, 85

symptoms, focusing on, 47
synthesis, 25, 138–139
synthesizing findings (PET process #9), 31
systematic approaches, reviews with, 83t–84t
systematic literature, searching, 93, 94–109

T

targeted searches (PET process #5), 29–30
targeted searches, conducting, 98
teams, 35, 69t
    content experts, 134
    designating leaders, 69
    dynamics, 68–69
    EBP questions, 60f
    effective teamwork, 70–73
    identifying impacted groups, 69–70
    interprofessional, 64, 65, 66 (*see also* interprofessional teams)
    selecting team members, 66–69
technology explosions, 6
teleconferencing, 10
TELOS (Technology and Systems, Economy, Legal, Operations, and Schedule) considerations, 152–153
terminology, 120
    evidence/considerations guide, 249–263
    frequently associated terms, 128t
    questions, 58f
    translation phase, 148
timelines, 35
    projects, 167
timing, dissemination, 172
titles, 112, 122
tools
    Anecdotal Evidence Appraisal Tool, 243–246
    Appraisal Tool Selection Algorithm, 225–227
    best-evidence searches, 135 (*see also* searching)
    Best-Evidence Summary Tool, 135, 265–268
    citation management, 108
    EBP Project Steps and Overview, 207–209
    Evidence Summary tools, 134, 135 (*see also* Evidence Summary tools)
    Evidence Terminology and Considerations Guide, 249–263
    feasibility, 152
    implementation, 165
    Implementation and Action Planning (A3) tool, 289–291
    Individual Evidence Summary Tool, 135, 137, 138, 139, 271–274
    Pre-Appraised Evidence Appraisal Tool, 229–232
    Quality Function Deployment (QFD), 152
    Question Development Tool, 95, 211–215
    Searching and Screening Tool, 217–223
    Single Study Evidence Appraisal Tool, 235–241
    Summary, Synthesis, & Best-Evidence Recommendations Tool, 139, 277–282
    translation, 152–153
    Translation Tool, 285–287
topics, 123–126
transformational learning, 23
transitions, managing, 173
translation, 32–34
    action items, 149–152
    definition of, 148
    implementation, 157, 158
    science, 148
    tools, 152–153
Translation Tool, 285–287
trials, controlled, 126–127
triggers
    knowledge-focused, 44, 45t
    problem-focused, 44, 45t
Trip database, 97t
types
    of action items by type of evidence, 121f
    of bias, 113
    of dissemination, 184
    of EBP questions, 56–57
    of evidence, 81–89
    of literature searches, 95t
    of translation, 148

U

University of Illinois Chicago College of Engineering, 10
unsystematic approaches, reviews with, 89t
updated EBP questions, 57–62. *See also* EBP questions
US Preventive Services Taskforce (USPSTF), 95, 96t

V

variables, 128
    dependent, 126
    independent, 126, 127
    manipulation of, 127
video calls, 10
vocabularies
    controlled vocabularies, 102t
    searching, 102

W–X–Y–Z

websites, journal repository, 182t
Work Breakdown Structure (WBS), 168, 168f
World Health Organization (WHO), 11, 95, 96t
Worldviews on Evidence-Based Nursing, 8
writing EBP questions (PET process #3), 28–29